Orbit, Eyelids, and Lacrimal System

Orbit, Eyelids, and Lacrimal System

Section 7

2004–2005

(Last major revision 2003–2004)

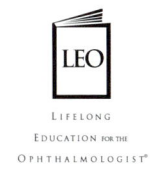

AMERICAN ACADEMY
OF OPHTHALMOLOGY
The Eye M.D. Association

LEO

LIFELONG
EDUCATION FOR THE
OPHTHALMOLOGIST

BASIC AND CLINICAL SCIENCE COURSE

LEO The Basic and Clinical Science Course is one component of the Lifelong Education for the Ophthalmologist (LEO) framework, which assists members in planning their continuing medical education. LEO includes an array of clinical education products that members may select to form individualized, self-directed learning plans for updating their clinical knowledge. Active members or fellows who use LEO components may accumulate sufficient CME credits to earn the LEO Award. Contact the Academy's Clinical Education Division for further information on LEO.

> The American Academy of Ophthalmology is accredited by the Accreditation Council for Continuing Medical Education to provide continuing medical education for physicians.
>
> The American Academy of Ophthalmology designates this educational activity for a maximum of 30 category 1 credits toward the AMA Physician's Recognition Award. Each physician should claim only those hours of credit that he/she actually spent in the activity.
>
> The American Medical Association has determined that non-U.S. licensed physicians who participate in this CME activity are eligible for AMA PRA category 1 credit.

The Academy provides this material for educational purposes only. It is not intended to represent the only or best method or procedure in every case, nor to replace a physician's own judgment or give specific advice for case management. Including all indications, contraindications, side effects, and alternative agents for each drug or treatment is beyond the scope of this material. All information and recommendations should be verified, prior to use, with current information included in the manufacturers' package inserts or other independent sources, and considered in light of the patient's condition and history. Reference to certain drugs, instruments, and other products in this course is made for illustrative purposes only and is not intended to constitute an endorsement of such. Some material may include information on applications that are not considered community standard, that reflect indications not included in approved FDA labeling, or that are approved for use only in restricted research settings. The FDA has stated that it is the responsibility of the physician to determine the FDA status of each drug or device he or she wishes to use, and to use them with appropriate patient consent in compliance with applicable law. The Academy specifically disclaims any and all liability for injury or other damages of any kind, from negligence or otherwise, for any and all claims that may arise from the use of any recommendations or other information contained herein.

Copyright © 2004
American Academy of Ophthalmology
All rights reserved
Printed in the United States of America

Basic and Clinical Science Course

Thomas J. Liesegang, MD, Jacksonville, Florida, *Senior Secretary for Clinical Education*
Gregory L. Skuta, MD, Oklahoma City, Oklahoma, *Secretary for Ophthalmic Knowledge*
Louis B. Cantor, MD, Indianapolis, Indiana, *BCSC Course Chair*

Section 7

Faculty Responsible for This Edition

Robert C. Kersten, MD, *Chair*, Cincinnati, Ohio
François Codère, MD, Montreal, Quebec
Roger A. Dailey, MD, Portland, Oregon
James A. Garrity, MD, Rochester, Minnesota
Jeffrey A. Nerad, MD, *Consultant*, Iowa City, Iowa
Jerry K. Popham, MD, Denver, Colorado
John Bryan Holds, MD, St. Louis, Missouri
   Practicing Ophthalmologists Advisory Committee for Education

The authors state the following financial relationships:

Dr. Holds: ad hoc consultant for Allergan Pharmaceuticals

The other authors state that they have no significant financial interest or other relationship with the manufacturer of any commercial product discussed in the Chapters that they contributed to this publication or with the manufacturer of any competing commercial product.

Recent Past Faculty

George B. Bartley, MD
Thomas L. Beardsley, MD
Kenneth V. Cahill, MD
Richard P. Carroll, MD
Richard K. Dortzbach, MD
Russell S. Gonnering, MD
James A. Katowitz, MD
Francis G. LaPiana, MD
Russell W. Neuhaus, MD
Thaddeus S. Nowinski, MD
William R. Nunery, MD
James R. Patrinely, MD
Priscilla E. Perry, MD
John W. Shore, MD
Francis C. Sutula, MD
Nicholas J. Vincent, MD
Darrell E. Wolfley, MD
Paul L. Wright, MD
Allan E. Wulc, MD

In addition, the Academy gratefully acknowledges the contributions of numerous past faculty and advisory committee members who have played an important role in the development of previous editions of the Basic and Clinical Science Course.

American Academy of Ophthalmology Staff

Richard A. Zorab, *Vice President, Ophthalmic Knowledge*
Hal Straus, *Director, Publications Department*
Carol L. Dondrea, *Publications Editor*
Christine Arturo, *Acquisitions Editor*
Maxine Garrett, *Administrative Coordinator*

Cover design: Paula Shuhert Design
Cover photograph: Choroidal folds, by Patrick J. Saine, MEd, CRA, Dartmouth-Hitchcock Medical Center

AMERICAN ACADEMY OF OPHTHALMOLOGY
The Eye M.D. Association

655 Beach Street
Box 7424
San Francisco, CA 94120-7424

Contents

General Introduction xiii

Objectives 1

PART I Orbit 3
Introduction 5

1 Orbital Anatomy 7
Dimensions 7
Topographic Relationships 7
    Roof of the Orbit 8
    Lateral Wall of the Orbit 8
    Medial Wall of the Orbit 9
    Floor of the Orbit 10
Apertures 11
    Ethmoidal Foramina 11
    Superior Orbital Fissure 11
    Inferior Orbital Fissure 11
    Zygomaticofacial and Zygomaticotemporal Canals 11
    Nasolacrimal Canal 11
    Optic Canal 11
Soft Tissues 12
    Periorbita 12
    Intraorbital Optic Nerve 12
    Extraocular Muscles and Orbital Fat 12
    Annulus of Zinn 14
    Vasculature System 15
    Nerves 15
    Lacrimal Gland 16
Periorbital Structures 20
    Nose and Paranasal Sinuses 20
    Fossae and Fissures 21

2 Evaluation of Orbital Disorders 23
The Six P's 23
    Pain 23
    Proptosis 23
    Progression 24
    Palpation 24
    Pulsation 24
    Periorbital Changes 24

Physical Examination and Laboratory Tests 24
    Inspection 24
    Palpation 26
    Auscultation 27
    Workup Checklist 27
Primary Studies 27
    Computed Tomography .29
    Three-Dimensional Computed Tomography 29
    Magnetic Resonance Imaging 30
    Comparison of CT and MRI. 31
    Ultrasonography 33
Secondary Studies 34
    Venography 34
    Arteriography 34
Pathology 35
Laboratory Studies 35

3 Congenital Orbital Anomalies 37
Anophthalmos 37
Microphthalmos 37
Craniofacial Clefting 38
Tumors 39

4 Infectious and Inflammatory Disorders 41
Infections 41
    Cellulitis 41
    Necrotizing Fasciitis 44
    Phycomycosis 45
    Aspergillosis 46
    Orbital Tuberculosis 47
    Parasitic Diseases 47
Inflammations 48
    Graves Ophthalmopathy .48
    Idiopathic Orbital Inflammation (Orbital Inflammatory
       Syndrome, Orbital Pseudotumor) 56
    Sarcoidosis 59
    Vasculitis 59

5 Orbital Neoplasms 63
Congenital Orbital Tumors 63
    Hamartomas and Choristomas 63
    Dermoid Cysts 63
    Lipodermoids 64
    Teratomas 64
Vascular Tumors 64
    Capillary Hemangiomas .64
    Cavernous Hemangiomas 67
    Hemangiopericytomas 67

Lymphangiomas 67
Masquerading Conditions. 69
Neural Tumors 72
Optic Nerve Gliomas 72
Neurofibromas 75
Neurofibromatosis Type 1. 75
Meningiomas 77
Schwannomas 79
Mesenchymal Tumors 79
Rhabdomyosarcomas 79
Miscellaneous Mesenchymal Tumors 81
Lymphoproliferative Disorders 81
Lymphoid Hyperplasias and Lymphomas 81
Plasma Cell Tumors 88
Histiocytic Disorders 88
Juvenile Xanthogranuloma 88
Lacrimal Gland Tumors 89
Epithelial Tumors of the Lacrimal Gland 89
Nonepithelial Tumors of the Lacrimal Gland 91
Secondary Orbital Tumors 92
Globe and Eyelid Origin 92
Sinus Origin 92
Brain Origin 93
Metastatic Tumors 94
Metastatic Tumors in Children 94
Metastatic Tumors in Adults 95
Management of Orbital Metastases 96

6 Orbital Trauma 97
Midfacial (Le Fort) Fractures 97
Orbital Fractures 97
Zygomatic Fractures 97
Orbital Apex Fractures 100
Orbital Roof Fractures 100
Medial Orbital Fractures 101
Orbital Floor Fractures 102
Intraorbital Foreign Bodies 106
Orbital Hemorrhage 106
Traumatic Visual Loss With Clear Media 106
Management 108

7 Orbital Surgery 109
Surgical Spaces 109
Anterior Orbitotomy 109
Superior Approach 109
Inferior Approach 110
Medial Approach 111
Lateral Orbitotomy 114

viii • Contents

    Orbital Decompression 115
    Postoperative Care 116
    Special Surgical Techniques in the Orbit 116
    Complications of Orbital Surgery 117

8 The Anophthalmic Socket 119
    Enucleation 119
        Guidelines for Enucleation 121
        Enucleation in Childhood 121
        Orbital Implants 121
        Prostheses 122
        Intraoperative Complications of Enucleation 123
    Evisceration 123
        Advantages of Evisceration 123
        Disadvantages of Evisceration 123
        Techniques of Evisceration 124
    Anophthalmic Socket Complications and Treatment 124
        Deep Superior Sulcus 124
        Contracture of Fornices 125
        Exposure and Extrusion of Implant 125
        Contracted Sockets 125
        Anophthalmic Ectropion 126
        Anophthalmic Ptosis 127
        Lash Margin Entropion 127
        Cosmetic Optics 127
    Exenteration 127
        Considerations for Exenteration 127
        Types of Exenteration 129

PART II Periocular Soft Tissues 131
    Introduction 133

9 Anatomy 135
    Face 135
    Eyelids 139
        Skin and Subcutaneous Tissue 139
        Protractors 139
        Orbital Septum 140
        Orbital Fat 141
        Retractors 142
        Tarsus 145
        Conjunctiva 145
        Other Anatomical Considerations 145

10 Principles of Facial and Eyelid Surgery 149
    Patient Preparation 149
    Anesthesia 150

11 Classification and Management of Eyelid Disorders 153
Congenital Anomalies 153
Blepharophimosis Syndrome. 153
Congenital Ptosis of the Upper Eyelid 154
Congenital Ectropion 154
Euryblepharon. 154
Ankyloblepharon. 154
Epicanthus 156
Epiblepharon 156
Congenital Entropion 156
Congenital Distichiasis 157
Congenital Coloboma 157
Congenital Eyelid Lesions 158
Cryptophthalmos. 158
Acquired Eyelid Disorders 158
Chalazion 158
Hordeolum (Stye) 160
Eyelid Edema 160
Floppy Eyelid Syndrome 160
Eyelid Imbrication Syndrome 161
Eyelid Neoplasms 162
Clinical Evaluation of Eyelid Tumors 162
Benign Eyelid Lesions 163
Benign Adnexal Lesions 166
Benign Melanocytic Lesions 169
Premalignant Epidermal Lesions 172
Premalignant Melanocytic Lesions 174
Malignant Eyelid Tumors 174
Masquerading Neoplasms 184
Eyelid Trauma 184
Blunt Trauma 184
Penetrating Trauma 184
Secondary Repair. 186
Dog and Human Bites 187
Burns 187
Eyelid and Canthal Reconstruction 188
Eyelid Defects Not Involving the Eyelid Margin . . . 188
Eyelid Defects Involving the Eyelid Margin. 189
Lateral Canthal Defects. 192
Medial Canthal Defects. 193

12 Periocular Malpositions and Involutional Changes . . 195
Ectropion 195
Congenital Ectropion 195
Involutional Ectropion 195
Paralytic Ectropion 199

- Cicatricial Ectropion ... 200
- Mechanical Ectropion ... 201
- Entropion ... 201
  - Congenital Entropion ... 201
  - Acute Spastic Entropion ... 201
  - Involutional Entropion ... 202
  - Cicatricial Entropion ... 205
- Symblepharon ... 207
- Trichiasis ... 207
  - Mechanical Epilation ... 207
  - Electrolysis ... 207
  - Cryotherapy ... 208
  - Argon Laser ... 208
  - Surgery ... 208
- Blepharoptosis ... 208
  - Evaluation ... 209
  - Physical Examination ... 209
  - Classification ... 213
  - Pseudoptosis ... 219
  - Treatment of Ptosis ... 220
- Eyelid Retraction ... 223
  - Treatment of Eyelid Retraction ... 224
- Facial Dystonia ... 226
  - Benign Essential Blepharospasm ... 226
  - Hemifacial Spasm ... 227
- Involutional Periorbital Changes ... 228
  - Dermatochalasis ... 228
  - Blepharochalasis ... 228
- Blepharoplasty ... 229
  - Upper Eyelid ... 229
  - Lower Eyelid ... 229
  - Technique ... 230
  - Complications ... 232
- Brow Ptosis ... 234
  - Treatment of Functional Brow Ptosis ... 235
  - Browpexy ... 235
- Cosmetic Facial Surgery ... 235
  - Pathogenesis of the Aging Face ... 236
  - Physical Examination of the Aging Face ... 236
- Facial Rejuvenation Surgery (Beyond Blepharoplasty) ... 237
  - Laser Skin Resurfacing ... 237
  - Cosmetic Uses of Botulinum Toxin ... 239
  - Upper Face Rejuvenation (Brow and Forehead Lift) ... 239
  - Midface Rejuvenation (Suborbicularis Oculi Fat/Midface Lift) ... 241
  - Lower Face and Neck Rejuvenation ... 244
- Conclusions ... 248

Contents • xi

PART III Lacrimal System 249
Introduction 251

13 Anatomy and Physiology 253
Normal Anatomy 253
    Secretory Apparatus 253
    Excretory Apparatus 254
Physiology 256
Developmental Abnormalities 257

14 Evaluation and Management of the Tearing
Patient 259
Congenital Tearing 259
    Evaluation 259
    Management 260
Acquired Tearing 267
    Evaluation 267
    Assessment 267
    Management 274
    Upper System Abnormalities 274
    Lower System Abnormalities 278

Basic Texts 285
Related Academy Materials 287
Credit Reporting Form 289
Study Questions 293
Answers 303
Index 307

General Introduction

The Basic and Clinical Science Course (BCSC) is designed to meet the needs of residents and practitioners for a comprehensive yet concise curriculum of the field of ophthalmology. The BCSC has developed from its original brief outline format, which relied heavily on outside readings, to a more convenient and educationally useful self-contained text. The Academy updates and revises the course annually, with the goals of integrating the basic science and clinical practice of ophthalmology and of keeping ophthalmologists current with new developments in the various subspecialties.

The BCSC incorporates the effort and expertise of more than 80 ophthalmologists, organized into 14 section faculties, working with Academy editorial staff. In addition, the course continues to benefit from many lasting contributions made by the faculties of previous editions. Members of the Academy's Practicing Ophthalmologists Advisory Committee for Education serve on each faculty and, as a group, review every volume before and after major revisions.

Organization of the Course

The Basic and Clinical Science Course comprises 14 volumes, incorporating fundamental, ophthalmic knowledge, subspecialty areas, and special topics:

1. Update on General Medicine
2. Fundamentals and Principles of Ophthalmology
3. Optics, Refraction, and Contact Lenses
4. Ophthalmic Pathology and Intraocular Tumors
5. Neuro-Ophthalmology
6. Pediatric Ophthalmology and Strabismus
7. Orbit, Eyelids, and Lacrimal System
8. External Disease and Cornea
9. Intraocular Inflammation and Uveitis
10. Glaucoma
11. Lens and Cataract
12. Retina and Vitreous
13. International Ophthalmology
14. Refractive Surgery

In addition, a comprehensive Master Index allows the reader to easily locate subjects throughout the entire series.

References

Readers who wish to explore specific topics in greater detail may consult the journal references cited within each chapter and the Basic Texts listed at the back of the book.

These references are intended to be selective rather than exhaustive, chosen by the BCSC faculty as being important, current, and readily available to residents and practitioners.

Related Academy educational materials are also listed in the appropriate sections. They include books, audiovisual materials, self-assessment programs, clinical modules, and interactive programs.

Study Questions and CME Credit

Each volume of the BCSC is designed as an independent study activity for ophthalmology residents and practitioners. The learning objectives for this volume are stated on page 1. The text, illustrations, and references provide the information necessary to achieve the objectives; the study questions allow readers to test their understanding of the material and their mastery of the objectives. Physicians who wish to claim CME credit for this educational activity may do so by mail, by fax, or online. The necessary forms and instructions are given at the end of the book.

Conclusion

The Basic and Clinical Science Course has expanded greatly over the years, with the addition of much new text and numerous illustrations. Recent editions have sought to place a greater emphasis on clinical applicability, while maintaining a solid foundation in basic science. As with any educational program, it reflects the experience of its authors. As its faculties change and as medicine progresses, new viewpoints are always emerging on controversial subjects and techniques. Not all alternate approaches can be included in this series; as with any educational endeavor, the learner should seek additional sources, including such carefully balanced opinions as the Academy's Preferred Practice Patterns.

The BCSC faculty and staff are continuously striving to improve the educational usefulness of the course; you, the reader, can contribute to this ongoing process. If you have any suggestions or questions about the series, please do not hesitate to contact the faculty or the editors.

The authors, editors, and reviewers hope that your study of the BCSC will be of lasting value and that each section will serve as a practical resource for quality patient care.

Objectives

Upon completion of BCSC Section 7, *Orbit, Eyelids, and Lacrimal System,* the reader should be able to:

- Describe the normal anatomy and function of orbital and periocular tissues

- Identify general and specific pathophysiological processes (including congenital, infectious, inflammatory, traumatic, neoplastic, and involutional) that affect the structure and function of these tissues

- Choose appropriate examination techniques and protocols for diagnosing disorders of the orbit, eyelids, and lacrimal system

- Select from among the various imaging and ancillary studies available those that are most useful for the particular patient

- Develop appropriate differential diagnoses for disorders of the orbital and periocular tissues

- Compare the indications for enucleation, evisceration, and exenteration

- Distinguish between functional and cosmetic indications in the surgical management of eyelid and periorbital conditions

- Outline the principles of medical and surgical management of conditions affecting the orbit, eyelids, and lacrimal system

- Recognize the major postoperative complications of orbital, eyelid, and lacrimal system surgery

PART I

Orbit

Introduction

Disorders of the orbit are uncommon. Orbital disorders may arise primarily within the orbit; alternatively, they may spread there from adjacent structures or from distant sources via vascular pathways, or these disorders may be manifestations of systemic diseases. The diagnosis and management of these conditions challenge the physician's knowledge and ingenuity. The incidence and prevalence of orbital disease vary with geographic location, sex, age, and race. Frequently, diagnosis requires the assistance of a pathologist skilled in the interpretation of abnormal orbital tissues. Consequently, the ability to obtain and prepare biopsy specimens is a part of both basic and advanced orbital surgical technique. Collaboration with neurosurgeons, otolaryngologists, plastic surgeons, neuroradiologists, neuroanesthesiologists, and endocrinologists is frequently required, adding to the complexity and interest of this field of study.

CHAPTER 1

Orbital Anatomy

Dimensions

The orbits are the bony cavities that contain the globes, extraocular muscles, nerves, fat, and blood vessels. Each bony orbit is pear-shaped, tapering posteriorly to the apex and the optic canal. The medial orbital walls are approximately parallel and are separated by 25 mm in the average adult. The widest dimension of the orbit is approximately 1 cm behind the anterior orbital rim. Approximate measurements of the adult orbit are shown in Table 1-1. The orbital segment of the optic nerve is slightly curved and can move with the eye. This curve allows the eye to move forward with proptosis without damaging the nerve.

Topographic Relationships

The orbital septum arises from the orbital rims anteriorly. The paranasal sinuses are either rudimentary or very small at birth, and they increase in size through adolescence. They lie adjacent to the floor, medial wall, and anterior portion of the orbital roof. The orbital walls are composed of seven bones: ethmoid, frontal, lacrimal, maxillary, palatine, sphenoid, and zygomatic. The composition of each of the four walls and the location in relation to adjacent extraorbital structures are shown in Figures 1-1, 1-2, and 1-3 and summarized below.

Table 1-1 Adult Orbital Dimensions

Volume	30 cc
Entrance height	35 mm
Entrance width	40 mm
Medial wall length	45 mm
Distance from posterior globe to optic foramen	18 mm
Length of orbital segment of optic nerve	25–30 mm

8 • Orbit, Eyelids, and Lacrimal System

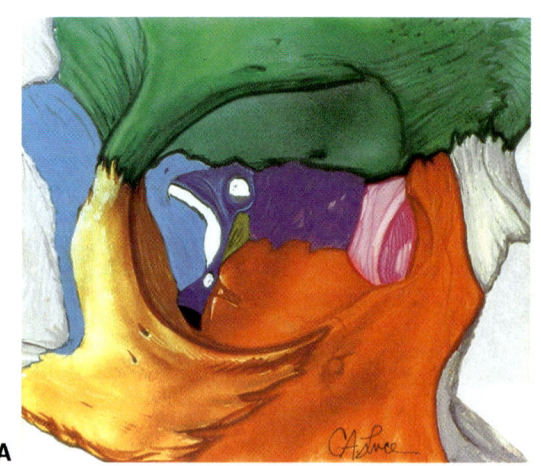

Figure 1-1 A, Bony components of the right orbit identified by color: maxilla *(orange)*, zygoma *(beige)*, sphenoid bone, greater wing *(light blue)*, lesser wing *(dark blue)*, palatine bone *(light green)*, ethmoid bone *(purple)*, lacrimal bone *(pink)*, frontal bone *(green)*. **B,** Lateral oblique view of right orbit. *(From Zide BM, Jelks GW, eds.* Surgical Anatomy of the Orbit. *New York: Raven; 1985:3.)*

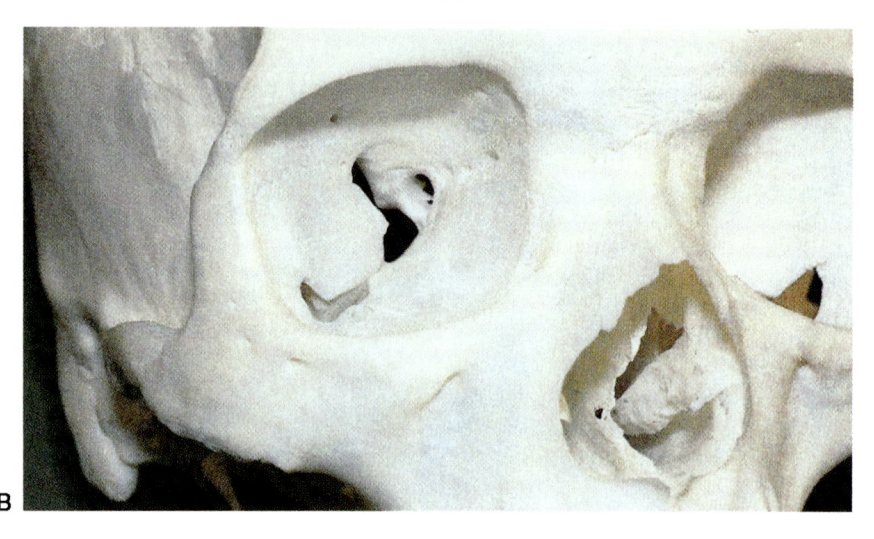

Roof of the Orbit

- Composed of the frontal bone and lesser wing of sphenoid.
- Important landmarks include the lacrimal gland fossa, fossa for the trochlea of the superior oblique tendon and muscle, and supraorbital notch or foramen.
- Located adjacent to anterior cranial fossa and frontal sinus.

Lateral Wall of the Orbit

- Composed of the zygomatic bone and greater wing of sphenoid. Separated from the lesser wing portion of the orbital roof by the superior orbital fissure.
- Important landmarks include the lateral orbital tubercle of Whitnall, to which the lateral canthal tendon is attached, and the frontozygomatic suture located 1 cm above the tubercle.
- Located adjacent to the middle cranial fossa and temporal fossa.

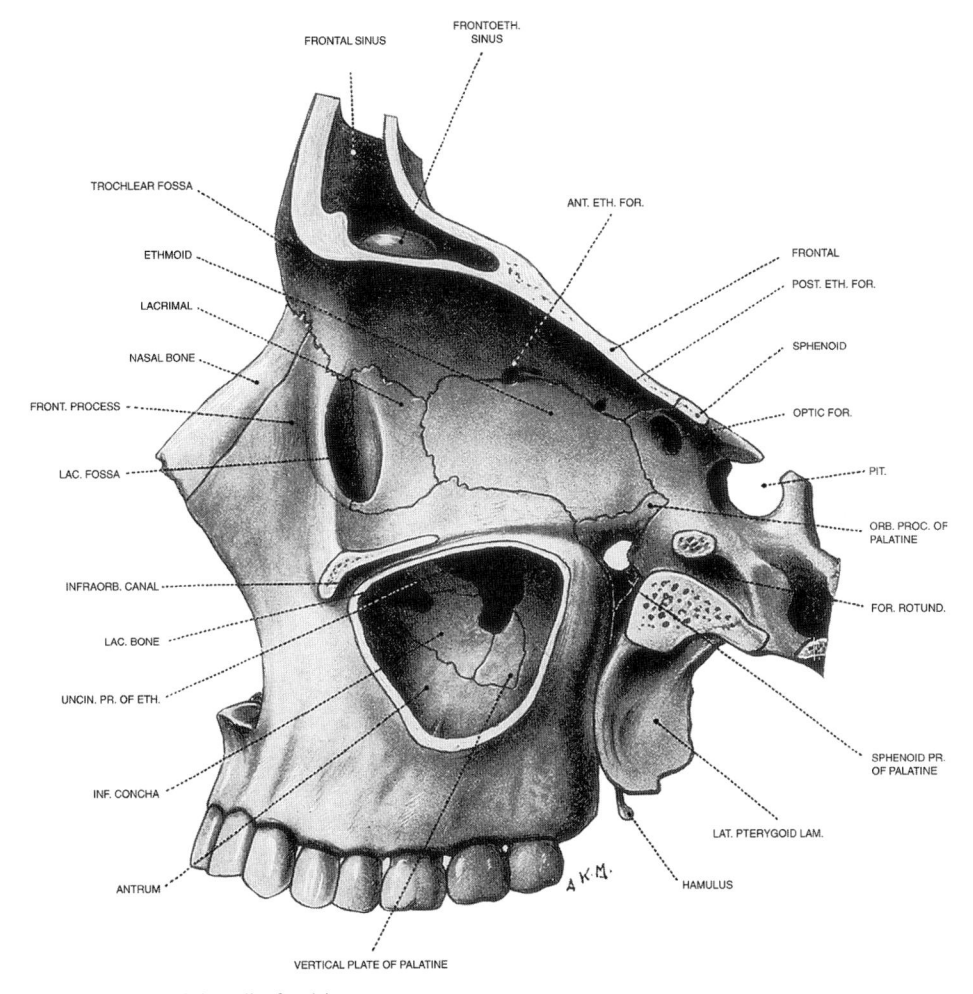

Figure 1-2 Medial wall of orbit. *(From Wolff E, Last RJ. Anatomy of the Eye and Orbit. 6th ed. Philadelphia: Saunders; 1968.)*

- The lateral orbital rim is usually at the equator of the eye, allowing wide peripheral vision.
- The globe is vulnerable to trauma laterally, where the lateral orbital wall protects approximately the posterior half of the eye.

Medial Wall of the Orbit

- Composed of the ethmoid, lacrimal, maxillary, and sphenoid bones.
- Important landmarks include the frontoethmoid suture. The anterior and posterior ethmoidal arteries enter the orbit in this suture. The cribriform plate lies at the level of the frontoethmoid suture.
- Located adjacent to the ethmoid and sphenoid sinuses and nasal cavity.
- Medial wall of the optic canal forms the lateral wall of the sphenoid sinus.

10 • Orbit, Eyelids, and Lacrimal System

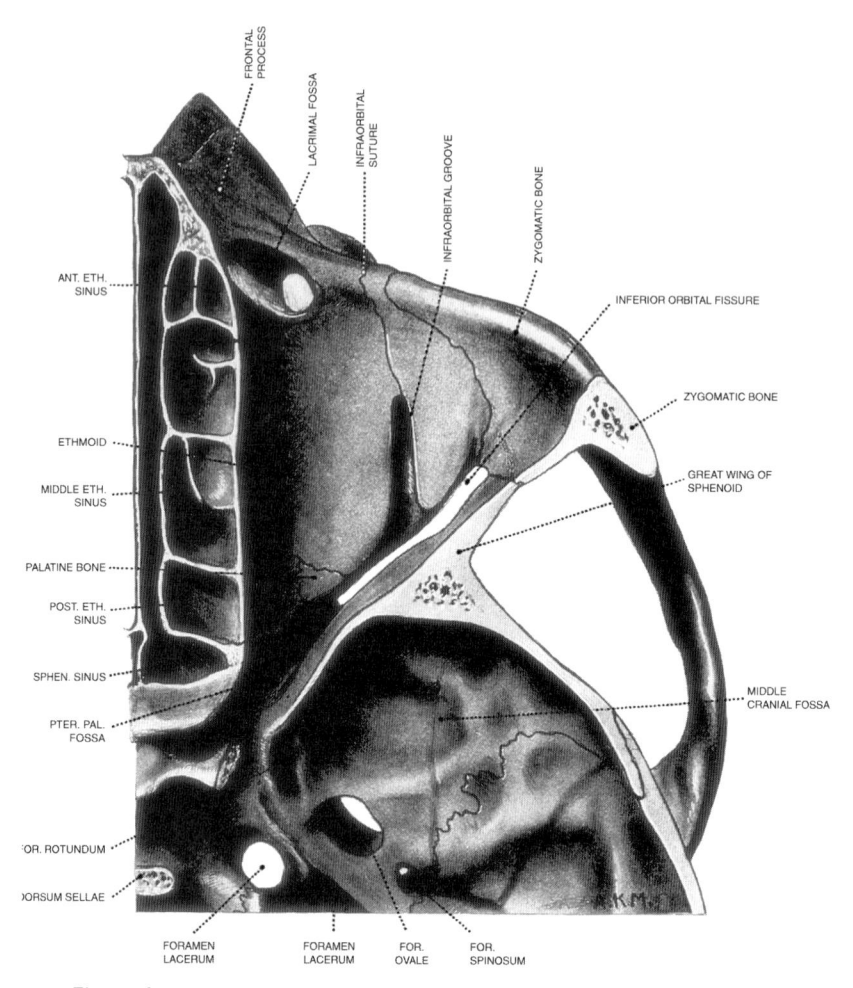

Figure 1-3 Floor of orbit. *(From Warwick R. Wolff's Anatomy of the Eye and Orbit. 7th ed. Philadelphia: Saunders; 1976.)*

The thinnest walls of the orbit are the *lamina papyracea*, which covers the ethmoid sinuses along the medial wall, and the *maxillary bone*, particularly in its posteromedial portion. These are the bones most frequently fragmented as a result of indirect blowout fractures (see Chapter 6). Among children, infections of the ethmoid sinuses commonly extend through the lamina papyracea to cause orbital cellulitis and proptosis.

Floor of the Orbit

- Composed of the maxillary, palatine, and zygomatic bones.
- Forms the roof of the maxillary sinus.
- Important landmarks are the infraorbital groove and canal.

Apertures

The orbital walls are perforated by several important apertures. (See Figs 1-1, 1-2, and 1-3.)

Ethmoidal Foramina

The anterior and posterior ethmoidal arteries pass through the corresponding ethmoidal foramina in the medial orbital wall along the frontoethmoidal suture. These foramina may provide a route of entry into the orbit for infections and neoplasms from the sinuses.

Superior Orbital Fissure

The superior orbital fissure separates the greater and lesser wings of the sphenoid and transmits cranial nerves III, IV, and VI; the first (ophthalmic) division of cranial nerve V; and sympathetic nerve fibers. Most of the venous drainage from the orbit passes through this fissure by way of the superior ophthalmic vein to the cavernous sinus.

Inferior Orbital Fissure

The inferior orbital fissure is bounded by the sphenoid, maxillary, and palatine bones and lies between the lateral orbital wall and orbital floor. It transmits the second (maxillary) division of cranial nerve V, including the zygomatic nerve and branches of the inferior ophthalmic vein leading to the pterygoid plexus. The infraorbital nerve, which is a branch of the maxillary nerve, leaves the skull through the foramen rotundum and travels through the pterygopalatine fossa to enter the orbit at the infra-orbital groove. The nerve travels anteriorly in the floor of the orbit through the infraorbital canal, emerging on the face of the maxilla 1 cm below the inferior orbital rim. The infraorbital nerve carries sensation from the lower eyelid, cheek, upper lip, upper teeth, and gingiva. Numbness in this distribution often accompanies blowout fractures of the orbital floor.

Zygomaticofacial and Zygomaticotemporal Canals

The zygomaticofacial canal and zygomaticotemporal canal transmit vessels and branches of the zygomatic nerve through the lateral orbital wall to the cheek and the temporal fossa, respectively.

Nasolacrimal Canal

The nasolacrimal canal extends from the lacrimal sac fossa to the inferior meatus beneath the inferior turbinate in the nose. Through this canal passes the nasolacrimal duct, which is continuous from the lacrimal sac to the mucosa of the nose. (See Part III, Lacrimal System.)

Optic Canal

The optic canal is 8–10 mm long and is located within the lesser wing of the sphenoid. This canal is separated from the superior orbital fissure by the bony optic strut. The optic nerve, ophthalmic artery, and sympathetic nerves pass through this canal. The orbital end of the canal is the optic foramen, which normally measures less than 6.5 mm in diameter (adult). Optic canal enlargement accompanies the expansion of the nerve seen with optic nerve gliomas. Blunt trauma may cause an optic canal fracture, hematoma at the orbital apex, or shearing of the nerve at the foramen, resulting in optic nerve damage.

Soft Tissues

Periorbita

The periorbita is the periosteal covering of the orbital bones. At the orbital apex, it fuses to the dura mater covering the optic nerve. Anteriorly, the periorbita is continuous with the orbital septum and the periosteum of the facial bones. The line of fusion of these layers at the orbital rim is called the *arcus marginalis*. The periorbita is loosely adherent to the bone except at the orbital margin, sutures, fissures, foramina, and canals. In an exenteration, the periorbita can be easily separated except where these firm attachments are present. Subperiosteal fluid, such as pus or blood, is usually loculated within these boundaries. The periorbita, supplied by the sensory nerves of the orbit, is quite sensitive.

Intraorbital Optic Nerve

The intraorbital portion of the optic nerve is about 30 mm long. The nerve is somewhat longer than the orbit, making an S-shaped curve to allow for movement with the eye. The optic nerve is 4 mm in diameter and surrounded by pia mater, arachnoid, and dura mater, which are continuous with the same layers covering the brain. The dura mater covering the posterior portion of the intraorbital optic nerve fuses with the annulus of Zinn at the orbital apex and is continuous with the periosteum of the optic canal.

Extraocular Muscles and Orbital Fat

The extraocular muscles are responsible for the movement of the eye and synchronous movements of the eyelids. All of the extraocular muscles, except the inferior oblique muscle, originate at the orbital apex and travel anteriorly to insert onto the eye or eyelid. The four rectus muscles (superior, medial, lateral, and inferior recti) originate from the annulus of Zinn. The levator muscle arises above the annulus on the lesser wing of the sphenoid. The superior oblique muscle originates slightly medial to the levator muscle and travels anteriorly through the trochlea on the superomedial orbital rim, where it turns posterolateral toward the eye. The inferior oblique muscle originates from the anterior orbital floor lateral to the lacrimal sac and travels posteriorly and laterally, within the lower eyelid retractors, to insert inferolateral to the macula.

In the anterior portion of the orbit, the rectus muscles are connected by a membrane known as the *intermuscular septum*. When viewed in the coronal plane, this membrane forms a ring that divides the orbital fat into the *intraconal fat (central surgical space)* and the *extraconal fat (peripheral surgical space)*. These anatomic designations on an MRI or a CT scan are helpful in describing the location of a mass. Surgeons operating in the orbit find that a knowledge of these spaces helps direct the orbital dissection to the mass. The orbit is further divided by many fine fibrous septa that unite and support the globe, optic nerve, and extraocular muscles (Fig 1-4). Accidental or surgical orbital trauma can disrupt this supporting system and contribute to globe displacement and restriction. In many cases of diplopia after fracture, restriction of eye movement is caused by the entrapment of the orbital connective tissue rather than by the muscles themselves.

Koornneef L. Orbital septa: anatomy and function. *Ophthalmology.* 1979;86:876–880.

Cranial nerves III, IV, and VI supply motor innervation to the extraocular muscles. The superior rectus and levator muscles are supplied by the superior division of cranial nerve III (oculomotor). The inferior rectus, medial rectus, and inferior oblique muscles are supplied by the inferior division of cranial nerve III. The lateral rectus is supplied by cranial nerve VI (abducens). The cranial nerves to the rectus muscles enter the orbit posteriorly and travel through the intraconal fat to enter the muscles from the undersurface at the junction of the posterior third and anterior two thirds. Cranial nerve IV (trochlear) crosses over the levator muscle and innervates the superior oblique on the superior surface at its posterior third. The nerve to the inferior rectus travels anteriorly on the lateral aspect of the inferior rectus to enter the muscle on its posterior surface.

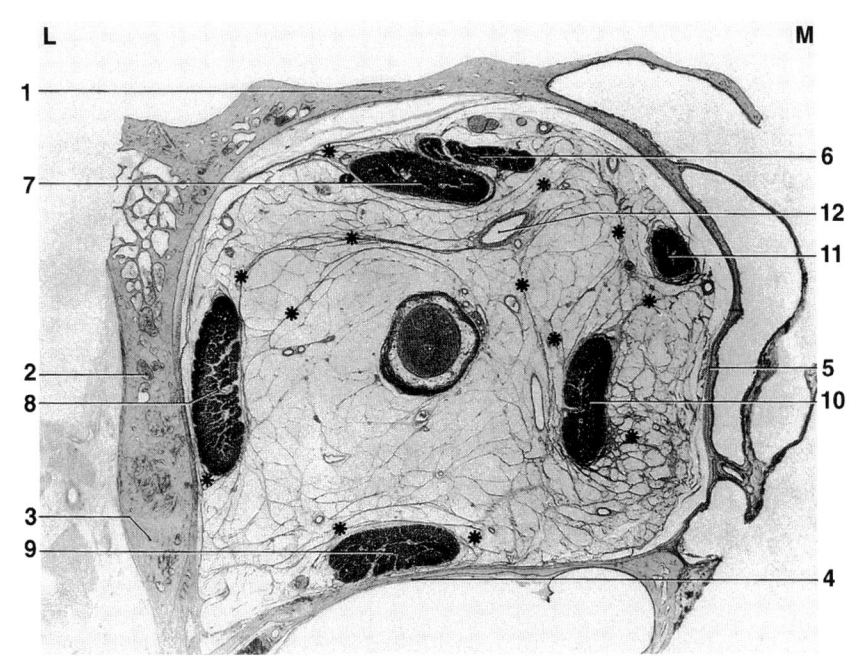

Figure 1-4 Frontal section (60 µm) of a right orbit in the retrobulbar area, 2.1 mm from the back of the eyeball: *1,* frontal bone; *2,* greater wing of sphenoid; *3,* zygomatic bone; *4,* maxilla; *5,* ethmoid; *6,* superior levator palpebrae muscle; *7,* superior rectus muscle; *8,* lateral rectus muscle; *9,* inferior rectus muscle; *10,* medial rectus muscle; *11,* superior oblique muscle; *12,* superior ophthalmic vein; *asterisks,* connective tissue septa. *M* indicates medial and *L,* lateral (hematoxylin-azophloxin/Mayer, ×3). *(From Koornneef L. New insights in the human orbital connective tissue. Result of a new anatomical approach.* Arch Ophthalmol. *1977;95:1269–1273.)*

14 • Orbit, Eyelids, and Lacrimal System

Annulus of Zinn

The annulus of Zinn is the fibrous ring formed by the common origin of the rectus muscles (Fig 1-5). The ring encircles the optic foramen and the central portion of the superior orbital fissure. The superior origin of the lateral rectus muscle separates the superior orbital fissure into two compartments. The portion of the orbital apex enclosed by the annulus is called the *oculomotor foramen*. This opening transmits cranial nerve III (upper and lower divisions), cranial nerve VI, and the nasociliary branch of the ophthalmic division of cranial nerve V (trigeminal). The superior and lateral aspect of the superior orbital fissure transmits cranial nerve IV as well as two other branches of the ophthalmic division of cranial nerve V: the frontal and lacrimal nerves. Cranial nerve IV is the only nerve innervating an extraocular muscle that does not pass directly into the muscle cone when entering the orbit. Cranial nerves III and VI pass directly into the muscle cone through the oculomotor foramen. The superior ophthalmic vein passes through the superior and lateral portion of the superior orbital fissure outside the oculomotor foramen.

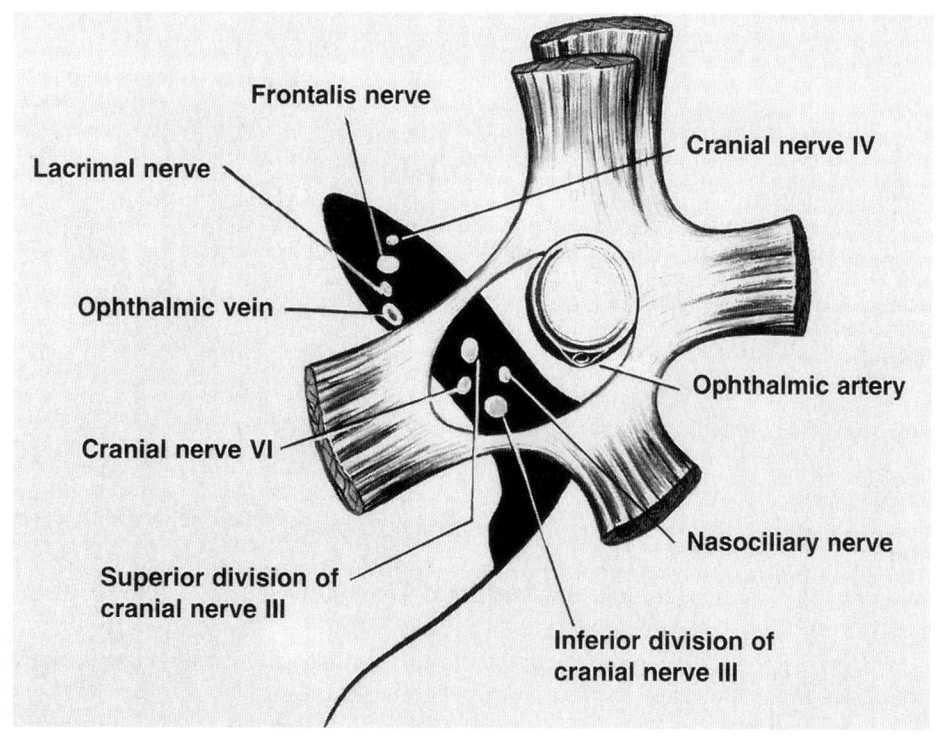

Figure 1-5 View of orbital apex, right orbit. The ophthalmic artery enters the orbit through the optic canal, whereas the superior and inferior divisions of cranial nerve III, cranial nerve VI, and the nasociliary nerve enter the muscle cone through the oculomotor foramen. Cranial nerve IV, the frontalis and lacrimal nerves, and the ophthalmic vein enter through the superior orbital fissure and thus lie within the periorbita but outside of the muscle cone. Note that the presence of many nerves and arteries along the lateral side of the optic nerve mandates a superonasal surgical approach to the optic nerve in the orbital apex. *(From Housepian EM. Intraorbital tumors. In: Schmidek HH, Sweet WH, eds. Current Techniques in Operative Neurosurgery. Orlando, FL: Grune & Stratton; 1976:148.)*

Vasculature System

The blood supply to the orbit arises primarily from the ophthalmic artery, which is a branch of the internal carotid artery. Smaller contributions come from the external carotid artery via the internal maxillary artery and the facial artery. The ophthalmic artery travels underneath the intracranial optic nerve through the dura mater along the optic canal to enter the orbit. The major branches of the ophthalmic artery are the

- Branches to the extraocular muscles
- Central retinal artery (to the optic nerve and retina)
- Posterior ciliary arteries (long to the anterior segment and short to the choroid)

Terminal branches of the ophthalmic artery travel anteriorly and form rich anastomoses with branches of the external carotid in the face and periorbital region.

The superior ophthalmic vein provides the main venous drainage of the orbit. This vein starts in the superonasal quadrant of the orbit and extends posteriorly through the superior orbital fissure into the cavernous sinus. Frequently, the superior ophthalmic vein appears on axial orbital CT scans as the only structure coursing diagonally through the superior orbit. Many anastomoses occur anteriorly with the veins of the face as well as posteriorly with the pterygoid plexus. See Figures 1-6 through 1-8.

Nerves

Sensory innervation to the periorbital area is provided by the ophthalmic and maxillary divisions of cranial nerve V (Fig 1-9). The ophthalmic division of cranial nerve V travels anteriorly from the ganglion in the lateral wall of the cavernous sinus, where it divides into three main branches: frontal, lacrimal, and nasociliary. The frontal and lacrimal nerves enter the orbit through the superior orbital fissure above the annulus of Zinn (see Fig 1-5) and travel anteriorly in the extraconal fat to innervate the medial canthus (supratrochlear branch), upper eyelid (lacrimal and supratrochlear branches), and forehead (supraorbital branch). The nasociliary branch enters the orbit through the superior orbital fissure within the annulus of Zinn, thus entering the intraconal space, where the nasociliary branch travels anteriorly to innervate the eye via the ciliary branches. The short ciliary nerves penetrate the sclera after passing through the ciliary ganglion without synapse. The long ciliary nerves pass by the ciliary ganglion and enter the sclera to extend anteriorly to supply the iris, cornea, and ciliary muscle.

Motor innervation to the extraocular muscles has already been outlined. The muscles of facial expression, including the orbicularis oculi, procerus, corrugator superciliaris, and frontalis muscles, receive their motor supply via branches of cranial nerve VII (the facial nerve) that penetrate the undersurface of each muscle.

The parasympathetic innervation, which allows accommodation, pupillary constriction, and lacrimal gland stimulation, follows a complicated course. Parasympathetic innervation enters the eye as the short posterior ciliary nerves after synapsing with the ciliary ganglion. Parasympathetic innervation to the lacrimal gland originates in the lacrimal nucleus of the pons and eventually joins the lacrimal nerve to enter the lacrimal gland.

The sympathetic innervation to the orbit provides for pupillary dilation, vasoconstriction, smooth muscle function of the eyelids and orbit, and hidrosis. The nerve fibers

16 • Orbit, Eyelids, and Lacrimal System

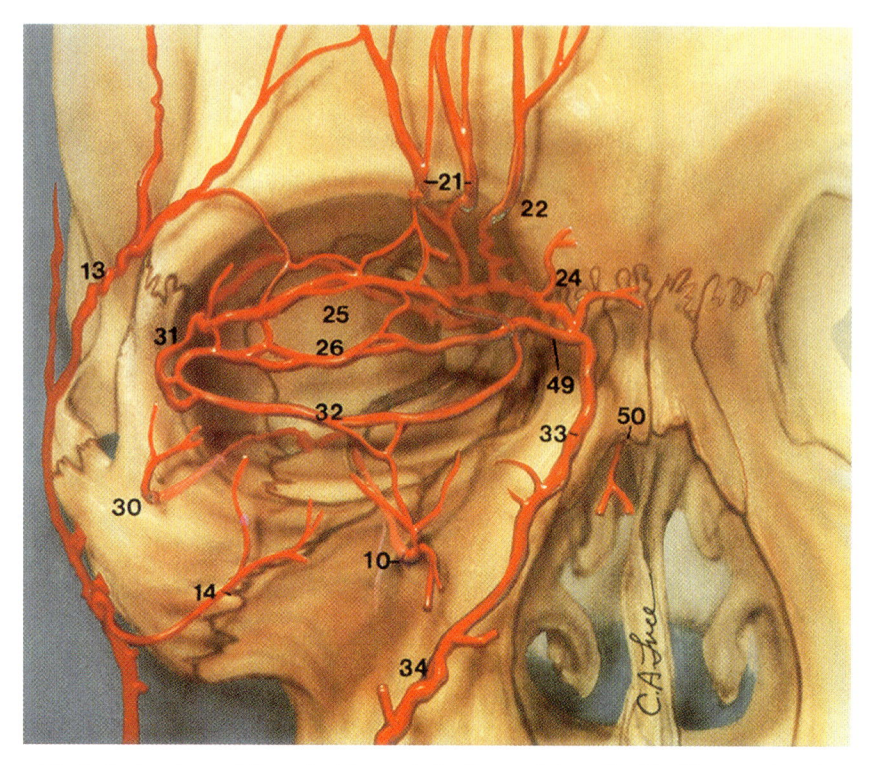

Figure 1-6 Anterior view of the arterial supply to the eyelids and orbit. The arteries shown are *10,* infraorbital; *13,* superficial temporal; *14,* transverse facial; *21,* supraorbital; *22,* supratrochlear; *24,* infratrochlear; *25,* superior peripheral arcade; *26,* superior marginal arcade; *30,* zygomaticofacial; *31,* lateral palpebral; *32,* inferior marginal arcade; *33,* angular; *34,* facial; *49,* medial palpebral; *50,* dorsal nasal. *(From Zide BM, Jelks GW, eds.* Surgical Anatomy of the Orbit. *New York: Raven; 1985:11.)*

follow the arterial supply to the pupil, eyelids, and orbit and travel anteriorly in association with the long ciliary nerves. Interruption of this innervation results in the familiar signs of Horner syndrome: ptosis of the upper eyelid, elevation of the lower lid, miosis, anhidrosis, and vasodilation.

Lacrimal Gland

The lacrimal gland is composed of a larger orbital lobe and a smaller palpebral lobe. The gland is located within a fossa of the frontal bone in the superior temporal orbit. Ducts from both lobes pass through the palpebral lobe and empty into the upper conjunctival fornix temporally. Frequently, a portion of the palpebral lobe is visible on slit-lamp examination with the upper eyelid everted. Biopsy is generally not performed on the palpebral lobe because it can interfere with drainage of the orbital lobe. Similarly, biopsy of the temporal fornix is avoided when possible. With age, the orbital lobe lacrimal gland may prolapse inferiorly out of the fossa and present as fullness or a mass in the lateral portion of the upper eyelid.

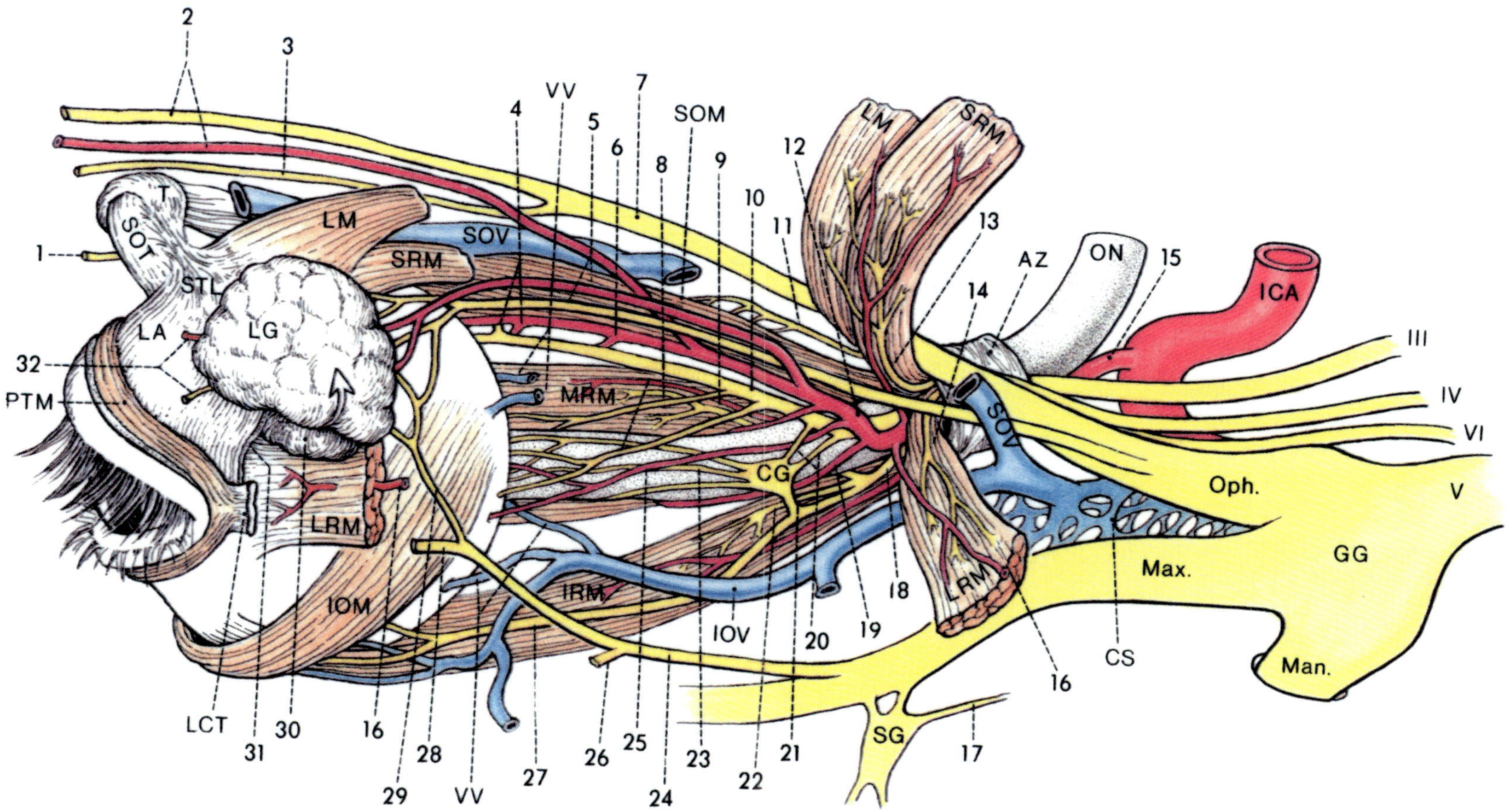

CHAPTER 1: Orbital Anatomy • 17

Figure 1-7 Side view of left orbit. *AZ,* annulus of Zinn; *CG,* ciliary ganglion; *CS,* cavernous sinus; *GG,* Gasserian ganglion; *ICA,* internal carotid artery; *IOM,* inferior oblique muscle; *IOV,* inferior ophthalmic vein; *IRM,* inferior rectus muscle; *LA,* levator aponeurosis; *LCT,* lateral canthal tendon; *LG,* lacrimal gland; *LM,* levator muscle; *LRM,* lateral rectus muscle; *Man.,* mandibular nerve; *Max.,* maxillary nerve; *MRM,* medial rectus muscle; *ON,* optic nerve; *Oph.,* ophthalmic nerve; *PTM,* pretarsal muscle; *SG,* sphenopalatine ganglion; *SOM,* superior oblique muscle; *SOT,* superior oblique tendon; *SOV,* superior ophthalmic vein; *SRM,* superior rectus muscle; *STL,* superior transverse ligament; *T,* trochlea; *VV,* vortex veins; *1,* infratrochlear nerve; *2,* supraorbital nerve and artery; *3,* supratrochlear nerve; *4,* anterior ethmoid nerve and artery; *5,* lacrimal nerve and artery; *6,* posterior ethmoid artery; *7,* frontal nerve; *8,* long ciliary nerves; *9,* branch of cranial nerve III to medial rectus muscle; *10,* nasociliary nerve; *11,* cranial nerve IV; *12,* ophthalmic (orbital) artery; *13,* superior ramus of cranial nerve III; *14,* cranial nerve VI; *15,* ophthalmic artery, origin; *16,* anterior ciliary artery; *17,* vidian nerve; *18,* inferior ramus of cranial nerve III; *19,* central retinal artery; *20,* sensory branches from ciliary ganglion to nasociliary nerve; *21,* motor (parasympathetic) nerve to ciliary ganglion from nerve to inferior oblique muscle; *22,* branch of cranial nerve III to inferior rectus muscle; *23,* short ciliary nerves; *24,* zygomatic nerve; *25,* posterior ciliary arteries; *26,* zygomaticofacial nerve; *27,* nerve to inferior oblique muscle; *28,* zygomaticotemporal nerve; *29,* lacrimal secretory nerve; *30,* lacrimal gland—palpebral lobe; *31,* lateral horn of levator aponeurosis; *32,* lacrimal artery and nerve-terminal branches. (From Stewart WB, ed. Ophthalmic Plastic and Reconstructive Surgery. 4th ed. San Francisco, American Academy of Ophthalmology Manuals Program; 1984.)

18 • Orbit, Eyelids, and Lacrimal System

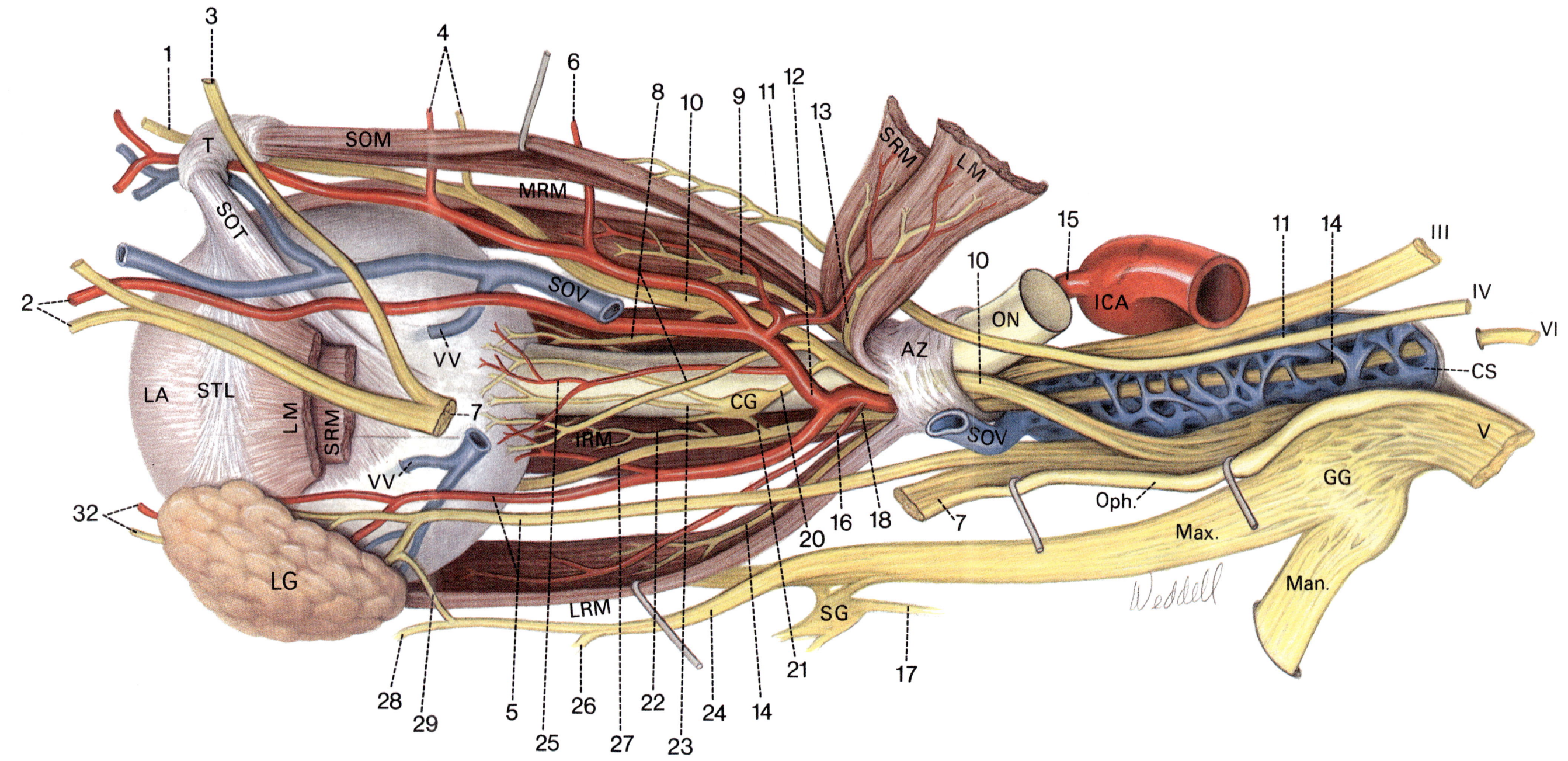

Figure 1-8 Top view of left orbit. *AZ,* annulus of Zinn; *CG,* ciliary ganglion; *CS,* cavernous sinus; *GG,* Gasserian ganglion; *ICA,* internal carotid artery; *IRM,* inferior rectus muscle; *LA,* levator aponeurosis; *LG,* lacrimal gland; *LM,* levator muscle; *LRM,* lateral rectus muscle; *Man.,* mandibular nerve; *Max.,* maxillary nerve; *MRM,* medial rectus muscle; *ON,* optic nerve; *Oph.,* ophthalmic nerve; *SG,* sphenopalatine ganglion; *SOM,* superior oblique muscle; *SOT,* superior oblique tendon; *SOV,* superior ophthalmic vein; *SRM,* superior rectus muscle; *STL,* superior transverse ligament; *T,* trochlea; *VV,* vortex veins; *1,* infratrochlear nerve; *2,* supraorbital nerve and artery; *3,* supratrochlear nerve; *4,* anterior ethmoid nerve and artery; *5,* lacrimal nerve and artery; *6,* posterior ethmoid artery; *7,* frontal nerve; *8,* long ciliary nerves; *9,* branch of cranial nerve III to medial rectus muscle; *10,* nasociliary nerve; *11,* cranial nerve IV; *12,* ophthalmic (orbital) artery; *13,* superior ramus of cranial nerve III; *14,* cranial nerve VI; *15,* ophthalmic artery, origin; *16,* anterior ciliary artery; *17,* vidian nerve; *18,* inferior ramus of cranial nerve III; *20,* sensory branches from ciliary ganglion to nasociliary nerve; *21,* motor (parasympathetic) nerve to ciliary ganglion from nerve to inferior oblique muscle; *22,* branch of cranial nerve III to inferior rectus muscle; *23,* short ciliary nerves; *24,* zygomatic nerve; *25,* posterior ciliary arteries; *26,* zygomaticofacial nerve; *27,* nerve to inferior oblique muscle; *28,* zygomaticotemporal nerve; *29,* lacrimal secretory nerve; *32,* lacrimal artery and nerve terminal branches. (From Stewart WB, ed. Ophthalmic Plastic and Reconstructive Surgery. 4th ed. San Francisco, American Academy of Ophthalmology Manuals Program; 1984.)

CHAPTER 1: Orbital Anatomy • 19

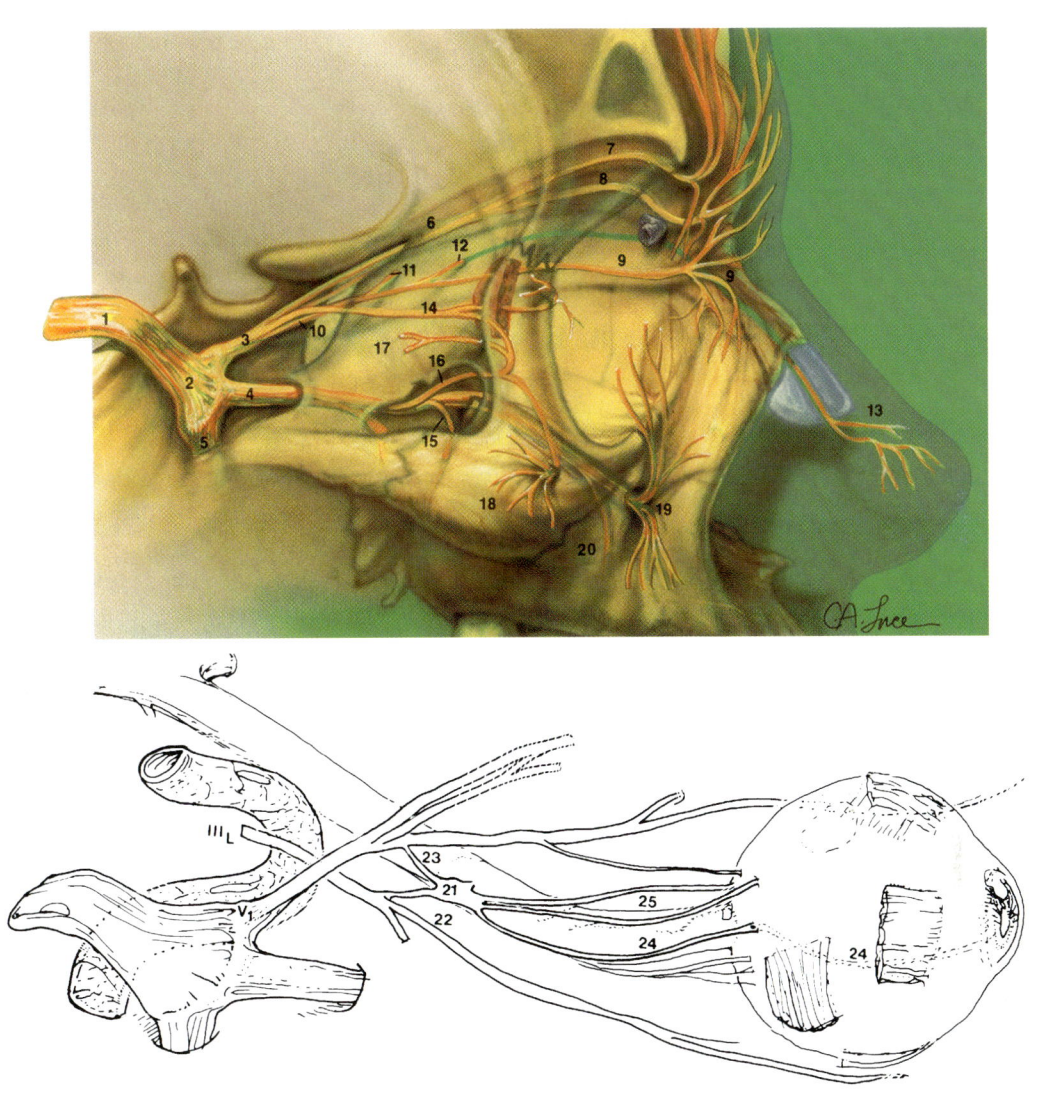

Figure 1-9 Sensory nerves. *1,* cranial nerve V; *2,* trigeminal ganglion; *3,* ophthalmic division of trigeminal nerve V_1; *4,* maxillary division of trigeminal nerve V_2; *5,* mandibular division of trigeminal nerve V_3; *6,* frontal nerve; *7,* supraorbital nerve; *8,* supratrochlear nerve (trochlea noted by *purple*); *9,* infratrochlear nerve; *10,* nasociliary nerve; *11,* posterior ethmoidal nerve; *12,* anterior ethmoidal nerve; *13,* external or dorsal nasal nerve; *14,* lacrimal nerve; *15,* posterior superior alveolar nerve; *16,* zygomatic nerve; *17,* zygomaticotemporal nerve; *18,* zygomaticofacial nerve; *19,* infraorbital nerve; *20,* anterior superior alveolar nerve; *21,* ciliary ganglion; *22,* nerve to inferior oblique; *23,* sensory root of ciliary ganglion; *24,* long ciliary nerves; *25,* short ciliary nerves. *(From Zide BM, Jelks GW, eds.* Surgical Anatomy of the Orbit. *New York: Raven; 1985:12.)*

Periorbital Structures

Nose and Paranasal Sinuses

The bones forming the medial, inferior, and superior orbital walls are close to the nasal cavity and are pneumatized by the paranasal sinuses, which arise from and drain into the nasal cavity. Ophthalmologists should be familiar with the anatomy and physiology of the nasal cavity and paranasal sinuses. Pathophysiologic processes common to these spaces that secondarily affect the orbit include sinonasal carcinomas, phycomycoses, Wegener granulomatosis, inverted papillomas, and sinusitis, which may cause orbital cellulitis or abscess.

The nasal cavity is divided into two nasal fossae by the nasal septum. The lateral wall of the nose has three bony projections: the superior, middle, and inferior conchae (turbinates). The conchae are covered by nasal mucosa, and they overhang the corresponding meatuses. Just cephalad to the superior concha is the sphenoethmoidal recess, into which the sphenoid sinus drains. The frontal sinus and the anterior and middle ethmoid air cells drain into the middle meatus. The nasolacrimal duct opens into the inferior meatus. The nasal cavity is lined by a pseudostratified, ciliated columnar epithelium with copious goblet cells. The mucous membrane overlying the lateral alar cartilage is hair-bearing and therefore less suitable for use as a composite graft in eyelid reconstruction than the mucoperichondrium over the nasal septum, which is devoid of hair.

The frontal sinuses develop from evaginations of the frontal recess and cannot be seen radiographically until the sixth year of life. Pneumatization of the frontal bone continues through childhood and is complete by early adulthood (Fig 1-10). The sinuses develop asymmetrically and vary greatly in size and shape. The two sinuses are almost always separated by the midline intersinus septum. Each sinus drains through separate frontonasal ducts and empties into the anterior portion of the middle meatus.

The ethmoid air cells are thin-walled cavities that lie between the medial orbital wall and the lateral wall of the nose. They can extend into the frontal, lacrimal, and maxillary bone and may extend into the orbital roof. Ethmoid air cells in this area are called *supraorbital ethmoids*. The numerous small, thin-walled air cells of the ethmoid sinus are divided into three groups: anterior, middle, and posterior. The anterior and middle air cells drain into the middle meatus; the posterior air cells drain into the superior meatus. The ethmoid air cells are present at birth and expand as the child grows. Orbital cellulitis is most frequently secondary to ethmoid sinusitis spreading into the orbit.

The sphenoid sinus evaginates from the posterior nasal roof to pneumatize the sphenoid bone and is divided into two cavities by a bony septum. Occasionally, pneumatization extends into the sphenoid, the pterygoid, and the occipital bone. The sphenoid sinus is rudimentary at birth and reaches full size after puberty. The sinus drains into the sphenoethmoid recess of each nasal fossa. The optic canal is located immediately superior and lateral to the sinus wall. Visual loss and visual field abnormalities can be direct sequelae of pathologic processes involving the sphenoid sinus.

The maxillary sinuses are the largest of the paranasal sinuses. Together, the roofs of each sinus form the floor of the orbit. The sinuses extend posteriorly in the maxillary bone to the inferior orbital fissure. The infraorbital nerve and artery travel along the roof

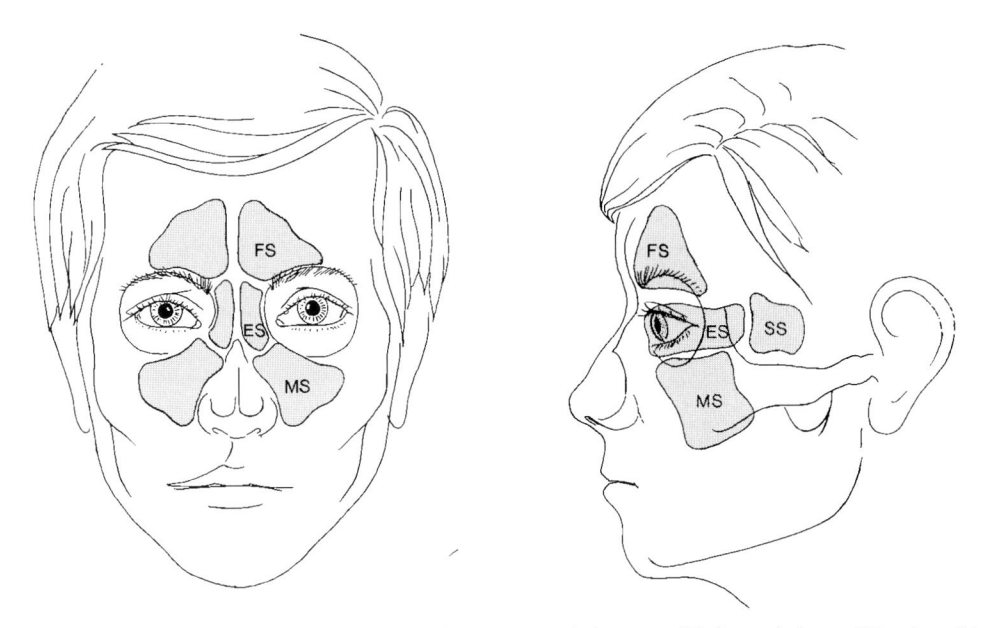

Figure 1-10 Relationship of the orbits to the paranasal sinuses: *FS*, frontal sinus; *ES*, ethmoid sinus; *MS*, maxillary sinus; *SS*, sphenoid sinus.

of the sinus from posterior to anterior. The bony nasolacrimal canal lies within the medial wall. The sinus drains into the middle meatus of the nose by way of the maxillary ostium. Orbital blowout fractures break the floor of the orbit medial to the infraorbital canal. These fractures frequently damage the infraorbital nerve, causing hypoesthesia of the cheek.

Fossae and Fissures

The orbit communicates with several fossae surrounding it. These spaces include the middle cranial fossa, the pterygopalatine fossa, and the infratemporal fossa. The middle cranial fossa lies posterior to the orbit. With the exception of the optic nerve, most nerves and vessels passing between the orbit and brain travel through the superior orbital fissure. The optic nerve passes through the optic canal. Inferior and posterior to the orbit, and posterior to the maxillary sinus, lies the pterygopalatine fossa. This fossa extends laterally to become the infratemporal fossa. These two fossae communicate with the orbit via the inferior orbital fissure.

The superior orbital fissure extends upward and outward from the orbital apex between the orbital roof and the lateral wall of the orbit. The superior orbital fissure is formed by the lesser wing of the sphenoid bone medially and the greater wing of the sphenoid laterally. The superior orbital fissure transmits cranial nerves III, IV, and VI; the ophthalmic division of cranial nerve V; and the superior ophthalmic vein. The optic canal is medial to the superior orbital fissure within the lesser wing of the sphenoid bone. A narrow segment of bone, the optic strut, separates the optic canal from the superior orbital fissure.

The inferior orbital fissure extends anteriorly and laterally between the lateral and inferior orbital walls. The inferior orbital fissure connects the orbit to the pterygopalatine fossa posteriorly and infratemporal fossa anteriorly. The maxillary division of cranial nerve V leaves the cranium through the foramen rotundum into the pterygopalatine fossa and then travels into the orbit through the inferior orbital fissure. The infraorbital vessels, the venous communications between the orbital veins and the pterygoid plexus, and the zygomatic branch of the maxillary nerve travel in through the inferior orbital fissure. The superior and inferior orbital fissures meet in the orbital apex.

For further discussion and illustrations of ocular anatomy, see BCSC Section 2, *Fundamentals and Principles of Ophthalmology.*

Dutton JJ. *Atlas of Clinical and Surgical Orbital Anatomy.* Philadelphia: Saunders; 1994.

Jordan DR, Anderson RA. *Surgical Anatomy of the Ocular Adnexa: A Clinical Approach.* Ophthalmology Monograph 9. San Francisco: American Academy of Ophthalmology; 1996.

Zide BM, Jelks GW, eds. *Surgical Anatomy of the Orbit.* New York: Raven; 1985.

CHAPTER 2

Evaluation of Orbital Disorders

The evaluation of an orbital disorder should distinguish orbital from periorbital and intraocular lesions. A detailed history is essential in establishing a probable diagnosis and in guiding the initial workup and therapy; such a history should include:

- Onset, course, and duration of symptoms (pain, diplopia, changes in vision) and signs (erythema, palpable mass, globe displacement)
- Prior disease (such as Graves ophthalmopathy or sinus disease) and therapy
- Injury (especially head or facial trauma)
- Systemic disease (especially carcinoma)
- Family history

Old photographs are frequently helpful.

The Six P's

It is helpful to remember the six P's: pain, proptosis, progression, palpation, pulsation, and periorbital changes.

Pain

Pain may be a symptom of inflammatory and infectious lesions, orbital hemorrhage, malignant lacrimal gland tumors, and nasopharyngeal carcinoma.

Proptosis

Proptosis often indicates the location of a mass because the globe is usually displaced away from the site of the mass. *Axial displacement* is caused by retrobulbar lesions such as cavernous hemangioma, glioma, meningioma, metastases, arteriovenous malformations, and any other mass lesion within the muscle cone. *Nonaxial displacement* is caused by lesions with a prominent component outside the muscle cone. *Superior displacement* is produced by maxillary sinus tumors invading and displacing the floor upward. *Inferomedial displacement* can result from dermoid cysts and lacrimal gland tumors. *Inferolateral displacement* can result from frontoethmoidal mucoceles, abscesses, osteomas, and sinus carcinomas. *Bilateral proptosis* can be produced by Graves ophthalmopathy, lymphoma, vasculitis, idiopathic orbital inflammatory disease (pseudotumor), metastatic tumors, carotid cavernous fistulas, cavernous sinus thrombosis, leukemia, and neuroblastoma. *Enophthalmos* can occur secondary to sclerosing tumors such as metastatic breast carcinoma or from expansion of the bony orbit as a result of fracture and displacement of the orbital walls.

Progression

The rate of progression can be a helpful diagnostic indicator. Disorders with onset occurring over days to weeks are usually caused by idiopathic orbital inflammatory disease, cellulitis, hemorrhage, thrombophlebitis, rhabdomyosarcoma, thyroid ophthalmopathy, neuroblastoma, metastatic tumors, or granulocytic sarcoma. Conditions with onset occurring over months to years are usually caused by dermoids, benign mixed tumors, neurogenic tumors, cavernous hemangiomas, lymphoma, fibrous histiocytoma, or osteomas.

Palpation

Masses palpable in the superonasal quadrant may be mucoceles, mucopyoceles, encephaloceles, neurofibromas, dermoids, or lymphomas. Masses palpable in the superotemporal quadrant include dermoids, a prolapsed lacrimal gland, lacrimal gland tumors, lymphomas, or idiopathic orbital inflammatory disease. Lesions behind the equator of the globe are usually not palpable.

Pulsation

Pulsation without bruits may be produced by neurofibromatosis or meningoencephaloceles, or it may result from surgical removal of the orbital roof. Pulsation with or without bruits may result from carotid cavernous fistulas, dural arteriovenous fistulas, and orbital arteriovenous fistulas.

Periorbital Changes

Periorbital changes may indicate underlying disorders. Table 2-1 lists various signs and their common causes.

Physical Examination and Laboratory Tests

Special attention to ocular motility, pupillary function, and ophthalmoscopy is necessary. Following the basic workup, radiologic studies are often required.

Inspection

Globe displacement is the most common clinical manifestation of an orbital abnormality. It usually results from a tumor, a vascular abnormality, or an inflammatory process.

Several terms are used to describe the position of the eye and orbit. *Proptosis* means a forward displacement or bulging of a body part and is commonly used to describe protrusion of the eye. *Exophthalmos* specifically describes proptosis of the eye and is sometimes used to describe the bulging of the eye associated with Graves ophthalmopathy. *Exorbitism* refers to an angle between the lateral orbital walls that is greater than

Table 2-1 Periorbital Changes Associated With Orbital Disease

Sign	Etiology
A salmon-colored mass in the cul-de-sac	Lymphoma (see Fig 5-16)
Eyelid retraction and eyelid lag	Graves ophthalmopathy
Vascular congestion over the insertions of the rectus muscles (particularly the lateral rectus)	Graves ophthalmopathy
Corkscrew conjunctival vessels	Arteriovenous fistula
Vascular anomaly of eyelid skin	Lymphangioma, varix, or capillary hemangioma
S-shaped eyelid	Plexiform neurofibroma
Anterior uveitis	Idiopathic orbital inflammatory syndrome or sarcoidosis
Eczematous lesions of the eyelids	Mycosis fungoides (T-cell lymphoma)
Ecchymoses of eyelid skin	Neuroblastoma, leukemia, or amyloidosis
Prominent temple	Sphenoid wing meningioma
Edematous swelling of lower eyelid	Meningioma, inflammatory tumor, metastases
Optociliary shunt vessels on disc	Meningioma
Frozen globe	Metastases or phycomycoses
Black-crusted lesions	Phycomycoses
Facial asymmetry	Fibrous dysplasia and neurofibromatosis
Gaze-evoked amaurosis	Optic nerve sheath meningioma or other orbital apex tumors

90°, which is usually associated with shallow orbital depth. This condition contrasts with *telorbitism (hypertelorism)*, which refers to a wider-than-normal separation of the medial orbital walls. Generally, exorbitism and hypertelorism refer to congenital abnormalities. *Telecanthus* refers to a wide intercanthal distance in the presence of a normal interpupillary distance (ie, the medial walls are normally positioned). Telecanthus can imply either a bony or a soft tissue abnormality and is used most commonly in describing acquired conditions. The eye may also be displaced vertically or horizontally by an orbital mass. Sinking of the eye, *enophthalmos*, may occur because of volume expansion of the orbit (fracture) or secondary to sclerosing orbital tumors (breast carcinoma).

Henderson JW, Campbell RJ, Farrow GM, et al. *Orbital Tumors*. 3rd ed. New York: Raven; 1994.

Rootman J, ed. *Diseases of the Orbit: A Multidisciplinary Approach*. Philadelphia: Lippincott; 1988.

Exophthalmometry usually proceeds from the lateral orbital rim to the anterior corneal surface. On average, the globes are more prominent in men than in women, and globes are more prominent in black patients than in white patients. An asymmetry of greater than 2 mm between the two eyes of a given patient suggests proptosis or enophthalmos. The Hertel exophthalmometer is generally used for adult patients. The accuracy of exophthalmometry with this instrument is enhanced when the examiner places his or her fifth finger in the patient's external auditory meatus for stabilization. Proptosis may best be appreciated clinically when the examiner looks up from below with the patient's head tilted back.

Bilateral proptosis in adults is caused most often by Graves ophthalmopathy and less frequently by other inflammations, such as idiopathic orbital inflammatory disease, Wegener granulomatosis, or neoplasms. *Unilateral proptosis* in adults is also most frequently caused by Graves ophthalmopathy. In children, bilateral proptosis may be caused by metastatic neuroblastoma, leukemia, or idiopathic orbital inflammatory disease.

Pseudoproptosis is either the simulation of abnormal prominence of the eye or a true asymmetry that is not the result of increased orbital contents. The diagnosis of pseudoproptosis should be postponed until a mass lesion has been ruled out. Causes of pseudoproptosis are

- Enlarged globe
- Extraocular muscle weakness or paralysis (allowing the eye to move forward)
- Contralateral enophthalmos
- Asymmetric orbital size
- Asymmetric palpebral fissures (usually caused by ipsilateral eyelid retraction or facial nerve paralysis or contralateral ptosis)

Ocular movements may be limited in a specific direction of gaze by neoplasms or inflammations that involve a single extraocular muscle. Graves ophthalmopathy usually involves multiple muscles bilaterally, although the bilaterality is often markedly asymmetric. Most commonly, Graves ophthalmopathy involves the inferior rectus muscle with fibrosis, which restricts globe elevation and in extreme cases may cause hypotropia in primary gaze. Upon attempted upgaze, intraocular pressure may rise. A large or rapidly enlarging orbital mass can also restrict ocular movements, even in the absence of direct muscle invasion.

Eyelid abnormalities are common in Graves ophthalmopathy. Retraction of the upper and lower eyelids and upper eyelid lag on downgaze are the most common physical signs of this condition. Capillary hemangiomas in the orbit often involve the skin of the eyelids, producing strawberry birthmarks that usually grow during the first year of life and then regress spontaneously. Plexiform neurofibromas frequently involve the lateral upper eyelids as well as the orbits and produce a "bag of worms" appearance and texture beneath the skin and conjunctiva. They may also cause an S-shaped curvature of the upper eyelids. Bilateral eyelid ecchymoses may occur in children with metastatic neuroblastoma.

Palpation

Palpation around the globe may disclose the presence of a mass in the anterior orbit, especially if the lacrimal gland is enlarged. Increased resistance to retrodisplacement of the globe is a nonspecific abnormality that may result from either a retrobulbar tumor or diffuse inflammation such as Graves ophthalmopathy. The physician should also palpate regional lymph nodes.

Pulsations of the eye are caused by transmission of the vascular pulse through the orbit. This may result from either abnormal vascular flow or transmission of normal intracranial pulsations through a bony defect in the orbital walls. Abnormal vascular flow may be caused by arteriovenous communication, such as carotid cavernous sinus fistulas. Defects in the bony orbital walls may result from sinus mucoceles, surgical removal of bone, trauma, or developmental abnormalities, including encephalocele, meningocele, or sphenoid wing dysplasia occurring in patients with neurofibromatosis.

Auscultation

Bruits may be detected with a stethoscope or be subjectively described by patients in cases of carotid cavernous fistulas. Patients with such arteriovenous communications often have tortuous dilated epibulbar vessels that characteristically stop short of the limbus.

Workup Checklist

Thorough ophthalmic examination of a patient with proptosis is complex, and thus, a checklist may be helpful to avoid omitting important observations (Fig 2-1). Such a list can also be used to record the findings of the examination in an organized format.

Primary Studies

Historically, plain-film radiography and tomography were used in evaluating patients with orbital disease (Fig 2-2). However, these techniques have been rendered largely obsolete by the widespread use of more current techniques, including computed tomography (CT) and magnetic resonance imaging (MRI). Ultrasonography may be helpful in some cases.

```
☐ Visual acuity                        ☐ Skin
☐ Refraction                           ☐ Oral and nasal examination
☐ Color vision                         ☐ Palpation
☐ Pupils                                   Orbit
☐ Extraocular motility                     Thyroid
☐ Anterior segment                         Regional lymph nodes
☐ Posterior segment                    ☐ Globe retropulsion
☐ Intraocular pressure                 ☐ Pulsation or thrill
☐ Anterior–posterior                   ☐ Bruit
     (exophthalmometry)                ☐ Valsalva
☐ Globe displacement                   ☐ Cranial nerves
     – Horizontal                            II        VI
     – Vertical                              III       VII
☐ Eyelids                                    IV        VIII
     Position                                V
     Margin–reflex distance (MRD)      ☐ Results of imaging
     Interpalpebral fissure                 Ultrasonography
     Lagophthalmos                          Computed tomography (CT) scan
                                            Magnetic resonance imaging (MRI)
```

Figure 2-1 Checklist for the evaluation of patients with proptosis.

28 • Orbit, Eyelids, and Lacrimal System

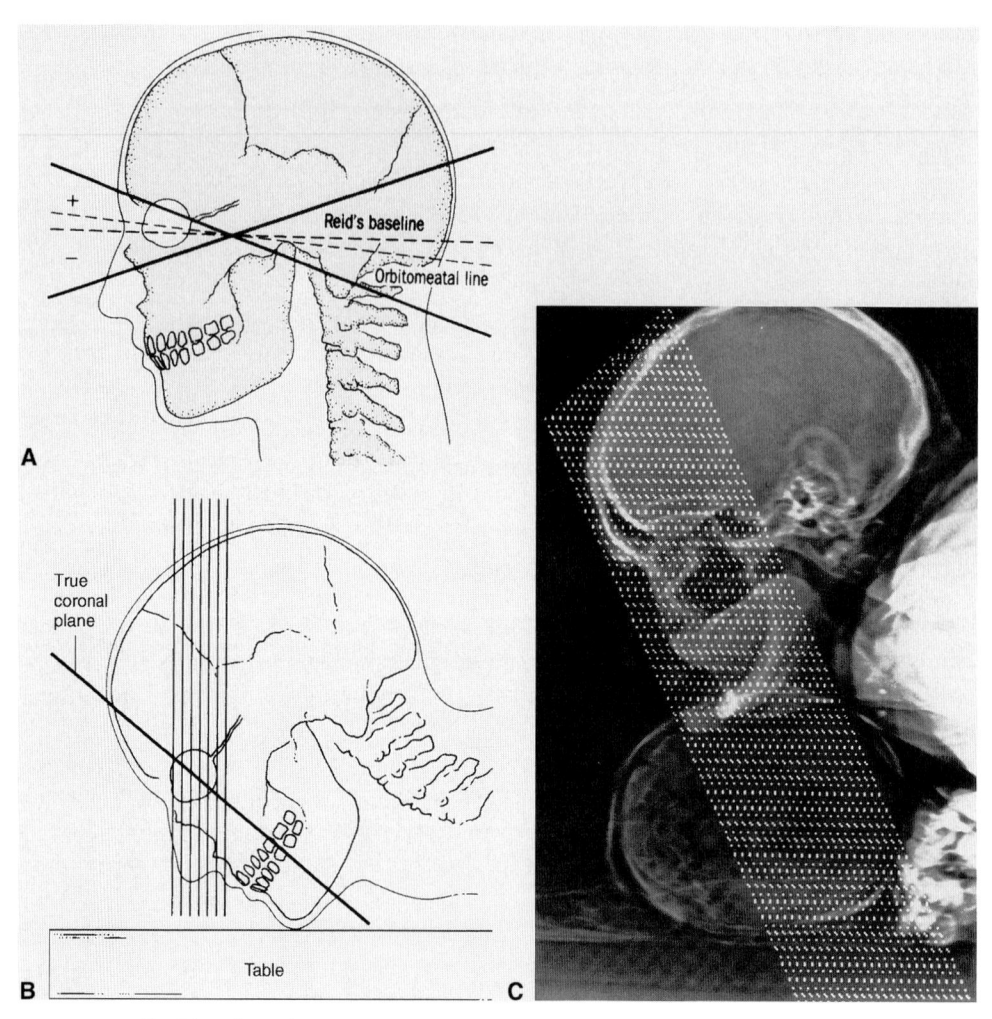

Figure 2-2 A, Direction of the x-ray beam in the axial plane. The orbitomeatal line extends from the lateral canthus to the center of the external auditory meatus and is the reference plane for positive (+) and negative (−) angulation. Reid's anatomic baseline extends from the inferior orbital rim to the upper margin of the external auditory meatus. Axial head scans are performed with positive angulation and may include the medulla oblongata and the base of the frontal lobe on the lowest slice; the orbit will be missed. Axial orbit scans are performed with negative angulation. Separate orbit and head sequences are usually required. **B,** Relative position of the head and the direction of the x-ray beam for direct coronal scanning of the orbit. Note that the neck scan cannot be extended sufficiently to achieve a true coronal plane. Moreover, the angulation may have to be further reduced from the direct coronal plane when the beam is directed anterior to the teeth to avoid artifacts from metallic fillings. Only MRI allows imaging in the true coronal plane. **C,** A scout CT for an almost true direct coronal series of scans in an edentulous patient. No compromise of angle was required to avoid the metallic artifacts caused by dental fillings. *(Reproduced by permission from Wirtschafter JD, Berman EL, McDonald CS.* Magnetic Resonance Imaging and Computed Tomography. Ophthalmology Monograph 6. *San Francisco: American Academy of Ophthalmology; 1992:40–41.)*

Computed Tomography

CT has revolutionized the management of orbital disorders. The tissues in a tomographic plane are assigned a density value proportional to their coefficient of absorption of x-rays. A two-dimensional image is electronically constructed from these density measurements. CT is the most valuable technique for delineating the shape, location, extent, and character of lesions in the orbit. CT helps to refine the differential diagnosis; moreover, when orbitotomy is indicated, CT guides the selection of the surgical approach by relating the lesion to the surgical space or spaces of the orbit.

Current CT scanners administer a dose of radiation of approximately 1–2 cGy per orbit scan. By comparison, a posteroanterior and lateral chest radiograph administers a dose of radiation of approximately 5 mGy.

The visualization of tumors that are well-supplied with blood vessels (eg, meningioma) or whose blood vessels leak is improved by the use of IV contrast-enhancing agents. CT has resolution and tissue-contrast capabilities allowing imaging of soft tissues, bones, contrast-containing blood vessels, and foreign bodies. Orbital images can be obtained in the axial plane, parallel to the course of the optic nerve, or in the coronal plane, viewing the eye, optic nerve, and extraocular muscles in cross-section. The simultaneous evaluation of axial and coronal views permits accurate three-dimensional assessment of orbital and periorbital tumors. Coronal CT is especially useful in evaluating orbital floor fractures and extraocular muscle size in Graves ophthalmopathy. Sinus anatomy, intracranial structures, and blood vessels can be examined at the same time as the orbits.

CT scanners allow the patient's head to be positioned for direct imaging in coronal and sagittal planes as well as axial planes. Although these direct views provide the highest resolution, they require additional scanning time and sometimes difficult patient positioning. To avoid such difficulties, CT techniques can be used to reconstruct (reformat) any section in any direction (axial, coronal, or sagittal), which may reduce the need for direct coronal and sagittal scanning. Reformatting can provide relatively clear images of the optic nerve, extraocular muscles, and bony structures, including the optic canals. However, the images obtained through direct scanning are sharper than those produced by reformatting.

The spiral CT technique, using new imaging hardware and software, moves the scanner in a "spiral" fashion around the patient, generating a continuous data set. Acquisition times are very short, making spiral CT especially good for use with children.

Three-Dimensional Computed Tomography

This technique allows reformatting of CT information into three-dimensional projections of the bony orbital walls. Because this type of imaging requires thin sections and additional computer time, three-dimensional CT is quite expensive. In some cases, three-dimensional CT may aid in the conceptualization of orbital bone changes and facilitate preparation for craniofacial surgical shifts or repairs of complex orbital fractures. Intraorbital contents cannot be visualized because of artifact.

Froula PD, Bartley GB, Garrity JA, et al. The differential diagnosis of orbital calcification as detected on computed tomographic scans. *Mayo Clin Proc.* 1993;68:256–261.

Magnetic Resonance Imaging

MRI is a noninvasive imaging technique that does not employ ionizing radiation and has no known adverse biological effects. MRI is based on the interaction of three physical components: atomic nuclei possessing an electrical charge, radiofrequency (RF) waves, and a powerful magnetic field.

Atoms with an unequal number of neutrons and protons possess an electrical charge and a nuclear spin, which generate a magnetic moment. These charged particles can be manipulated to interact with a magnetic field and RF waves. Under normal conditions, the charged nuclei spin about axes that point in random directions. Although many elements are capable of generating magnetic resonance signals, the hydrogen atom was selected for use because it is the most abundant element in the body.

The magnetic field must be extremely powerful (2,000–15,000 times greater than the earth's magnetic field) to affect the spinning hydrogen protons. The strength of the magnetic field is measured in tesla (T) or gauss (G) units (1 T = 10 kG). Current magnets in clinical use vary in strength from 0.1 to 1.5 T.

When a tissue containing hydrogen atoms is placed in the magnetic field, individual nuclei align themselves in the direction of the magnetic field. These aligned nuclei can be excited by an RF pulse emitted from a coil lying within the magnetic field. Excited nuclei align themselves against the static magnetic field; as the RF pulse is terminated, the nuclei flip back to their original magnetized position. As this occurs, the nuclei emit radiomagnetic energy that can be detected, processed, and imaged. The time it takes for this realignment to occur can be measured; it is called the *relaxation time.*

Each orbital tissue has specific magnetic resonance parameters that provide the information used to generate an image. (Figure 2-3 is an example of orbital MRI.) These parameters include tissue proton density and relaxation times. *Proton density* is determined by the number of protons per unit volume of tissue. Fat has greater proton density per unit volume than bone and, therefore, has greater signal intensity. T1, or *longitudinal relaxation time,* is the time required for the net bulk magnetization to realign itself along

Figure 2-3 Magnetic resonance scan of the orbit. *(From Edelstein WA, Schneck JF, Hart HR, et al. Surface coil magnetic resonance imaging. JAMA. 1985;253:828.)*

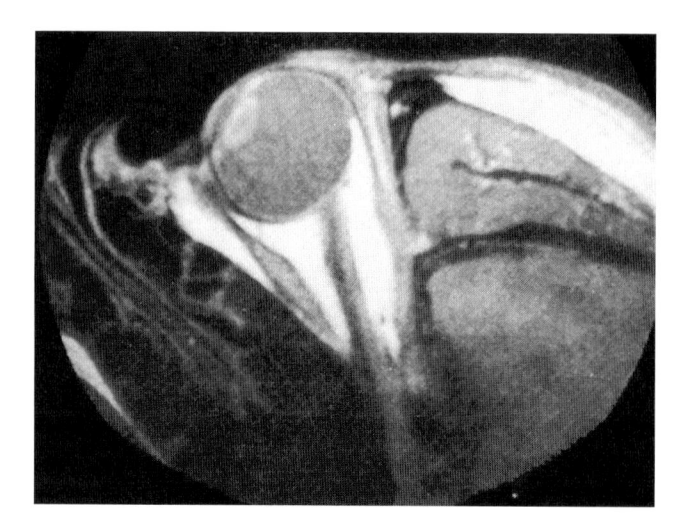

the original axis. T2, or *transverse relaxation time,* is the mean relaxation time based on the interaction of hydrogen nuclei within a given tissue, an indirect measure of the effect the nuclei have on each other. Each tissue has different proton density and T1 and T2 characteristics, providing the image contrast necessary to differentiate tissues. Healthy tissues can have imaging characteristics different from those of diseased tissue, a good example being the bright signal associated with tissue edema seen on T2-weighted scans.

MRI is usually performed with images created from both T1 and T2 parameters. T1-weighted images generally offer the best anatomical detail of the orbit. They require a shorter acquisition time than the T2-weighted images and therefore reduce the potential for motion artifact. T2-weighted images have the advantage of showing methemoglobin brighter than melanin, whereas these two substances have the same signal intensity on T1-weighted images. The difference in brightness seen on T2 images can be helpful in differentiating melanotic lesions from hemorrhagic processes of the choroid. Intravenous gadolinium enhancement brightens vascularized lesions so that they exhibit the same density as fat. Fat-suppression techniques in the computer software can be used to further improve the imaging of these enhanced lesions.

Comparison of CT and MRI

Although both CT and MRI are important modalities for the detection and characterization of orbital and ocular diseases, CT is currently the primary imaging technique. In general, CT provides better spatial resolution, whereas MRI provides better tissue contrast. Nevertheless, in most orbital conditions, the orbital fat provides sufficient natural tissue contrast to allow ready visualization of orbital tumors on CT. The bright T1 signal of orbital fat on MRI requires fat suppression, which may degrade image quality. MRI also remains significantly more expensive than CT. However, each of the techniques has advantages in specific situations, some of which are discussed below.

MRI resolution has been improved through the use of small-diameter surface coils and updated computer software (eg, fat suppression in the orbit). MRI offers advantages over CT in some situations. It allows the direct display of anatomical information in multiple planes (sagittal, axial, coronal, and any oblique plane) without repositioning the patient. Direct CT in the coronal plane requires hyperextension of the neck, which is impossible in some clinical settings. Although computer reformatting allows CT in any selected plane, image degradation occurs, limiting the usefulness of this technique. MRI provides better soft tissue definition than CT does. This advantage is especially helpful in the evaluation of demyelination and in vascular and hemorrhagic lesions. As with CT, contrast agents are available to improve MRI detail in selected cases.

Compared with CT, MRI also provides better tissue contrast of structures in the orbital apex, intracanalicular portion of the optic nerve, structures in periorbital spaces, and orbitocranial tumors, as there is no artifact from the skull base bones. Bone and calcification produce low signal on MRI. Bony structures may be evaluated by visualization of the signal void left by the bone. However, this is not possible when the bone is adjacent to structures that also create a signal void, such as air, rapidly flowing blood, calcification, and dura mater. Thus, CT is superior to MRI for the evaluation of fractures, bone destruction, and tissue calcification.

32 • Orbit, Eyelids, and Lacrimal System

Motion artifact remains a problem in MRI, which requires more time to perform than CT does. Patient anxiety and claustrophobia are also a problem because of the tighter confines of the MRI equipment. The use of magnetic resonance surface coils further aggravates this problem.

MRI is contraindicated in patients who have ferromagnetic metallic foreign bodies in the orbit or periorbital soft tissue, ferromagnetic vascular clips from previous surgery, magnetic intravascular filters, and electronic devices in the body such as cardiac pacemakers. If necessary, such foreign material can be ruled out with plain films or CT. Certain types of eye makeup can produce artifacts and should be removed prior to MRI. Dental amalgam is not a ferromagnetic substance and is not a contraindication to MRI, but this material does produce artifacts and degrades the images to some degree. Medical monitoring of a patient with serious health problems is easier in the environment of the CT room than in the MRI chamber. Because patients with acute head trauma are usually being evaluated for bone fractures, acute hemorrhagic problems, and possible foreign bodies, CT is usually the best choice in such cases, especially because it can be performed more quickly. For subacute trauma, MRI may be preferable because all planes of imaging can be obtained without hyperextension of the neck and because MRI is better at differentiating between fresh and old hemorrhages (Fig 2-4).

Although CT and MRI yield different images, it is unusual for both techniques to be required in the evaluation of an orbital disorder. The choice between these modalities

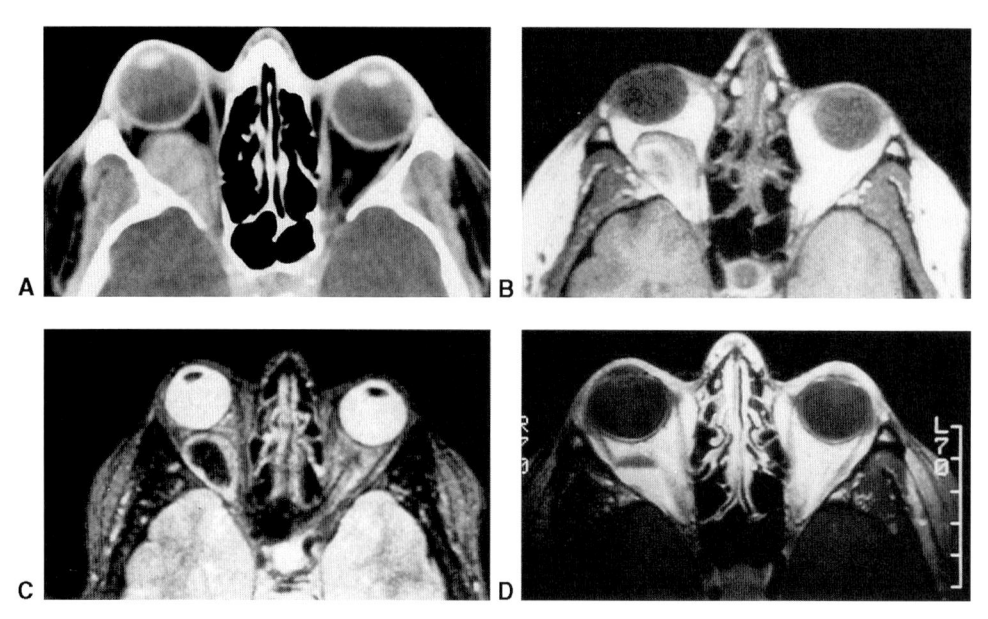

Figure 2-4 A, A CT scan of a patient with acute right exophthalmos as a result of a spontaneous orbital hemorrhage. The hematoma exhibits discrete margins, homogeneous consistency, and a radiodensity similar to blood vessels and muscle. **B,** A T1 MR scan obtained 4 days after the hemorrhage demonstrates the transient "bull's-eye" pattern characteristic of a hematoma beginning to undergo physical changes and biochemical hemoglobin degradation. **C,** A T2 MR scan obtained the same day as the T1 study shows a characteristic ring pattern. **D,** A T1 MR scan performed 3 months later shows that the hematoma has decreased in size. There is layering of the degraded blood components.

should be based on the specific patient's condition. In most cases, CT is the more effective and economical choice (Table 2-2). When the orbitocranial junction or brain is involved, CT scanning and MRI may be complementary.

> Davis PC, Newman NJ. Advances in neuroimaging of the visual pathways. *Am J Ophthalmol.* 1996;121:690–705.
>
> Ellis BD, Hogg JP. Neuroimaging for the general ophthalmologist. In: *Focal Points: Clinical Modules for Ophthalmologists.* San Francisco: American Academy of Ophthalmology; 1998: vol 16, no 8.
>
> Mukherji SK, Tart RP, Fitzsimmons J, et al. Fat-suppressed MR of the orbit and cavernous sinus: comparison of fast spin-echo and conventional spin-echo. *Am J Neuroradiol.* 1994; 15:1707–1714.
>
> Newton TH, Bilaniuk LT, eds. *Radiology of the Eye and Orbit (Modern Neuroradiology.* Vol 4). New York: Raven; 1990.
>
> Trobe JD, Gebarski SS. Looking behind the eyes. The proper use of modern imaging [editorial]. *Arch Ophthalmol.* 1993;111:1185–1186.
>
> Wirtschafter JD, Berman EL, McDonald CS. *Magnetic Resonance Imaging and Computed Tomography.* Ophthalmology Monograph 6. San Francisco: American Academy of Ophthalmology; 1992.

Ultrasonography

Orbital ultrasonography is sometimes used to examine patients with orbital disorders. The size, shape, and position of normal and abnormal orbital tissues can be determined by means of contemporary ultrasound techniques. Two-dimensional images of these tissues can be obtained with B-scan ultrasonography. Standardized A-scan ultrasonography provides unidimensional images of the orbital soft tissues characterized by a series of spikes of varying height and width that demonstrate the particular echogenic characteristics of each tissue.

Table 2-2 Comparison of CT Scan and MRI in Orbital Disease

CT Scan	MRI
Good for most orbital conditions, especially fractures and Graves ophthalmopathy	Better of orbitocranial junction or intracranial problems
Good view of bone and calcium	No view of bone or calcium
Degraded image of orbital apex because of bony artifact	Good view of orbital apex unimpeded by bony artifacts
Better spatial resolution	More soft tissue detail
Reformatting or rescanning required to image and multiple planes	Multiple planes can be imaged at once
Contrast improves imaging in many cases	Contrast improves imaging in many cases
Less motion artifact because of shorter scanning time	More motion artifact because of longer scanning time
Less claustrophobic	Difficult for claustrophobic patients
Good for metallic foreign bodies	Contraindicated for patients with ferromagnetic metallic foreign bodies, aneurysm clips, and pacemakers
Less expensive	More expensive

When used appropriately, ultrasonography is valuable to the orbital surgeon. Specific tissues, echo characteristics, and dynamic tissue manipulation techniques, such as compression, can be helpful in the diagnosis and localization of lesions. The levels of edema sometimes can be used to discern the degree of disease activity. Intraoperative localization of foreign bodies is possible.

Specific information regarding blood flow can be obtained using Doppler ultrasonography. For example, in patients with occlusive vascular disease or vascular abnormalities associated with increased blood flow, the velocity and direction of blood flow can be determined.

However, analysis of orbital disease requires specialized equipment and experienced personnel. In general, office-based ultrasound equipment is not suitable for the evaluation of orbital tissues. Ultrasonography is of limited value in assessing lesions of the posterior orbit (because of sound attenuation) or the sinuses or intracranial space (because sound does not pass well through air or bone). For these reasons, CT is used in evaluating the majority of orbital processes.

Aburn NS, Sergott RC. Orbital colour Doppler imaging. *Eye.* 1993;7:639–647.

Secondary Studies

Secondary studies that are performed for specific indications include venography and arteriography. These studies are rarely used but may be helpful in specific cases.

Venography

Before the age of CT and MRI, orbital venography was used in the diagnosis and management of orbital varices and in the study of the cavernous sinus. Contrast material is injected into the frontal or the angular vein to reveal a venous abnormality. Subtraction and magnification techniques have been used to increase the resolution of venography.

Arteriography

Arteriography should be used only in patients with a high probability of an arterial lesion such as an aneurysm or arteriovenous malformation. Retrograde catheterization of the cerebral vessels is accomplished through the femoral artery. There is a small risk of serious neurologic and vascular complications because the technique requires installation of the catheter and injection of radiopaque dye into the arterial system.

Visualization can be maximized by use of selective injection of the internal and external carotid arteries, magnification to allow viewing of the smaller caliber vessels, and subtraction techniques to radiographically eliminate bone.

Images can be obtained and stored using conventional sequential filming techniques or newer digital systems. Although digital systems are more economical, they currently do not provide the same degree of resolution as conventional film techniques. Newer techniques involving magnetic resonance angiography (MRA) allow noninvasive visualization of large and medium-size vessels of the arterial system but do not provide as fine detail as direct angiography.

Pathology

The diagnosis of an orbital lesion usually requires analysis of tissue obtained through an orbitotomy. Appropriate handling of the tissue specimen is necessary to ensure an accurate diagnosis. The majority of tissue samples are placed in formalin for permanent-section analysis. Frozen-section analysis is generally not used for definitive diagnosis of an orbital tumor. However, when the area of proposed biopsy is not obvious, frozen sections are helpful to confirm that appropriate tissue has been obtained for permanent-section analysis. Frozen-section analysis is also used intraoperatively to determine tumor margins, ensuring complete tumor removal. Tissue removed for frozen-section analysis should be placed in a dampened saline gauze and promptly sent to the frozen-section laboratory.

Because of the vast array of possible unusual tumor types in the orbit, preoperative consultation with a pathologist familiar with orbital disease may be helpful to maximize the information gained from any orbital biopsy. In many cases, fresh tissue should be obtained and frozen for cell-surface marker studies. Cell-marker studies are required in the analysis of all orbital lymphoid lesions. These studies may permit differentiation of reactive lymphoid hyperplasia from lymphoma. Such studies may also indicate the presence of estrogen receptors in cases of metastatic prostate or breast carcinoma and thus provide useful information regarding sensitivity to hormonal therapy. Marker studies are also useful in the diagnosis of poorly differentiated tumors when light microscopy alone cannot yield a definitive diagnosis. Although cell-marker studies have largely replaced electron microscopy in the diagnosis of very undifferentiated tumors, it may nevertheless be worthwhile in these cases to preserve fresh tissue in glutaraldehyde for possible electron microscopy. In cases of noncohesive tumors (hematologic or lymphoid), a touch prep may permit a diagnosis.

All biopsy specimens must be treated delicately to minimize crush artifact, which can confuse interpretation. Permanent tissue biopsy specimens must be placed in fixatives immediately. If fine-needle aspiration biopsy is planned, a cytologist or trained technician must be available to handle the aspirate. In special cases, the biopsy can be performed under either ultrasonographic or CT control. Although a fine-bore needle occasionally yields a sufficient cell block, the specimen is usually limited to cytologic study. This technique may not permit as firm a diagnosis as is possible with larger biopsy specimens in which the histologic pattern can be evaluated by use of light and electron microscopy.

See BCSC Section 4, *Ophthalmic Pathology and Intraocular Tumors*, for more extensive discussion of pathology.

Laboratory Studies

Screening for abnormal thyroid function commonly includes T_3, T_4, and thyroid-stimulating hormone. These serum test results are abnormal in 90% of patients with thyroid ophthalmopathy. However, if thyroid disease is strongly suspected and these results are normal, additional endocrine studies, including studies of thyroid-stimulating immunoglobulins, can be considered.

Wegener granulomatosis should be suspected in patients with sclerokeratitis or coexisting sinus disease and orbital mass lesions. The antineutrophil cytoplasmic antibody serum assay is a very sensitive test for this uncommon disease. Wegener granulomatosis may present as a chronic orbital inflammation. Biopsy of affected tissues classically shows vasculitis, granulomatous inflammation, and tissue necrosis, although necrotizing vasculitis is not always present in orbital biopsies. The disease affects the upper and lower respiratory tracts, the kidney, and the orbit, but limited forms may lack renal involvement. Early diagnosis and treatment of this disorder with cyclophosphamide and prednisone may be lifesaving.

Testing for angiotensin-converting enzyme may be helpful in the diagnosis of sarcoidosis. This multisystem granulomatous inflammatory condition may present with lacrimal gland enlargement, conjunctival granulomas, extraocular muscle or optic nerve infiltration, or solitary orbital granulomas. Diagnosis is confirmed through biopsy of one or more affected organs.

CHAPTER 3

Congenital Orbital Anomalies

Although most common anomalies of the eye and orbit are apparent before birth, developmental defects can manifest at any time from conception until late in life. If an anomaly is caused by a slowing or cessation of a normal stage, the resulting deformity can be considered a pure arrest. An example is microphthalmos. However, a superimposed aberrant growth usually follows the original arrest, and the resulting deformity does not represent any previous normal stage of development. An example of this latter condition is formation of an orbital cyst following incomplete closure of the fetal fissure. As a general rule, the more gross the abnormality, the earlier in development it occurred. For further discussion, including illustrations, see also Embryology, in BCSC Section 2, *Fundamentals and Principles of Ophthalmology*; and BCSC Section 6, *Pediatric Ophthalmology and Strabismus*.

Anophthalmos

True congenital anophthalmos is rare and occurs when the primary optic vesicle fails to grow out from the cerebral vesicle during embryonic development. In most cases in which a baby is born with a unilateral small orbit and no visible eye, a small microphthalmic globe is present in the orbital soft tissues. All such children have hypoplastic orbits, and treatment should consist of socket expansion with progressively enlarging conformers until a prosthesis can be fitted. Tissue expanders placed beneath the periosteum may be progressively inflated to enlarge the hypoplastic orbit in cases of severe bony asymmetry. Enucleation is usually not necessary for the fitting of conformers or an ocular prosthesis, and enucleation is usually avoided because it may worsen the bony hypoplasia. However, success has been reported with the use of dermis-fat grafts as orbital implants following early enucleation. These grafts appear to grow along with the patient, producing progressive socket expansion.

Microphthalmos

Microphthalmos is a developmental defect that causes reduction in the size of the eye and is usually associated with structural abnormalities. Eyes vary in size depending on the severity of the defect. *Microphthalmos with orbital cyst* results from the failure of the choroidal fissure to close in the embryo. This condition is usually unilateral but may be bilateral. The presence of an orbital cyst may be beneficial for stimulating normal growth of the involved orbital bone and eyelids. In some cases, the orbital cyst may have to be removed to allow for fitting of an ocular prosthesis.

Craniofacial Clefting

A craniofacial cleft occurs when normal development is arrested. Facial clefts in the skeletal structures are oriented around the orbit and maxilla. Facial clefts in the soft tissues are distributed around the eyelids and the lips. Examples of clefting syndromes that affect the orbit and eyelids are mandibulofacial dysostosis (Treacher Collins–Franceschetti syndrome—Fig 3-1), oculoauricular dysplasia (Goldenhar syndrome), and some forms of midline clefts with hypertelorism.

The bones of the skull or orbit may also have congenital clefts through which the intracranial contents can herniate. These protruding contents can be the meninges *(meningocele)*, brain tissue *(encephalocele)*, or both meninges and brain tissue *(meningoencephalocele)*, as illustrated in Figure 3-2. When these herniations involve the orbit, they most commonly present anteriorly with a protrusion subcutaneously near the medial canthus over the bridge of the nose. Straining or crying may produce an increase in the size of the mass, and the globe may be displaced temporally and downward. Such herniations less commonly move into the posterior orbit; these lesions may cause anterior displacement and pulsation of the globe. Meningoceles and encephaloceles adjacent to the orbit are frequently associated with anomalies of the optic disc. Treatment is surgical and should be carried out in collaboration with a neurosurgeon.

Craniosynostosis, the premature closure of one or more sutures in the bones of the skull, results in various skeletal deformities. Hypertelorism and proptosis are frequently observed in craniosynostosis syndromes such as Crouzon syndrome (craniofacial dysostosis—Fig 3-3) and Apert syndrome (acrocephalosyndactyly).

The severe orbital defects associated with craniofacial deformities can sometimes be corrected with osteoplastic surgery. Such operations usually require the joint efforts of neurosurgeons, general plastic surgeons, and otolaryngologists, as well as ophthalmologists.

Figure 3-1 Treacher Collins–Franceschetti syndrome (mandibulofacial dysostosis). *(Photograph courtesy of James Garrity, MD.)*

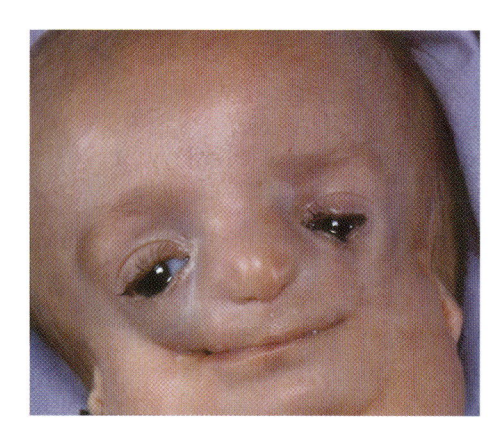

CHAPTER 3: Congenital Orbital Anomalies • 39

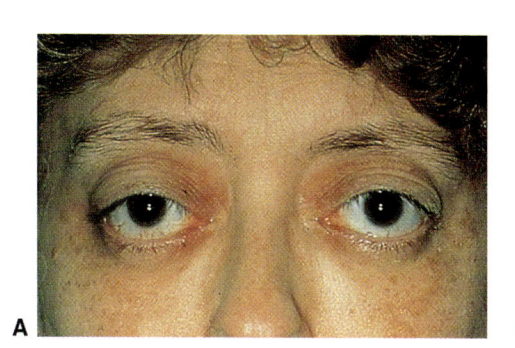

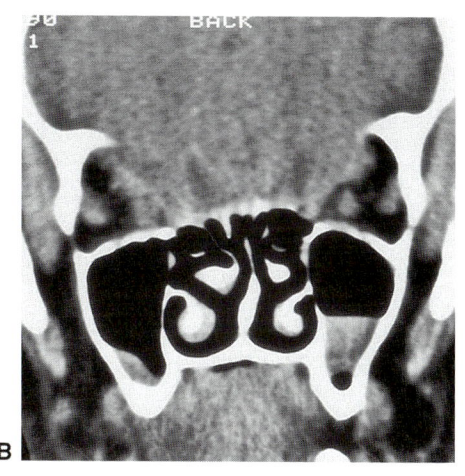

Figure 3-2 A, Patient with telecanthus and bilateral pulsatile proptosis. **B,** CT scan of large orbital meningoencephalocele through congenital cleft of skull base.

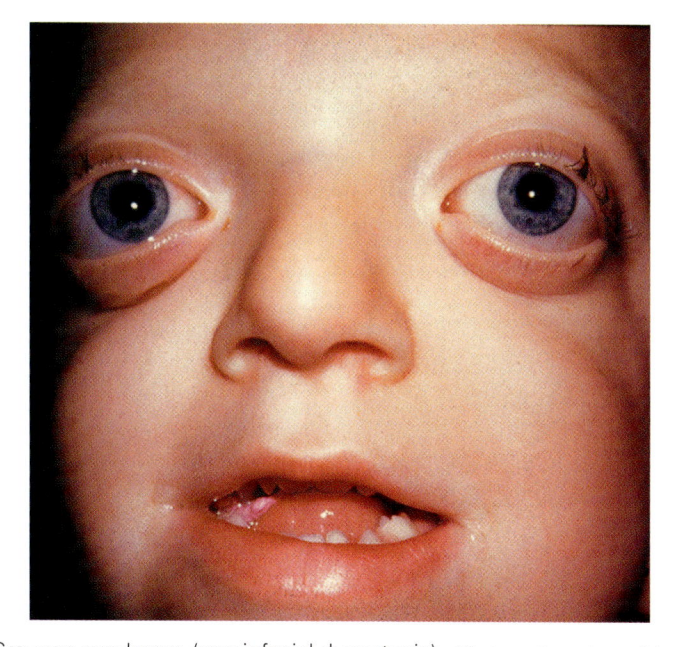

Figure 3-3 Crouzon syndrome (craniofacial dysostosis). *(Photograph courtesy of James Garrity, MD.)*

Tumors

For a discussion of *dermoid cysts, lipodermoids, teratomas,* and *developmental vascular malformations and neoplasms,* see Chapter 5, Orbital Neoplasms.

CHAPTER 4

Infectious and Inflammatory Disorders

Infections

Cellulitis

Bacterial infections of the orbit or periorbital soft tissues occur from three primary sources:

- Direct spread from an adjacent sinusitis (the large majority of cases)
- Direct inoculation following trauma or skin infection
- Bacteremic spread from a distant focus (otitis media, pneumonia)

Although periorbital infections are typically classified as being either preseptal or orbital cellulitis, they often represent a continuum, with common underlying causes requiring similar treatment regimens. It must be emphasized that in cellulitis—whether preseptal or orbital—underlying sinusitis is most likely if no obvious source of inoculation is noted.

Preseptal cellulitis

Preseptal cellulitis is defined as inflammation and infection confined to the eyelids and periorbital structures anterior to the orbital septum. The orbital structures posterior to the septum are not infected but may be secondarily inflamed. Eyelid edema, erythema, and inflammation may be severe. Usually, the globe is uninvolved. Pupillary reaction, visual acuity, and ocular motility are not disturbed. Pain on eye movement and chemosis are absent.

Designating the cellulitis as preseptal implies an infective process superficial to the orbital septum, one thought to require less intensive treatment than orbital cellulitis. Although preseptal cellulitis in adults is usually due to penetrating trauma or a cutaneous source of infection, in children the most common cause is underlying sinusitis. Historically, preseptal cellulitis in infants and children younger than 5 years was often associated with bacteremia, septicemia, and meningitis caused by *Haemophilus influenzae*. This cause of preseptal and orbital cellulitis has virtually been eliminated by the introduction of the HiB vaccine. However, some cases of preseptal and orbital cellulitis in children may still be associated with bacteremia, usually of gram-positive cocci. Workup should proceed quickly and include CT of the orbit and sinuses if no direct site of inoculation is identified. The patient should be treated in consultation with a pediatrician, and hospitalization and intravenous antibiotics are indicated if there is underlying sinusitis.

In teenagers and adults, preseptal cellulitis usually arises from a superficial source (eg, traumatic inoculation, infected chalazion or epidermal inclusion cyst) and responds quickly to appropriate oral antibiotics. Initial antibiotic selection is based on the history, clinical findings, and initial laboratory studies. Prompt sensitivity studies are indicated so that the antibiotic selection can be revised, if necessary. *Staphylococcus aureus* is the most common pathogen in patients with preseptal cellulitis resulting from trauma. The infection usually responds quickly to a penicillinase-resistant penicillin, such as methicillin or ampicillin-sulbactam. However, methicillin-resistant *S aureus* is increasingly encountered.

Imaging studies should be performed to rule out underlying sinusitis if no direct inoculation site is identified. If the patient does not respond quickly to oral antibiotics or if orbital involvement becomes evident, prompt hospital admission, CT, and intravenous antibiotics are usually indicated.

Surgical drainage may be necessary if preseptal cellulitis progresses to a localized abscess. Incision and drainage can usually be performed directly over the abscess, but care should be taken to avoid damaging the levator aponeurosis in the upper eyelid. The orbital septum should not be opened to avoid contaminating the orbital soft tissue.

Orbital cellulitis

In orbital cellulitis (Fig 4-1), active infection of the orbital soft tissue is present posterior to the orbital septum. In more than 90% of cases, orbital cellulitis occurs as a secondary extension of acute or chronic bacterial sinusitis (Table 4-1). Clinical findings that suggest orbital cellulitis include fever (present along with leukocytosis in 75% of cases), proptosis, chemosis, restriction of ocular motility, and pain on movement of the globe. Decreased vision and pupillary abnormalities suggest involvement of the orbital apex and demand immediate investigation and aggressive management. Delay in treatment may result in progression of the infection and development of an orbital apex syndrome or cavernous sinus thrombosis. Blindness, cranial nerve palsies, brain abscess, and even death can result. Such devastating consequences are best avoided by aggressive management. Orbital extension of a preexisting periorbital cellulitis is sometimes difficult to diagnose clinically.

Because orbital cellulitis is a manifestation of underlying sinusitis in more than 90% of cases, evaluation of the paranasal sinuses, preferably by CT, is essential. Identification of sinusitis mandates otolaryngologic consultation. Antibiotic therapy should provide broad-spectrum coverage because infections in adults usually grow multiple organisms that may include gram-positive cocci, *H influenzae* and *M catarrhalis*, and anaerobes. Although nasal decongestants may help spontaneous drainage of the infected sinus, early surgical intervention to drain the involved sinuses is usually indicated, especially if orbital findings progress during intravenous antibiotic therapy. In contrast, orbital cellulitis in children is more often caused by a single organism and is less likely to require surgical drainage of the infected sinus.

Orbital cellulitis following blowout fractures is generally limited to patients with underlying sinus disease. Prophylactic antibiotics are recommended if CT scans of orbital fractures identify pansinusitis. The risk of orbital cellulitis is increased if the medial wall is fractured.

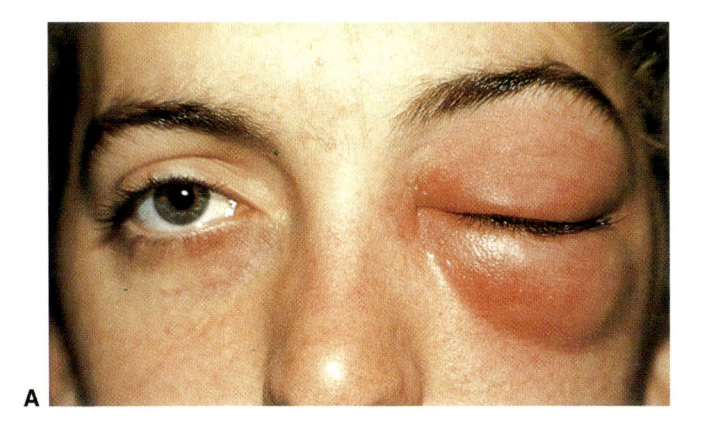

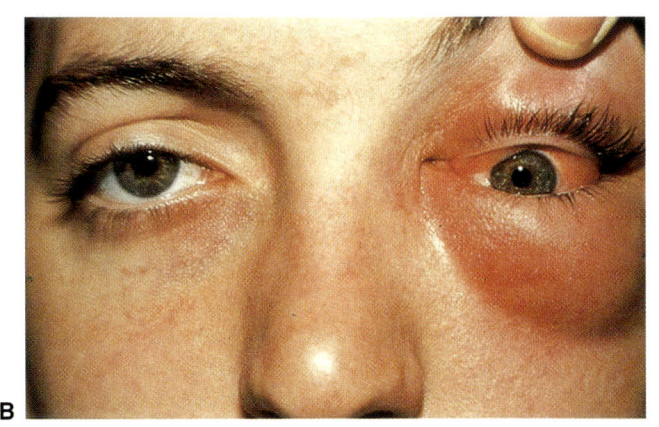

CHAPTER 4: Infectious and Inflammatory Disorders • 43

Figure 4-1 A, Orbital cellulitis with marked erythema, proptosis, and ptosis. **B,** Chemosis and hypo-ophthalmia are present. **C,** Vertical ductions are impaired OS. *(Photographs courtesy of Jeffrey A. Nerad, MD.)*

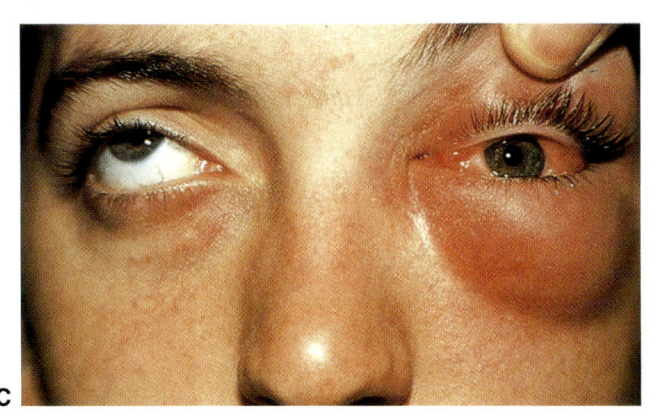

A significant percentage of cases of orbital cellulitis proceed to abscess formation, which may present as progressive proptosis or globe displacement. Progression of infection and clinical deterioration can occur even in patients on appropriate antibiotics. Abscesses usually localize in the subperiosteal space, adjacent to the infected sinus, but may occur within the orbital soft tissue or in the preaponeurotic space (Fig 4-2). Such abscesses should be suspected if patients on intravenous antibiotics do not show daily improvement. Serial clinical examinations coupled with good-quality CT scans are in-

Table 4-1 Causes of Orbital Cellulitis

Extension from periorbital structures
Paranasal sinuses
Face and eyelids
Dacryocystitis
Dental infection
Intracranial

Exogenous
Trauma (rule out foreign bodies)
Postsurgical (any orbital or periorbital surgery)

Endogenous
Bacteremia with septic embolization

Intraorbital
Endophthalmitis
Dacryoadenitis

---

valuable in detecting abscess localization and in planning the surgical approach for drainage.

Not all subperiosteal abscesses require surgical drainage. Isolated medial or inferior subperiosteal orbital abscesses in children under age 9 with underlying isolated ethmoid sinusitis and intact vision and moderate proptosis have been reported to respond to medical therapy alone. However, surgical drainage coupled with appropriate antibiotic therapy is recommended in older patients or more severe presentation and usually leads to dramatic clinical improvement within 24–48 hours. Concomitant sinus surgery is indicated if sinusitis is present. The refractory nature of orbital abscesses in adolescents and adults is thought to be usually due to the multiple pathogens, including anaerobic bacteria.

The majority of patients with orbital cellulitis and abscesses respond to appropriate medical and surgical treatment. These orbital infections rarely spread posteriorly to the cavernous sinus. Cavernous sinus thrombosis is often heralded by the rapid progression of proptosis and changes in mental status. Meningitis may develop, and a lumbar puncture may show acute inflammatory cells and yield a positive cerebrospinal fluid culture.

Harris GJ. Subperiosteal abscess of the orbit: age as a factor in the bacteriology and response to treatment. *Ophthalmology.* 1994;101:585–595.

Harris GJ. Subperiosteal abscess of the orbit: computed tomography and the clinical course. *Ophthal Plast Reconstr Surg.* 1996;12:1–8.

Necrotizing Fasciitis

Necrotizing fasciitis is an uncommon, severe bacterial infection involving the subcutaneous soft tissues, particularly the superficial and deep fascia. Although a variety of organisms, including aerobic and anaerobic gram-positive and gram-negative bacteria, may cause this disorder, recent attention has focused on group A *Streptococcus* because of the number of well-publicized cases of the "flesh-eating disease."

This disorder develops quickly and is potentially fatal. It may occur in previously healthy persons, without a history of trauma, but many patients are relatively immu-

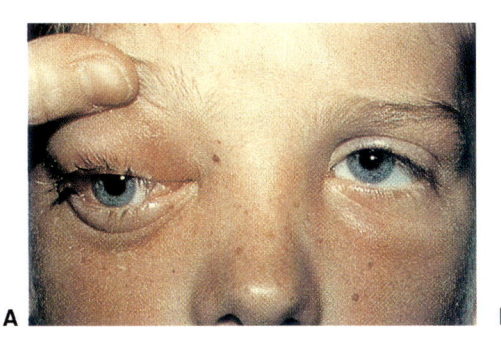

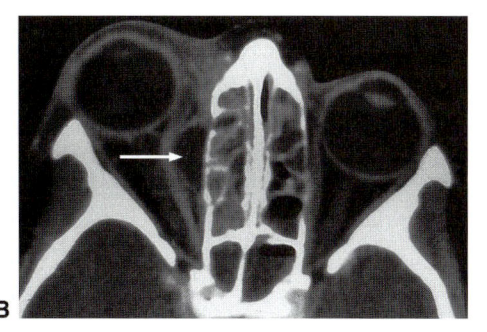

Figure 4-2 A, Right orbital cellulitis. Note proptosis and exotropia. **B,** CT scan of right orbital subperiosteal abscess. Note medial rectus displaced by abscess. Fine line of extraconal fat between periorbita and medial rectus demonstrates that the abscess is subperiosteal. *(Photographs courtesy of Robert C. Kersten, MD.)*

nocompromised by such conditions as diabetes and alcoholism. These infections may be accompanied by a shocklike syndrome. Typically, the initial clinical presentation is similar to that of orbital or preseptal cellulitis, with swelling, erythema, and pain. Because necrotizing fasciitis tends to track along avascular tissue planes, an early sign may be anesthesia over the affected area owing to involvement of deep cutaneous nerves. In addition, disproportionate complaints of pain may suggest the possibility of necrotizing fasciitis, as do typical changes in skin color progressing from rose coloration to blue-gray with bullous formation and frank necrosis. This disease has been reported following minor trauma.

Treatment includes early surgical debridement along with intravenous antibiotics. If the involved pathogen is unknown, then broad-spectrum coverage for gram-positive and gram-negative as well as anaerobic organisms is indicated. Some cases of necrotizing fasciitis limited to the eyelids can be cautiously followed with systemic antibiotic therapy and little or no debridement; this is considered only in cases that rapidly demarcate in the periorbital skin and show no signs of toxic shock.

Patients may experience rapid deterioration, culminating in hypotension, renal failure, and adult respiratory distress syndrome. Reported clinical series from all body sites have shown up to a 30% mortality rate, usually due to a toxic-shock syndrome, but this appears uncommon in the periocular region.

> Luksich JA, Holds JB, Hartstein ME. Conservative management of necrotizing fasciitis of the eyelids. *Ophthalmology*. 2002;109:2118–2122.
> Marshall DH, Jordan DR, Gilberg SM, et al. Periocular necrotizing fasciitis: a review of five cases. *Ophthalmology*. 1997;104:1857–1862.

Phycomycosis

Phycomycosis (also known as *mucormycosis*) is the most common and the most virulent fungal disease involving the orbit. The specific fungal genus involved is usually *Mucor* or *Rhizopus*. These fungi, belonging to the class Phycomycetes, almost always extend into the orbit from an adjacent sinus or the nasal cavity. These fungi can invade blood vessel walls and produce thrombosing vasculitis.

Patients commonly present with proptosis and an orbital apex syndrome (internal and external ophthalmoplegia, ptosis, decreased corneal sensation, and decreased vision). Predisposing factors are systemic disability with metabolic acidosis, often associated with diabetes, malignant tumors, and treatment with antimetabolites or steroids. Diagnosis is confirmed by a biopsy of the involved necrotic-appearing tissues in the nasopharynx. The positive biopsy shows nonseptate large branching hyphae that stain well with hematoxylin-eosin (unlike most fungi). Therapeutic measures consist of control of the underlying metabolic abnormality, local surgical excision of infected tissues, and administration of amphotericin B. Some authors have proposed adjunctive hyperbaric oxygen therapy. The role of primary exenteration has decreased recently, but it is unclear whether patient survival (typically poor) has been adversely affected by less-aggressive surgical excision.

> Ferry AP, Abedi S. Diagnosis and management of rhinoorbitocerebral mucormycosis (phycomycosis). A report of 16 personally observed cases. *Ophthalmology*. 1983;90:1096–1104.
>
> Kronish JW, Johnson TE, Gilberg SM, et al. Orbital infections in patients with human immunodeficiency virus infection. *Ophthalmology*. 1996;103:1483–1492.

Aspergillosis

The fungus *Aspergillus* can affect the orbit in several distinct clinical entities. Acute aspergillosis is a fungal disease characterized by fulminant sinus infection with secondary orbital invasion. Patients present with severe periorbital pain, decreased vision, and proptosis. Diagnosis is confirmed by one or more biopsies. Gomori methenamine–silver nitrate stain shows septate branching hyphae of uniform width. Therapy consists of aggressive surgical excision of all infected tissues and administration of amphotericin B, flucytosine, rifampin, or a combination thereof.

In addition to acute fulminant fungal sinusitis with orbital invasion, aspergillosis can cause chronic indolent infection resulting in slow destruction of the sinuses and adjacent structures. Although the prognosis is much better than for acute fulminant disease, intraorbital and intracranial extension can occur in the chronic invasive form of fungal sinusitis as well and result in significant morbidity.

The sinuses can also be involved by chronic localized noninvasive aspergillosis that occurs in immunocompetent patients who may not have a history of atopic disease. A history of chronic sinusitis is often elicited, and proliferation of saprophytic organisms results in a tightly packed fungus ball. This type of aspergillosis is characterized by a lack of inflammation or bone erosion.

A newer entity, *allergic aspergillosis sinusitis,* occurs in immunocompetent patients with nasal polyposis and chronic sinusitis. Patients may have peripheral eosinophilia, an elevated total immunoglobulin E level, fungus-specific immunoglobulin E and immunoglobulin G, and positive skin test results for fungal antigens. CT reveals thick allergic mucin within the sinus as mottled areas of increased attenuation on nonenhanced images. Bone erosion and remodeling are frequently present but do not signify actual tissue invasion. Magnetic resonance imaging may be more specific, showing signal void areas on T2-weighted scans. Sinus biopsy reveals thick, peanut butter–like or green mucus, pathological study of which reveals numerous eosinophils and eosinophil degradation products and extramucosal fungal hyphae. Definitive surgical treatment is usually described through an endoscopic approach with extirpation of allergic mucin and aeration and drainage of the involved sinuses. Treatment with systemic and topical corticosteroids is also recommended. Orbital problems have been responsible for presentation in up to 17% of patients with allergic fungal sinusitis.

> Como JA, Dismukes WE. Oral azole drugs as systemic antifungal therapy. *N Engl J Med.* 1994;330:263–272.
>
> Klapper SR, Lee AG, Patrinely JR, et al. Orbital involvement in allergic fungal sinusitis. *Ophthalmology.* 1997;104:2094–2100.
>
> Levin LA, Avery R, Shore JW, et al. The spectrum of orbital aspergillosis: a clinicopathological review. *Surv Ophthalmol.* 1996;41:142–154.

Orbital Tuberculosis

Although not uncommon in endemic areas of the developing world, tuberculosis has reemerged as a public health threat in developed countries in recent years. It affects the orbit as a chronic inflammatory process, as a periostitis, or as a so-called cold abscess. The predominant route of spread to the orbit is hematogenous from a pulmonary focus, which is often subclinical. Less often, spread occurs from an adjacent tuberculous sinusitis. Proptosis, motility dysfunction, bone destruction, and chronic draining fistulas may be the presenting findings. HIV immunosuppression and inner-city poverty are most often associated with this disease in the developed world. The majority of recent orbital cases have been reported to occur in children, and the infection is often mistaken for an orbital malignancy. The disease is usually unilateral. Acid-fast bacilli may be difficult to detect in pathological specimens, which usually show caseating necrosis, epithelioid cells, and Langhans giant cells. Skin testing and fine-needle aspiration biopsy with culture early in the course of the disease may help establish the diagnosis. Antituberculous therapy is usually curative.

> Khalil M, Lindley S, Matouk E. Tuberculosis of the orbit. *Ophthalmology.* 1985;92:1624–1627.

Parasitic Diseases

Parasitic diseases of the orbit are generally limited to developing countries and include trichinosis and echinococcosis. *Trichinosis* is caused by ingestion of the nematode *Trichinella spiralis.* The eyelids and extraocular muscles may be inflamed by migration of the larvae. *Echinococcosis* is caused by the dog tapeworm *Echinococcus granulosus.* A hydatid cyst containing tapeworm larvae may form in the orbit. Rupture of such a cyst may cause progressive inflammation and a severe immune response. *Taenia solium*, the pork tapeworm, may also encyst and progressively enlarge in the orbital tissues, causing a condition known as *cysticercosis.*

Inflammations

Graves Ophthalmopathy

Graves ophthalmopathy (also known as *thyroid-associated ophthalmopathy, dysthyroid ophthalmopathy, thyroid eye disease, thyroid orbitopathy, thyrotoxic exophthalmos,* and other terms) is an autoimmune inflammatory disorder whose underlying cause continues to be elucidated. The clinical signs, however, are characteristic and include a combination of eyelid retraction, lid lag, proptosis, restrictive extraocular myopathy, and optic neuropathy (Figs 4-3 through 4-8). It has been recognized for many years that the various signs and symptoms of Graves ophthalmopathy may progress and abate independently of other clinical features and that disease activity in the two eyes may be remarkably asymmetric. Although typically associated with hyperthyroidism, Graves ophthalmopathy may accompany hypothyroidism or Hashimoto thyroiditis; in some patients, characteristic eye findings occur in the absence of objective evidence of thyroid dysfunction *(euthyroid Graves disease)*. The course of ophthalmopathy does not necessarily parallel the activity of the thyroid gland or the treatment of thyroid abnormalities.

Diagnosis

The diagnosis of Graves ophthalmopathy is straightforward when a patient with hyperthyroidism has eyelid retraction, proptosis, restrictive myopathy, chemosis, conjunctival

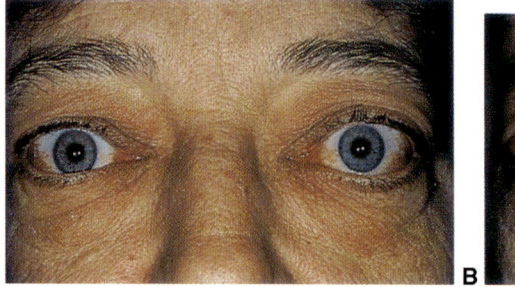

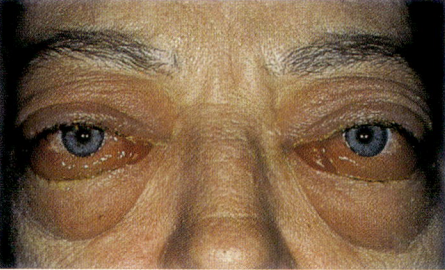

Figure 4-3 A, Bilateral proptosis and upper eyelid retraction in a middle-aged woman with Graves ophthalmopathy. Note minimal signs of active inflammation. **B,** Marked inflammation 3 months later, with chemosis, eyelid swelling, and increased proptosis. *(Photographs courtesy of Jeffrey A. Nerad, MD.)*

Figure 4-4 Graves ophthalmopathy, with proptosis, eyelid retraction, and hypotropia resulting from fibrosis of the medial and inferior rectus muscles. *(Photograph courtesy of George B. Bartley, MD.)*

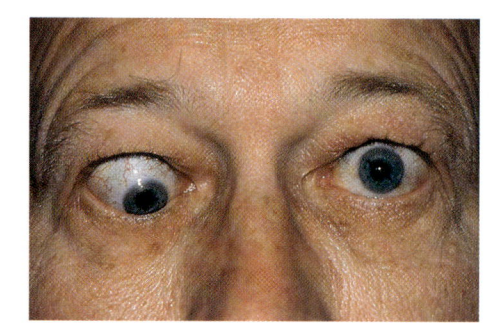

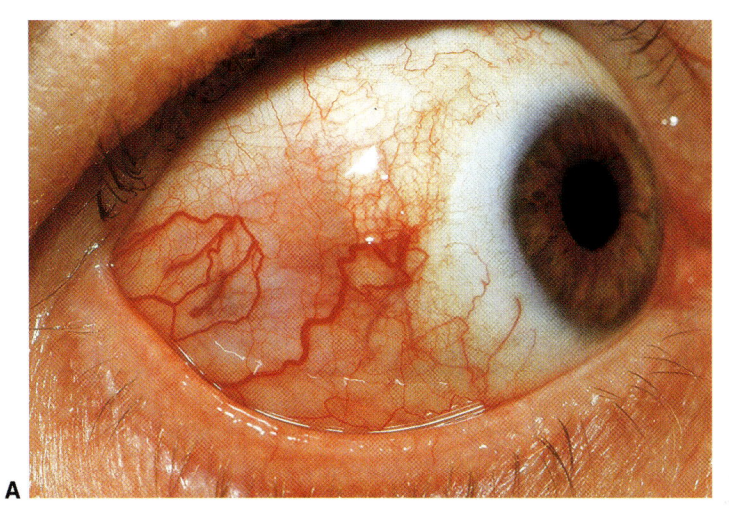

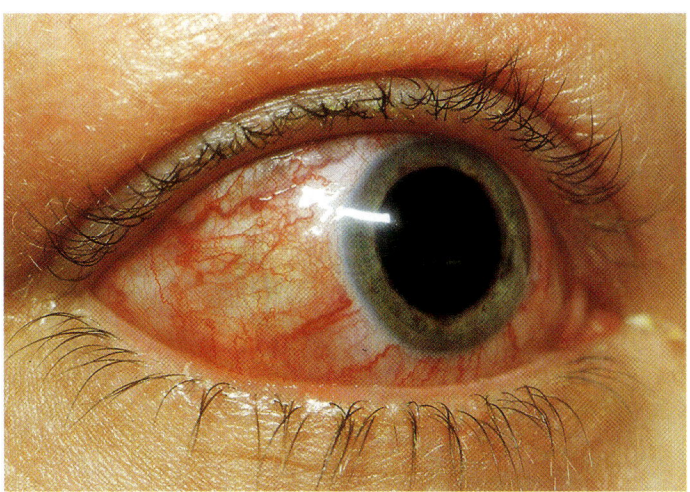

CHAPTER 4: Infectious and Inflammatory Disorders • 49

Figure 4-5 A, Conjunctival erythema over the insertions of the horizontal rectus muscles is a frequent sign of Graves ophthalmopathy. Typically, there is a clear zone between the anterior extent of the abnormally dilated blood vessels and the corneoscleral limbus. **B,** In contrast, the arterialization of blood vessels that occurs with a dural shunt is usually more diffuse and extends to the limbus. *(Photographs courtesy of George B. Bartley, MD.)*

erythema over the insertions of the horizontal recti, eyelid fullness, superior limbic keratoconjunctivitis, and decreased vision from corneal exposure or optic neuropathy. In patients who lack such clinical signs and in whom the thyroid status is unknown or thought to be normal, the diagnosis may be problematic. Graves hyperthyroidism is caused by TSH-receptor (TSH-R) stimulating immunoglobulins, and the ophthalmopathy of Graves disease may relate to antibodies to cross-reactive TSH-R antigens expressed on orbital fibroblasts. Recent interest has focused on testing for circulating TSH-R antibody (thyroid-stimulating immunoglobulin) levels whose presence correlates strongly with the clinical activity score of the eye disease.

50 • Orbit, Eyelids, and Lacrimal System

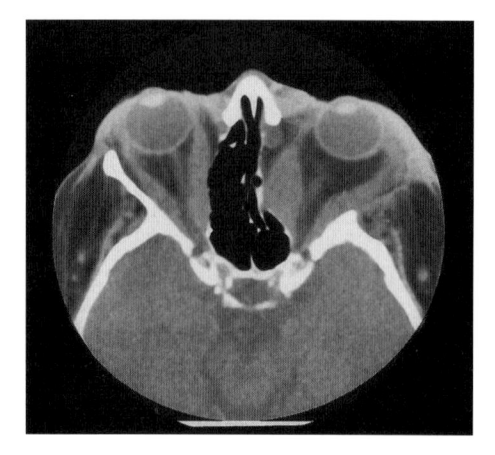

Figure 4-6 Extraocular muscle enlargement in Graves ophthalmopathy characteristically is fusiform and spares the tendons. Note that this patient had undergone a unilateral medial and lateral orbital decompression. *(Photograph courtesy of George B. Bartley, MD.)*

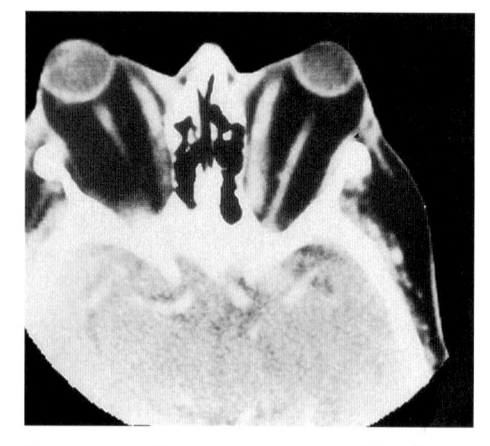

Figure 4-7 Some patients with Graves ophthalmopathy have relatively modest enlargement of the extraocular muscles but a marked increase in orbital fat, as demonstrated here. Note severe proptosis with stretching of the optic nerves. *(Photograph courtesy of Jeffrey A. Nerad, MD.)*

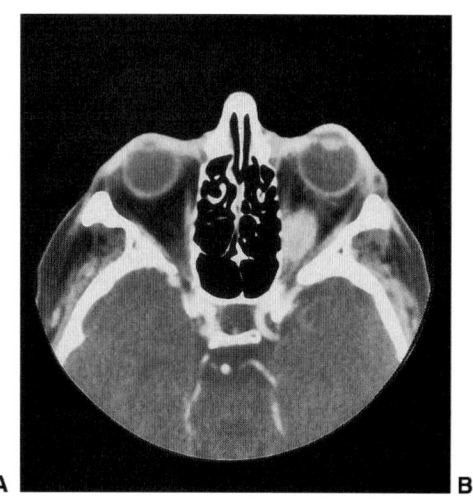

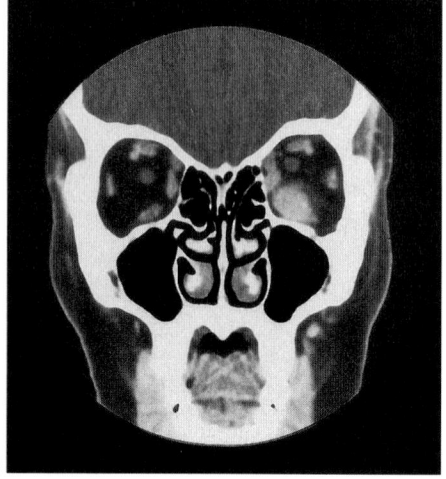

Figure 4-8 A, A tumor in the orbital apex is occasionally misdiagnosed on axial CT sections in patients with Graves ophthalmopathy. **B,** A coronal section demonstrates that the "tumor" actually is enlargement of the inferior rectus muscle. *(Photographs courtesy of George B. Bartley, MD.)*

Graves ophthalmopathy is considered to be present if eyelid retraction (upper eyelid position at or above the superior corneoscleral limbus) occurs together with objective evidence of thyroid dysfunction (preferably including, but not limited to, serum thyroid-stimulating immunoglobulins), or exophthalmos (exophthalmometry measurement ≥20 mm), or optic nerve dysfunction, or extraocular muscle involvement (either restrictive myopathy or enlarged muscles as determined by CT, MRI, or ultrasonography). The clinical features may be unilateral or bilateral, and masquerading entities must be excluded (eg, inflammatory myositis or lymphoma). If eyelid retraction is absent, then Graves ophthalmopathy may be diagnosed only if exophthalmos, optic nerve involvement, or restrictive extraocular myopathy coexists with thyroid dysfunction and no other causes for the ophthalmic features are apparent. The above diagnostic criteria for Graves ophthalmopathy are summarized in Figure 4-9.

> Gerding MN, van der Meer JWC, Broenink M, et al. Association of thyrotropin receptor antibodies with the clinical features of Graves' ophthalmopathy. *Clin Endocrinol.* 2000; 52:267–271.
>
> Mourits MP, Prummel MF, Wiersinga WM, et al. Clinical activity score as a guide in the management of patients with Graves ophthalmopathy. *Clin Endocrinol.* 1997:47;9–14.

Pathogenesis

Mechanically speaking, we know that many of the symptoms and signs of Graves ophthalmopathy result from a discrepancy between the fixed volume of the bony orbit and the increased volume of the swollen retrobulbar tissues. Glycosaminoglycans expressed from fibroblasts, with secondary water retention, had always been presumed to be the operative mechanism for the retrobulbar swelling; now, however, adipogenesis is thought to play a major role as well. It is not known what initiates the immune response, but most evidence points to TSH-R as the antigen. Subsequent events involve activation of T cells, antigen recognition, cytokine release, and disease expression involving the target cell. Studies have shown a predominance of T cell activity early in the course of the disease. The myocyte and the fibroblast (more specifically the preadipocyte fibroblast) have been mentioned as possible target cells. Recent reports argue against the myocyte as a target cell. Evidence against the myocyte includes:

- There are more lymphocytes in the orbital fat than in the extraocular muscles.
- Histologically, the muscle remains normal until late in the course of the disease.
- Reported and measured extraocular muscle antibodies are probably secondary to late degeneration.

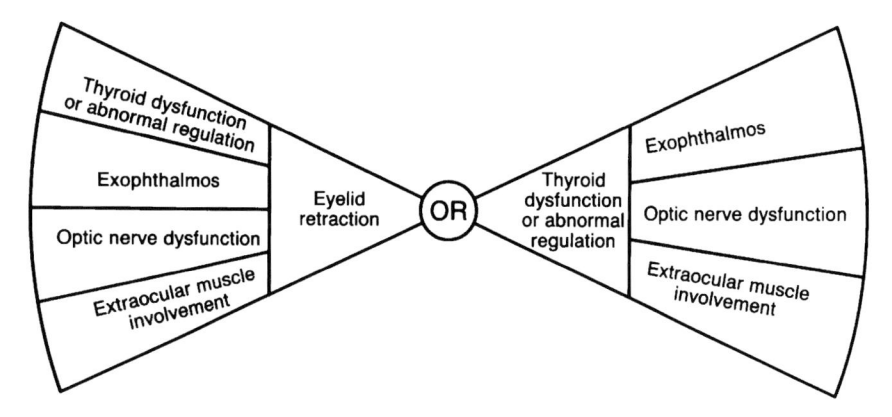

Figure 4-9 Diagram of diagnostic criteria for Graves ophthalmopathy; see text for details. *(Reprinted by permission from Bartley GB, Gorman CA. Diagnostic criteria for Graves' ophthalmopathy. Am J Ophthalmol. 1995;119:792–795.)*

- The myocyte lacks significant TSH-R.
- The myocyte shows no immunoreactivity for adhesion molecules.

Reactivity for adhesion molecules and TSH-R has been detected in the perimysial connective tissue, however. Arguments for the fibroblast as a more suitable target cell include:

- Expression of TSH-R on the fibroblast and an increased number of TSH-R on the adipocytes
- Identification of a preadipocyte fibroblast
- Ability to induce preadipocyte fibroblasts to be transformed into adipocytes
- Ability to induce increased numbers of TSH-R on cultured fibroblasts and increased levels of adiponectin (a product of adipocyte cell differentiation) in patients with Graves ophthalmopathy

Fibroblasts throughout the body express TSH-R, but what accounts for site-specific differences in fibroblast activity (eg, ophthalmopathy and pretibial dermopathy) is not known. Cytokines are expressed both locally and systemically. Local cytokines include interferon-γ, tumor necrosis factor α, and interleukin-2; systemic levels of interleukin-6 are also increased in patients with Graves ophthalmopathy. There may be a systemic connective tissue response associated with the fibroblast, the TSH-R, and interleukin-6.

There are probably three different, interrelated aspects to consider in the pathogenesis of Graves ophthalmopathy:

- A cellular response manifested through the fibroblasts and adipocytes
- An immunologic response mediated through the antigen, the target cell, and cytokines
- A mechanical contribution to account for site-specific differences of fibroblastic response and orbital asymmetry

Mechanical contributions may include some type of local trauma (eg, myxedematous responses are known to occur in surgical scars) or effects of local pressure increases. Theoretically, intervention at any point in the cycle could influence the course of the disease.

For extensive discussion of immunology, see Part I of BCSC Section 9, *Intraocular Inflammation and Uveitis*.

Bahn RS. Understanding the immunology of Graves' ophthalmopathy. Is it an autoimmune disease? *Endocrinol Metab Clin.* 2000;29:287–296.

Wiersinga WM, Prummel MF. Pathogenesis of Graves' ophthalmopathy—current understanding [editorial]. *J Clin Endocrinol Metab.* 2001;86:501–503.

Epidemiology

A recent (1996) epidemiologic study of white American patients with Graves ophthalmopathy determined that the overall age-adjusted incidence rate for women was 16 cases per 100,000 population per year, whereas the rate for men was 3 cases per 100,000 population per year. Graves ophthalmopathy affected women approximately six times more frequently than men (86% versus 14% of cases, respectively). The peak incidence rates occurred in the age groups 40–44 years and 60–64 years in women and 45–49 years and 65–69 years in men. The median age at the time of diagnosis of Graves ophthalmopathy was 43 years (range, 8–88 years).

Clinical features
Among patients with Graves ophthalmopathy in the incidence cohort, approximately 90% had Graves hyperthyroidism, 1% had primary hypothyroidism, 3% had Hashimoto thyroiditis, and 6% were euthyroid. There was a close temporal relationship between the development of hyperthyroidism and Graves ophthalmopathy: in about 20% of patients, the diagnoses are made at the same time; in approximately 60% of patients, the eye disease occurred within 1 year of onset of the thyroid disease. Of those patients who had no history of abnormal thyroid function or regulation at the time of diagnosis of ophthalmopathy, the risk of thyroid disease was about 25% within 1 year and 50% within 5 years. Although the large majority of patients with Graves ophthalmopathy have or will develop hyperthyroidism, only about 30% of patients with autoimmune hyperthyroidism have or will develop ophthalmopathy.

Eyelid retraction was the most common ophthalmic feature of Graves ophthalmopathy, being present either unilaterally or bilaterally in more than 90% of patients at some point in their clinical course. Exophthalmos of one or both eyes affected approximately 60% of patients, restrictive extraocular myopathy was apparent in about 40% of patients, and optic nerve dysfunction occurred in one or both eyes in 6% of patients with Graves ophthalmopathy. Only 5% of patients had the complete constellation of classic findings: eyelid retraction, exophthalmos, optic nerve dysfunction, extraocular muscle involvement, and hyperthyroidism.

Upper eyelid retraction, either unilateral or bilateral, was documented in approximately 75% of patients at the time of diagnosis of Graves ophthalmopathy. Lid lag in downgaze also was a frequent early sign, being present either unilaterally or bilaterally in 50% of patients at the initial examination. The most frequent ocular symptom when ophthalmopathy was first confirmed was pain or discomfort, which affected 30% of patients and often was the result of dry eyes. Some degree of diplopia was noted by approximately 17% of patients, lacrimation or photophobia by about 15%–20% of patients, and blurred vision by 7.5% of patients. Decreased vision attributable to optic neuropathy was present in less than 2% of eyes at the time of diagnosis of Graves ophthalmopathy.

Thyroid dermopathy and acropachy accompanied Graves ophthalmopathy in approximately 4% and 1% of patients, respectively, and myasthenia gravis occurred in less than 1% of patients.

Treatment and prognosis
Graves ophthalmopathy is presumed to be self-limiting but may run an active course of exacerbations and remissions with a duration varying from months to years. After the active disease plateaus, a quiescent burnt-out phase ensues, although late reactivation of inflammation may rarely occur. Cigarette smoking has been shown to increase the likelihood of ophthalmopathy, and heavy smoking increases the severity of ophthalmopathy. Most patients with Graves ophthalmopathy require only supportive care, such as topical ocular lubricants for irritative symptoms. However, if orbital inflammation is severe,

emergent intervention may be necessary to prevent or ameliorate corneal exposure, globe subluxation, or optic neuropathy. Therapy usually is directed toward either decreasing orbital congestion and inflammation (by systemic corticosteroids, colchicine, or radiotherapy) or expanding the orbital bony volume (by surgical orbital decompression).

The correction of thyroid function abnormalities is an important part of the overall care of patients with Graves ophthalmopathy. Hyperthyroidism usually is treated with radioactive iodine, antithyroid drugs, or thyroidectomy. In some studies, ophthalmopathy has been demonstrated to worsen transiently after radioactive iodine has been administered, presumably as a result of the release of TSH-R antigens, which incite an enhanced immune response. In addition, allowing a period of post-treatment hypothyroidism following radioactive iodine treatment may exacerbate ophthalmopathy via stimulation of the TSH-R. Hyperthyroid patients with active ophthalmopathy, those with elevated T_3 levels, and smokers appear to be at greatest risk for exacerbation of ophthalmopathy when iodine 131 (^{131}I) is used. Many endocrinologists recommend concurrent prednisone treatment in these patients. In addition, block-and-replace therapy with ^{131}I, methimazole, and thyroxine may prevent exacerbation of eye findings by limiting posttreatment TSH spikes. All patients should be strongly counseled to stop smoking because cessation may limit the severity and activity of the ophthalmopathy.

Ophthalmopathy often improves with reestablishment of the euthyroid state, but eye disease may continue to progress. Ophthalmopathy tends to stabilize over a course of months, and most patients require only nonspecific medical management and reassurance. Roughly 20% of patients with Graves ophthalmopathy undergo surgical treatment. Men and older patients are more likely to have more severe orbitopathy requiring surgical intervention. Surgery should be delayed until the disease has plateaued, unless urgent intervention is required to reverse visual loss due to compressive optic neuropathy or corneal exposure. Elective orbital decompression, strabismus surgery, and eyelid retraction repair usually are not considered until a euthyroid state has been maintained and the ophthalmic signs have been confirmed to be stable for 6–9 months. In a recent review, 7% of patients underwent orbital decompression, 9% strabismus surgery, and 13% eyelid surgery. Only 2.5% required all three types of surgery. Orbital decompression, although historically indicated to treat optic neuropathy, severe orbital congestion, or advanced proptosis, has been used increasingly in recent years as an elective procedure to enhance cosmesis in patients without sight-threatening ophthalmopathy. If intractable diplopia in primary gaze or in the reading position persists, then strabismus surgery may be helpful in restoring single vision. Similarly, procedures to correct eyelid retraction may improve ocular comfort and help to restore a more normal appearance. Orbital decompression may alter extraocular motility and, if indicated, should precede strabismus surgery. Because extraocular muscle surgery may affect eyelid retraction, eyelid surgery should be undertaken last.

Some authors have advocated orbital radiotherapy (2000 cGy) as treatment for Graves ophthalmopathy. A presumed therapeutic effect is lympholysis. Theoretically, however, because lymphocytes should quickly repopulate the orbit, any true benefits from radiotherapy must result from other mechanisms. A recent prospective clinical trial designed to assess the treatment results in patients with congestive orbitopathy followed six separate parameters (volume of muscle, volume of fat, proptosis, eyelid fissures, monocular range of motion, and diplopia fields). The treatment showed no statistically significant effect compared with the natural history of the disease. This trial excluded patients with optic neuropathy. Some critics of the study have noted that the lack of apparent benefit can be ascribed to the inclusion of patients with inactive disease because the median time from onset of orbitopathy to radiation therapy was 1.3 years. However, the average clinical activity score at the time of radiation therapy was 6.2, suggesting moderate disease. Additionally, whether the interval between disease onset and radiotherapy was less than or greater than 1.3 years, treatment results were not significantly different. At present, there is no universally accepted means to assess disease activity or severity. Radiation therapy should not be considered in patients with diabetes because this technique may exacerbate retinopathy.

> Gorman CA, Garrity JA, Fatourechi V, et al. A prospective, randomized, double-blind, placebo-controlled study of orbital radiotherapy for Graves' ophthalmopathy. *Ophthalmology.* 2001;108:1523–1534.
>
> Mourits MP, van Kempen-Harteveld ML, Garcia MB, et al. Radiotherapy for Graves' orbitopathy: randomized placebo-controlled study. *Lancet.* 2000;355:1505–1509.

A long-term follow-up study of patients in an incidence cohort demonstrated that visual loss from optic neuropathy was uncommon and that persistent diplopia usually

KEY POINTS

Graves ophthalmopathy The following list highlights the essential points for the ophthalmologist to remember about Graves ophthalmopathy.

- Eyelid retraction is the most common clinical feature (and Graves ophthalmopathy is the most common cause of eyelid retraction).
- Graves ophthalmopathy is the most common cause of unilateral or bilateral proptosis.
- Graves ophthalmopathy is six times more common in women than in men.
- This condition is associated with hyperthyroidism in 90% of patients, but 6% are euthyroid.
- Severity of ophthalmopathy usually does not parallel serum levels of T_4 or T_3 but is closely related to thyroid-stimulating immunoglobulin.
- Ophthalmopathy may be markedly asymmetric.
- Urgent care may be required for optic neuropathy or severe proptosis with corneal exposure.
- If surgery is needed, the usual order is orbital decompression, followed by strabismus surgery, followed by eyelid retraction repair (see Chapter 7).
- Smoking is associated with increased risk and severity of Graves ophthalmopathy.
- Systemic corticosteroid treatment is usually reserved for patients with compressive optic neuropathy to reduce dysfunction while awaiting orbital decompression.

could be treated with prism spectacles. Subjectively, however, more than 50% of patients perceived that their eyes looked abnormal, and 38% of patients were dissatisfied with the appearance of their eyes. Thus, although few patients experience long-term functional impairment from Graves ophthalmopathy, the psychological and aesthetic sequelae of the disease are considerable. Orbital decompression is discussed in Chapter 7.

> Bartalena L, Marcocci C, Bogazzi F, et al. Relation between therapy for hyperthyroidism and the course of Graves' ophthalmopathy. *N Engl J Med.* 1998;338:73–78.
>
> Bartley GB, Fatourechi V, Kadrmas EF, et al. Clinical features of Graves' ophthalmopathy in an incidence cohort. *Am J Ophthalmol.* 1996;121:284–290.
>
> Bartley GB, Fatourechi V, Kadrmas EF, et al. Long-term follow-up of Graves ophthalmopathy in an incidence cohort. *Ophthalmology.* 1996;103:958–962.
>
> Bartley GB, Gorman CA. Diagnostic criteria for Graves' ophthalmopathy. *Am J Ophthalmol.* 1995;119:792–795.
>
> Burch HB, Wartkowski L. Graves ophthalmopathy: current concepts regarding pathogenesis and management. *Endocrinol Rev.* 1993;14:747–793.

Idiopathic Orbital Inflammation (Orbital Inflammatory Syndrome, Orbital Pseudotumor)

Orbital inflammations usually occur as a nonspecific idiopathic inflammatory process; they may also be caused by a number of specific local or systemic disease entities.

Both children and adults may be afflicted by idiopathic inflammations of the orbital tissues (Fig 4-10) that are unrelated to Graves ophthalmopathy or to any other systemic or local disorder. The current concept of inflammatory orbital pseudotumor defines it as an idiopathic tumorlike inflammation made up of a pleomorphic inflammatory cellular response and a fibrovascular tissue reaction. The pseudotumor is usually confined to orbital structures and has a variable but limited course.

Idiopathic orbital inflammation is often subclassified on the basis of the anatomic target area within the orbit. Clinically, the inflammation may present primarily as dacryoadenitis, myositis, sclerotenonitis, perioptic nerve inflammation, or an inflammatory process restricted to the vicinity of the superior orbital fissure and cavernous sinus (the Tolosa-Hunt syndrome of painful ophthalmoplegia) or as diffuse anterior soft tissue inflammation. Symptoms depend on the involved tissue.

Typically, patients present with acute onset of orbital pain, restricted eye movement, and proptosis. Conjunctival vascular injection and chemosis are common, as are eyelid erythema and soft tissue swelling. Pain associated with extraocular muscle excursions is highly suggestive of idiopathic orbital inflammatory syndrome—especially myositis. Visual acuity may be impaired if the optic nerve or posterior sclera is involved. Occasionally, systemic signs and symptoms, including leukocytosis and fever, suggest an infectious process. Exudative fluid in the adjacent sinuses may further complicate the picture.

A typical clinical presentation is often diagnostic and may be confirmed by orbital imaging. Prompt response to systemic steroids helps to confirm the diagnosis, although the physician must be aware that the inflammation associated with other orbital processes (eg, metastases, ruptured dermoid cysts, cellulitis) may also improve with systemic steroid administration. However, not all patients with orbital inflammatory pseudotumor pres-

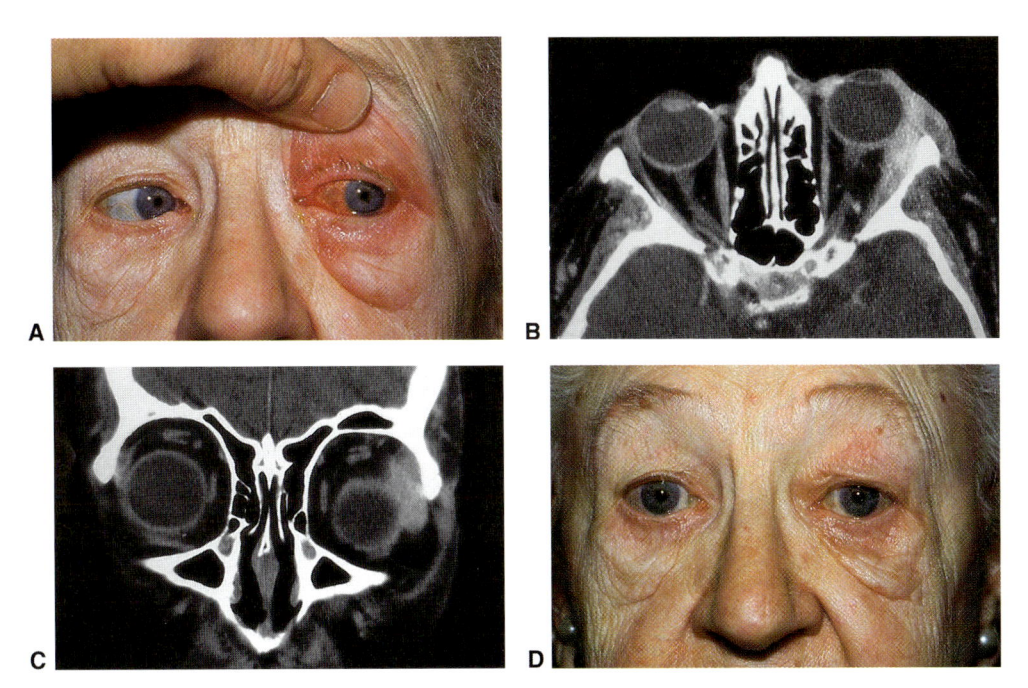

Figure 4-10 A, Acute onset of left eyelid inflammation, proptosis, pain, and left lateral rectus paresis. **B,** Axial CT scan demonstrating left eye proptosis and hazy inflammatory swelling of lateral rectus and lacrimal gland consistent with the diagnosis of orbital inflammatory disease. **C,** Coronal CT scan demonstrating inflammatory myositis of the lateral rectus. **D,** Marked improvement of inflammatory changes following a 48-hour course of oral prednisone. *(Photographs courtesy of Robert C. Kersten, MD.)*

ent with the classic signs and symptoms. For example, some patients do not experience the typical pain. Some may have minimal inflammatory signs and may present with a totally fibrotic scarred lesion *(idiopathic sclerosing inflammation of the orbit)*. Such lesions may require biopsy for diagnosis. Bilateral idiopathic inflammation in adults suggests the possibility of systemic vasculitis. In children, however, approximately one third of cases of idiopathic orbital inflammation are bilateral and are rarely associated with systemic disorders, even though half of the children have headache, fever, vomiting, abdominal pain, and lethargy.

Biopsy is not necessary in all cases because the findings on clinical, ultrasonographic, and radiologic (including CT) examination may be sufficiently diagnostic to permit therapy to be initiated. Peripheral blood eosinophilia, elevated erythrocyte sedimentation rate and antinuclear antibody levels, and mild cerebrospinal fluid pleocytosis can be found. In dacryoadenitis, CT reveals diffuse enlargement of the lacrimal gland (which is the most common anatomic target area to be affected). Both CT and ultrasonography reveal thickening of the extraocular muscles if the inflammatory response has a myositic component. The extraocular muscle tendons of insertion may be thickened in up to 50% of patients with orbital inflammatory syndrome, in contrast with Graves ophthalmopathy, in which the muscle insertions are generally spared. An inflammatory infiltrate of the retrobulbar fat pad is commonly seen, and contrast enhancement of the sclera may be caused by tenonitis (producing the *ring sign*). B-scan ultrasonography often shows an acoustically hollow area corresponding to an edematous Tenon's capsule.

Histopathologically, orbital inflammatory syndrome is characterized by a pleomorphic cellular infiltrate consisting of lymphocytes, plasma cells, and eosinophils with variable degrees of reactive fibrosis. The fibrosis becomes more marked as the process becomes more chronic, and early or acute cases are usually more responsive to steroids than the advanced stages associated with fibrosis. Although, historically, there was a tendency to group hypercellular lymphoid proliferations with the pseudotumors, hypercellular lymphoid proliferations are now recognized as very different clinical and histopathologic entities.

Treatment

Initial therapy consists of systemic corticosteroids in doses adjusted to the individual patient's needs. Beginning daily adult doses are generally 60–80 mg of prednisone. Acute cases generally respond rapidly. Steroids should be tapered more slowly below about 40 mg/day and very slowly below 20 mg/day, generally over a period of several months. Rapid reduction of systemic steroids may cause a recurrence of inflammatory symptoms and signs. Bilateral cases may require more prolonged courses of steroids than unilateral cases. Topical corticosteroid eyedrops may be helpful in decreasing the superficial inflammatory reaction and the anterior chamber reaction seen in some patients. Some investigators think that the combined use of intravenous dexamethasone along with oral prednisone may produce clinical improvement when oral prednisone alone fails to control the inflammation. Because many other orbital pathologic processes may be masked by steroids, an incomplete therapeutic response suggests the need for orbital biopsy for histopathologic confirmation and to rule out specific inflammatory diseases. After the diagnosis is confirmed, orbital irradiation, antimetabolites or alkylating agents such as methotrexate or cyclophosphamide, and continued steroid therapy may be useful in controlling the disease. Rarely, orbital decompression is necessary if optic nerve compression is progressive.

Although orbital inflammation is rarely associated with peritoneal or mediastinal fibrosis, it is quite unusual to find other associated systemic autoimmune disorders in these patients, and routine clinical and laboratory investigations are usually not productive. However, systemic evaluation may very rarely uncover an underlying collagen disease, such as systemic lupus erythematosus, dermatomyositis, retroperitoneal fibrosis, or periarteritis nodosa.

Recently, a distinct syndrome with predominant fibrosis and minimal cellular inflammation has been described as *idiopathic sclerosing inflammation*. It responds poorly to steroids or radiotherapy and may require aggressive immunosuppression with cyclosporine, methotrexate, or cyclophosphamide.

Mannor GE, Rose GE, Moseley IF, et al. Outcome of orbital myositis: clinical features associated with recurrence. *Ophthalmology.* 1997;104:409–414.

Mombaerts I, Goldschmeding R, Schlingemann RO, et al. What is orbital pseudotumor? *Surv Ophthalmol.* 1996;41:66–78.

Mombaerts I, Koornneef L. Current status in the treatment of orbital myositis. *Ophthalmology.* 1997;104:402–408.

Rootman J, McCarthy M, White V, et al. Idiopathic sclerosing inflammation of the orbit: a distinct clinicopathologic entity. *Ophthalmology*. 1994;101:570–584.

Sarcoidosis

Sarcoidosis is a multisystem disease that occurs most commonly in persons of African or Scandinavian descent. Histopathologically, the lesions are composed of noncaseating collections of epithelioid histiocytes in a granulomatous pattern. A mononuclear inflammation often appears at the periphery of the granuloma. The lacrimal gland is the site most frequently affected within the orbit, and the inflammation is typically bilateral. Gallium scanning of the lacrimal glands is nonspecific but has been reported to demonstrate lacrimal gland involvement in 80% of patients with systemic sarcoidosis, although only 7% of patients have clinically detectable enlargement of the lacrimal glands. Other orbital soft tissues, including the extraocular muscles and optic nerve, may very rarely be involved. Infrequently, sinus involvement with adjacent lytic bone lesions allows spillover into the orbit.

A biopsy specimen of the affected lacrimal gland or a suspicious conjunctival lesion may establish the diagnosis. Random conjunctival biopsies have a low yield. Chest radiography or CT to detect hilar adenopathy or pulmonary infiltrates, blood testing for angiotensin-converting enzyme, and measurement of serum lysozyme and calcium may be used to establish the diagnosis of sarcoidosis. Gallium scanning of the lacrimal glands may be nonspecific, and bronchoscopy with washings and biopsy may be necessary to confirm the diagnosis.

Isolated orbital lesions demonstrating noncaseating granulomas can occur without associated systemic disease. This condition is termed *orbital sarcoid*.

See BCSC Section 9, *Intraocular Inflammation and Uveitis*, for a more extensive discussion (including clinical photographs) of sarcoidosis.

Vasculitis

The vasculitides are inflammatory conditions in which the vessel walls are actually infiltrated by inflammatory cells. These lesions represent a type III hypersensitivity reaction to circulating immune complexes and usually lead to significant ocular or orbital morbidity. They are often associated with systemic vasculitis. The following discussion focuses primarily on the orbital manifestations of the vasculitides; their systemic and neuro-ophthalmic features are discussed in BCSC Section 1, *Update on General Medicine*, and Section 5, *Neuro-Ophthalmology*.

Giant cell arteritis

Although the orbital vessels are inflamed in giant cell arteritis (also known as *temporal arteritis*), it is not typically thought of as an orbital disorder. The vasculitis affects the aorta and branches of the external and internal carotid arteries and vertebral arteries but usually spares the intracranial carotid branches, which lack an elastic lamina. Symptoms of visual loss are caused by central retinal artery occlusion or ischemic optic neuropathy, and diplopia may result from ischemic dysfunction of other cranial nerves. Symptoms of headache, scalp tenderness, jaw claudication, or malaise are often present. The erythrocyte sedimentation rate is markedly elevated in 90% of patients, and diagnostic confidence is increased if the C-reactive protein is also elevated. Temporal artery biopsy usually provides a definitive diagnosis, although bilateral biopsies at multiple sites are sometimes necessary. Giant cell arteritis should be managed as an ophthalmic emergency. Failure to diagnose and treat giant cell arteritis immediately after loss of vision in one eye is particularly tragic because timely treatment with corticosteroids usually prevents an attack in the second eye.

> Goodwin JA. Temporal arteritis: diagnosis and management. In: *Focal Points: Clinical Modules for Ophthalmologists.* San Francisco: American Academy of Ophthalmology; 1992: vol 10, no 2.

Polyarteritis nodosa

Like giant cell arteritis, polyarteritis nodosa is a type of vasculitis that sometimes affects orbital vessels but does not usually cause orbital disease. Instead, the ophthalmic manifestations are the result of retinal and choroidal infarction. In this multisystem disease, small and medium-size arteries are affected by inflammation characterized by the presence of neutrophils and eosinophils with necrosis of the muscularis layer.

Vasculitis associated with connective tissue disorders

A number of connective tissue disorders may be associated with systemic vasculitis, most commonly systemic lupus erythematosus, dermatomyositis, and rheumatoid arthritis. Vasculitis primarily affects retinal vessels and less often may affect conjunctival vessels. Symptomatic orbital vasculitis is rare.

Wegener granulomatosis

In Wegener granulomatosis, the disease process is characterized by necrotizing granulomatous vasculitis, lesions of the upper and lower respiratory tract, necrotizing glomerulonephritis, and a small-vessel vasculitis that may affect any organ system including the orbit. Clinically, the full-blown syndrome includes sinus mucosa involvement with bone erosion, tracheobronchial necrotic lesions, cavitary lung lesions, and glomerulonephritis (Fig 4-11). The orbit and nasal lacrimal drainage system may be involved through extension from the surrounding sinuses. Up to 25% of patients with Wegener granulomatosis have associated scleritis. Limited forms of the disease have been described in which the renal component is absent or in which there is solitary orbital involvement by a granulomatous and lymphocytic vasculitis. Such isolated orbital involvement may be unilateral or bilateral, may lack frank necrotizing vasculitis on histopathologic examination, and, in the absence of respiratory tract and renal findings, may be difficult to diagnose.

Characteristic pathological findings consist of the triad of vasculitis, granulomatous inflammation (with or without giant cells), and tissue necrosis. Often only one or two of these three are present on extrapulmonary biopsies. Antineutrophil cytoplasmic antibodies (ANCA) measured by serum immunofluorescence have been shown to be associated with certain systemic vasculitides. The test distinguishes two types of immunofluorescence patterns. Diffuse granular fluorescence within the cytoplasm (C-ANCA) is highly specific for Wegener granulomatosis. This is caused by autoantibodies directed

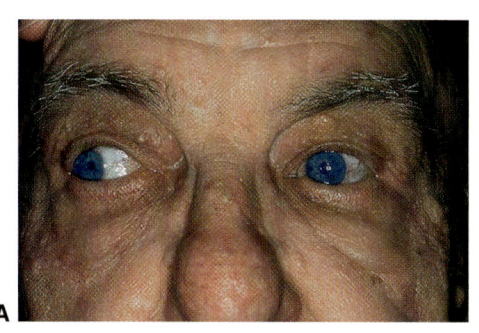

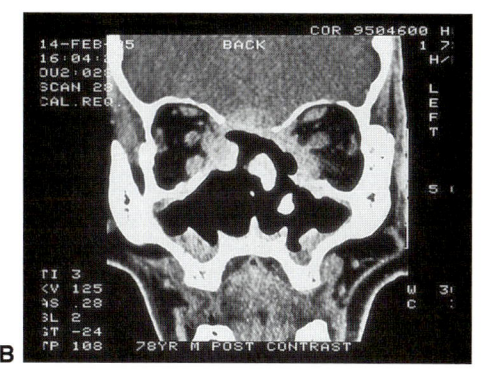

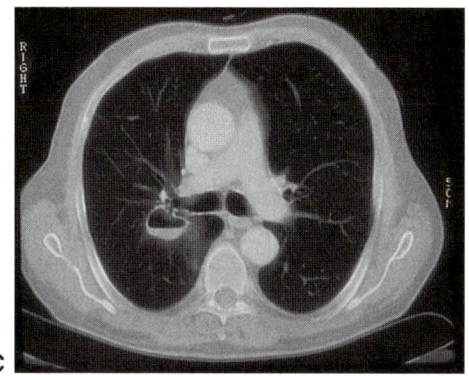

CHAPTER 4: Infectious and Inflammatory Disorders • 61

Figure 4-11 Wegener granulomatosis. **A,** Restrictive strabismus due to inflammatory tissue extending into medial aspects of orbit. **B,** Coronal CT scan showing extensive destruction of the nasal and sinus cavities with tissue extending into orbits and brain. **C,** CT of chest showing cavitary lung lesions. *(Photographs courtesy of Jeffrey Nerad, MD.)*

against proteinase 3, which can also be detected by enzyme-linked immunosorbent assay (ELISA). Fluorescence surrounding the nucleus (P-ANCA) is an artifact of ethanol fixation and can be caused by autoantibodies against many different target antigens. This finding is therefore nonspecific and needs to be confirmed by ELISA for ANCA reacting with myeloperoxidase (MPO-ANCA). MPO-ANCA testing has a high specificity for small-vessel vasculitis. Absolute levels of ANCA do not imply disease severity or activity, but changing titers can give a general idea of disease activity or response to therapy. C-ANCA findings may be negative early in the course of the disease, especially in the absence of multi-system involvement.

Wegener granulomatosis may proceed to a fulminant, life-threatening course. Treatment generally relies on immunosuppressives, usually cyclophosphamide, and should be coordinated with an immunologist. Chronic treatment with trimethoprim-sulfamethoxazole (Bactrim) appears to suppress disease activity in some patients.

Thrombophlebitis

Thrombophlebitis of the orbital vein is an unusual condition characterized by conjunctival congestion, pain, and occasional varicosities of the eyelids. Motility disturbances and decreased vision may result from inflammation of the veins supplying the extraocular muscle and optic nerve. The condition may be idiopathic or associated with spread of a periorbital infection through the angular vein or from the cavernous sinus forward via the supraorbital veins.

CHAPTER 5

Orbital Neoplasms

Congenital Orbital Tumors

Hamartomas and Choristomas

Hamartomas are anomalous growths of tissue consisting only of mature cells normally found at the involved site. Classic examples are capillary hemangiomas and the characteristic lesions of neurofibromatosis. *Choristomas* are tissue anomalies characterized by types of cells not normally found at the involved site. Classic examples are dermoid cysts, epidermoid cysts, lipodermoids, and teratomas. These congenital and juvenile tumors are discussed further in BCSC Section 6, *Pediatric Ophthalmology and Strabismus*.

Dermoid Cysts

Dermoid and epidermoid cysts are among the most common orbital tumors of childhood. These cysts are present congenitally and enlarge progressively. The more superficial cysts usually become symptomatic in childhood, but deeper orbital dermoids may not become clinically evident until adulthood. Dermoid cysts are lined by keratinizing epidermis with dermal appendages, such as hair follicles and sebaceous glands. They contain an admixture of oil and keratin. In contrast, epidermoid cysts are lined by epidermis only, are usually filled with keratin, and do not contain dermal appendages.

Preseptal orbital dermoid cysts occur most commonly in the area of the lateral brow adjacent to the frontozygomatic suture; less often they may be found in the medial upper eyelid adjacent to the frontoethmoidal suture. Dermoid cysts commonly present as palpable smooth, painless, oval masses that enlarge slowly. They may be freely mobile or may be fixed to periosteum at the underlying suture. If the dermoid occurs more posteriorly, in the temporal fossa, CT is often indicated to rule out dumbbell expansion through the suture into the underlying orbit. Medial lesions in the infant should be distinguished from congenital encephaloceles.

Dermoid cysts that do not present until adulthood often are not palpable because they are situated posteriorly in the orbit, usually in the superior and temporal portions adjacent to the bony sutures. The globe and adnexa may be displaced, causing progressive proptosis, and erosion or remodeling of bone can occur. Long-standing dermoids in the superior orbit may completely erode the orbital roof and become adherent to the dura mater. Less commonly, the clinical presentation may be orbital inflammation, which is incited by leakage of oil and keratin from the cyst. Expansion of the dermoid cyst and inflammatory response to leakage may result in an orbital cutaneous fistula, usually following incomplete surgical removal.

Management

Dermoid cysts are usually removed surgically. Because dermoids that present in childhood are often superficial, they can be excised through an incision placed in the upper eyelid crease or directly over the lesion (Fig 5-1). It is important to keep the cyst wall intact during surgery; rupture of the cyst can lead to an acute inflammatory process if part of the cyst wall or the irritating contents are allowed to remain within the eyelid or orbit. Surgical removal may be difficult if the cyst has leaked and adhesions have developed.

> Kersten RC. The eyelid crease approach to superficial lateral dermoid cysts. *J Pediatr Ophthalmol Strabismus.* 1988;25:48–51.
>
> Shields JA, Kaden IH, Eagle RC, et al. Orbital dermoid cysts: clinicopathologic correlations, classification, and management. *Ophthal Plast Reconstr Surg.* 1997;13:265–276.

Lipodermoids

Lipodermoids are solid tumors that are usually located beneath the conjunctiva over the lateral surface of the globe (Fig 5-2). These benign lesions may have deep extensions that lie near the levator and extraocular muscles. They usually require no treatment. If the lesion is very large and cosmetically objectionable, only the anterior portion that is visible should be excised; the surgeon should preserve the overlying conjunctiva if at all possible. Care must be taken to avoid damaging lacrimal gland ducts, extraocular muscles, and the levator aponeurosis. Lesions that may simulate lipodermoids are prolapsed orbital fat, prolapsed palpebral lobe of the lacrimal gland, and lymphomas (such processes are generally found only in adults).

> Fry CL, Leone CR Jr. Safe management of dermolipomas. *Arch Ophthalmol.* 1994;112:1114–1116.

Teratomas

Teratomas are rare tumors that arise from two or more germinal layers, including ectoderm and endoderm or mesoderm (or both). These tumors are usually cystic and can cause dramatic proptosis at birth. Exenteration is sometimes performed because of the fear of malignancy. However, in some cases, cystic teratomas can be removed without an exenteration, and ocular function may be preserved.

Vascular Tumors

Capillary Hemangiomas

Capillary hemangiomas are common primary benign tumors of the orbit in children (Fig 5-3). They should be distinguished from cavernous hemangiomas (discussed below), which are the most common benign orbital tumors in adults. Capillary hemangiomas

CHAPTER 5: Orbital Neoplasms • 65

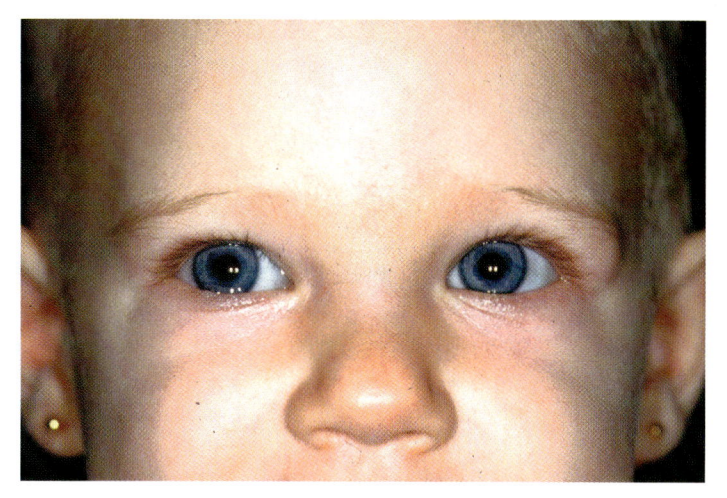

Figure 5-1 A 2-year-old child with a typical laterally located dermoid tumor (epithelial choristoma). *(Photograph courtesy of John B. Holds, MD.)*

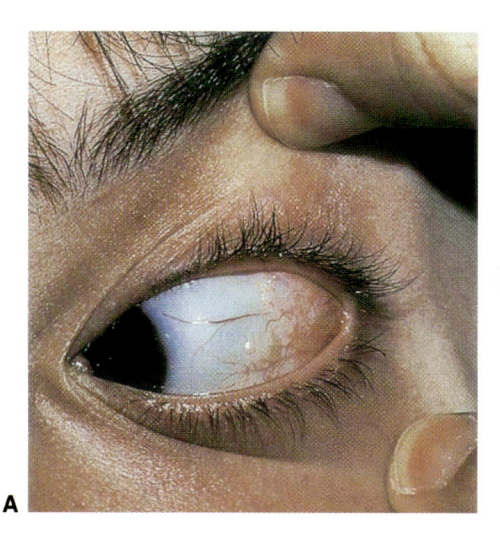

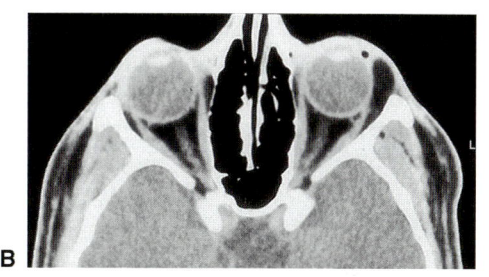

Figure 5-2 A, Lipodermoid of left lateral orbit. **B,** CT scan demonstrating lipodermoid, largely fat density in this case. *(Photographs courtesy of Jeffrey A. Nerad, MD.)*

are seen primarily in children in the first year of life, often appearing in the first week or two after birth and enlarging dramatically over the first 6 months to 1 year of age. After the first year, these vascular tumors begin to involute; 75% of lesions resolve during the next 4 years of life.

The clinical appearance of a periorbital hemangioma depends on the depth of the tumor under the skin. The majority of capillary hemangiomas are superficial and involve the skin, producing an elevated strawberry discoloration with a dimpled texture. Hemangiomas located deeper within the orbit may cause a bluish discoloration or may present merely as a progressively enlarging mass without any overlying skin change. The rapid growth in this circumstance may suggest a rhabdomyosarcoma. CT, although often helpful, cannot always distinguish between these two entities.

66 • Orbit, Eyelids, and Lacrimal System

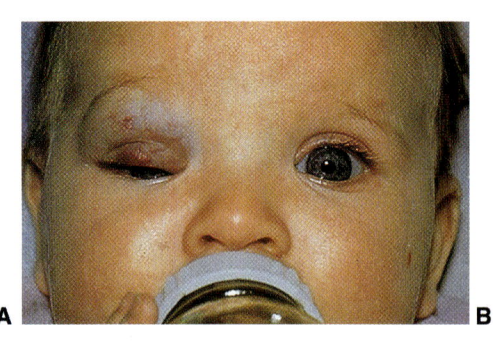

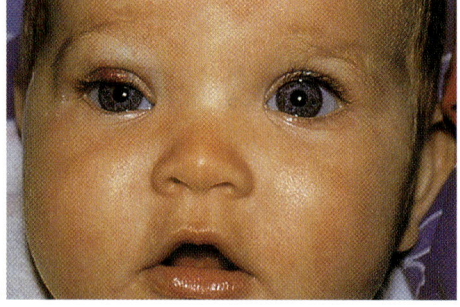

Figure 5-3 A, Capillary hemangioma of right upper eyelid. **B,** Marked regression of capillary hemangioma, 1 week after injection of steroid into lesion. *(Photographs courtesy of Robert C. Kersten, MD.)*

Capillary hemangiomas have a propensity for the head and neck region and, in particular, the superonasal quadrant of the orbit and medial upper eyelid. Periocular hemangiomas are commonly associated with hemangiomas on other parts of the body. Capillary hemangiomas that involve the neck can compromise the airway and lead to respiratory obstruction. Multiple large visceral capillary hemangiomas can also be related to thrombocytopenia (Kasabach-Merritt syndrome). Capillary hemangiomas of the eyelids and orbit may cause anisometropia, strabismus, or deprivation amblyopia. Cosmetic deformity is often significant. Capillary hemangiomas usually have high blood flow derived from multiple fine feeder vessels.

Management

Patients with capillary hemangiomas should undergo close monitoring of visual acuity, with prompt amblyopia therapy as indicated. Ophthalmic indications for treatment of capillary hemangiomas are anisometropia, strabismus, and amblyopia. Severe disfigurement may necessitate therapy, but it should be deferred until it is clear that the natural course of the lesion will not lead to the desired result.

When therapy is indicated, initial treatment consists of local steroid injection, usually an equal mixture of betamethasone, 6 mg/mL, and triamcinolone, 40 mg/mL. This therapy is often dramatically successful. However, side effects include necrosis of the skin overlying the hemangioma, subcutaneous fat atrophy, systemic growth retardation, and embolic visual loss. Repeated injections may be necessary. Systemic steroids have also been used, but they may cause rebound growth of the tumor when discontinued and have greater risks of systemic side effects. Smaller lesions that are refractory to steroids can be managed with surgical excision, but meticulous hemostasis must be maintained. The use of systemic interferon-α has been reported in the management of massive steroid-resistant capillary hemangiomas. Radiation therapy has also been used, but it has the potential to cause cataract formation, bony hypoplasia, and future malignancy. Pulsed-dye laser therapy has also been advocated, but its use is controversial. Although this therapy causes blanching of superficial lesions, it is unclear that large treated lesions fare better than untreated ones. Sclerosing solutions are not recommended because of severe scarring.

Haik BG, Karcioglu ZA, Gordon RA, et al. Capillary hemangioma (infantile periocular hemangioma). *Surv Ophthalmol.* 1994;38:399–426.

Walker RS, Custer PL, Nerad JA. Surgical excision of periorbital capillary hemangiomas. *Ophthalmology.* 1994;101:1333–1340.

Cavernous Hemangiomas

Cavernous hemangiomas (Fig 5-4) are the most common benign neoplasms of the orbit in adults. Middle-aged women are most commonly affected. Proptosis is usually slowly progressive, although growth may accelerate if the patient is pregnant. Retinal striae, hyperopia, optic nerve compression, increased intraocular pressure, and strabismus may develop. Diagnosis can usually be established by CT demonstrating a homogeneously enhanced, well-encapsulated mass. Arteriography and venography usually are not useful in diagnosis because the lesion has a very limited communication with the systemic circulation.

Histopathologically, the lesions are encapsulated and are composed of large cavernous spaces containing red blood cells. The walls of the spaces contain smooth muscle.

Management

Treatment consists of surgical excision if the lesion compromises ocular function. Lateral orbitotomy may be required because the lesions commonly lie in the retrobulbar space within the muscle cone. Coronal CT may be important in determining the position of the cavernous hemangioma relative to the optic nerve and planning the optimal surgical approach. These tumors rarely undergo spontaneous involution.

Hemangiopericytomas

Hemangiopericytomas are uncommon encapsulated, hypervascular, hypercellular lesions that appear in middle age. They may restrict ocular motility and cause conjunctival prolapse and engorgement of vessels in the conjunctival cul-de-sac. Hemangiopericytomas resemble cavernous hemangiomas on contrast-enhanced CT and may look blue in surgery. They are composed of plump pericytes that surround a rich capillary network. These lesions must be completely excised because they may recur, undergo malignant degeneration, and metastasize. Histopathologically, these lesions are unique in that microscopically "benign" lesions may recur and metastasize, whereas microscopically "malignant" lesions may remain localized.

Lymphangiomas

Lymphangiomas are relatively uncommon tumors that usually become apparent in the first decade of life. These lesions may occur in the conjunctiva, eyelids, orbit, oropharynx, and sinuses. Lymphangiomas often enlarge during upper respiratory tract infections, probably because of the response within the lymphoid tissues of the lesion. They may present with sudden proptosis caused by spontaneous hemorrhage. The histogenesis of lymphangiomas remains unclear, but they are thought to represent combined vascular malformations with both venous and lymphatic components.

Histologically, these tumors are characterized by large, serum-filled spaces that are lined by flattened, delicate endothelial cells. The endothelial spaces have no pericytes or

68 • Orbit, Eyelids, and Lacrimal System

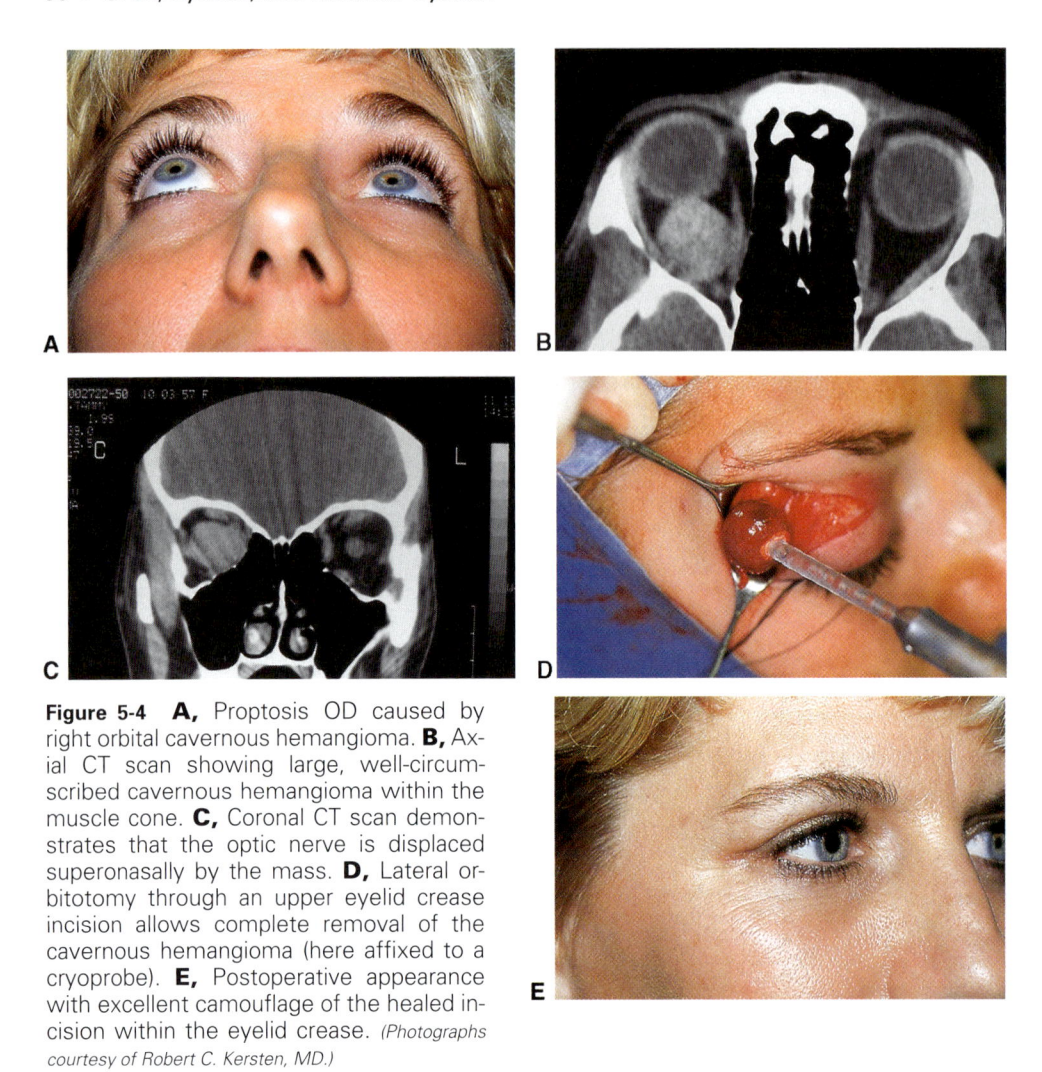

Figure 5-4 A, Proptosis OD caused by right orbital cavernous hemangioma. **B,** Axial CT scan showing large, well-circumscribed cavernous hemangioma within the muscle cone. **C,** Coronal CT scan demonstrates that the optic nerve is displaced superonasally by the mass. **D,** Lateral orbitotomy through an upper eyelid crease incision allows complete removal of the cavernous hemangioma (here affixed to a cryoprobe). **E,** Postoperative appearance with excellent camouflage of the healed incision within the eyelid crease. *(Photographs courtesy of Robert C. Kersten, MD.)*

smooth muscle in their walls. Scattered follicles of lymphoid tissues are found in the interstitium. The tumors have an infiltrative growth pattern and are not encapsulated.

The natural history of lymphangiomas varies and is unpredictable. Some are localized and slowly progressive, whereas many diffusely infiltrate orbital structures and may inexorably enlarge. Lymphangiomas can present abruptly as a mass lesion if there is hemorrhage from interstitial capillaries. Blood may become loculated, leading to the formation of chocolate cysts containing old, dark blood. Ultrasonography, CT, or MRI may be useful for localizing these cysts.

Management

In the case of blood cysts associated with lymphangiomas, spontaneous regression is common; thus, surgical intervention should be deferred unless vision is being damaged. In emergency situations, aspiration of blood through a hollow-bore needle or by open surgical exploration can be attempted. Unfortunately, there is a high incidence of recurrent hemorrhage within lymphangiomas. Whenever possible, orbital hemorrhage from a lymphangioma is allowed to resorb spontaneously. Surgery is generally ungratifying but may be considered when recurrent orbital hemorrhage compromises the globe or optic nerve or when cosmetic deformity is significant.

Although lymphangiomas, especially those located anteriorly, often diffusely infiltrate the orbital structures, some posterior orbital lymphangiomas remain more localized and thus are amenable to total or subtotal surgical excision. In more diffuse lesions, surgical debulking may be necessary to reduce the mass effect. Unfortunately, the lesion often does not respect tissue planes; in such cases, abnormal tissue must be left in the orbit in order to avoid sacrificing important structures.

The carbon dioxide and contact Nd:YAG lasers have proved to be useful adjuncts for surgery of lymphangiomas. Laser therapy provides good hemostasis and also can be used to cause shrinkage and scarring of some unresectable areas of tumor. Bipolar cautery can also be applied to shrink the tumor during surgical excision.

In more extensive diffuse lesions of the orbit, a transcranial approach with removal of the orbital roof provides wide exposure and may better allow total or subtotal excision. In some patients, performing an orbital decompression to allow the globe to return to a more normal position may be preferable to attempting to excise an infiltrative vascular lesion.

It has been reported that noncontiguous intracranial vascular malformation may occur in up to 25% of patients with orbital lymphangiomas. Prospective imaging of the intracranial vasculature is recommended to detect asymptomatic intracranial lesions because they may subsequently bleed.

> Harris GJ. Orbital vascular malformations: a consensus statement on terminology and its clinical implications. Orbital Society. *Am J Ophthalmol.* 1999;127:453–455.
>
> Harris GJ, Sakol PJ, Bonavolontù G, et al. An analysis of 30 cases of orbital lymphangioma: pathophysiological considerations and management recommendations. *Ophthalmology.* 1990;97:1583–1591.
>
> Kazim M, Kennerdell JS, Rothfus W, et al. Orbital lymphangioma: correlation of magnetic resonance images and intraoperative findings. *Ophthalmology.* 1992;99:1588–1594.
>
> Rootman J, Hay E, Graeb D, et al. Orbital-adnexal lymphangiomas. A spectrum of hemodynamically isolated vascular hamartomas. *Ophthalmology.* 1986;93:1558–1570.
>
> Wright JE, Sullivan TJ, Garner A, et al. Orbital venous anomalies. *Ophthalmology.* 1997; 104:905–913.

Masquerading Conditions

A variety of vascular disorders that are not neoplasms can mimic them by causing proptosis and other abnormalities. Among these are arteriovenous malformations, arteriovenous fistulas, orbital varices, and orbital hemorrhages.

Arteriovenous malformations

Arteriovenous malformations are developmental anomalies composed of abnormally formed anastomosing arteries and veins without an intervening capillary bed. Dilated corkscrew episcleral vessels may be prominent. Exsanguinating arterial hemorrhage may be possible with surgical intervention. After these lesions are studied by arteriography, they may be treated by selective occlusion of the feeding vessels, followed by surgical excision of the malformations.

Arteriovenous fistulas

As shown in Figures 5-5 and 5-6, arteriovenous fistulas are abnormal communications between previously normal arteries and veins that may be caused by trauma or degeneration. Basal skull fracture is the type of trauma that most commonly produces an arteriovenous fistula. Spontaneous fistula formation occurs most often as a degenerative process in older patients with systemic hypertension and atherosclerosis. The cavernous sinus is usually the venous structure involved. The internal carotid artery is the most common source of arterial blood for an arteriovenous fistula communicating with the cavernous sinus. This type of fistula is called a *carotid cavernous fistula.*

Carotid cavernous fistulas may produce characteristic tortuous epibulbar vessels and are often accompanied by a bruit that is audible to the examiner, the patient, or both. Pulsating proptosis may also be present. Ischemic ocular damage may result from diversion of arterialized blood into the venous system, and increased pressure in the cavernous sinus frequently causes compression of cranial nerve VI, producing a lateral rectus muscle palsy.

Selective arteriography is usually necessary to evaluate arteriovenous fistulas of the orbit and cavernous sinus. Treatment is difficult. Various types of embolic material have been used in interventional radiography to obstruct the involved artery. These treatment modalities are reserved for patients who are experiencing significant symptoms.

Small meningeal arterial branches that supply the dural walls of the cavernous sinus may rupture spontaneously into the sinus, creating a low-flow *dural sinus fistula.* Because this type generally produces less blood flow than a carotid cavernous fistula, its onset can be insidious; and orbital congestion, proptosis, and pain may be mild. Arterialization of the conjunctival veins causes chronic red eye. Increased episcleral venous pressure results in asymmetric elevation of intraocular pressure on the ipsilateral side, a key sign, and patients with chronic fistulas are at risk for glaucomatous optic disc damage. CT shows diffuse enlargement of all the extraocular muscles resulting from venous engorgement and a characteristically enlarged superior ophthalmic vein. Small fistulas often close spontaneously. Angiography and embolization are less frequently needed for dural sinus fistulas than for high-flow carotid cavernous fistulas.

Orbital varices

Orbital varices (Fig 5-7) can occur primarily as dilations of preexisting venous channels. Proptosis that increases when the patient's head is dependent or after a Valsalva maneuver suggests the presence of orbital varices, and the diagnosis can be confirmed via contrast-enhanced spiral CT. Rapid spiral CT during the Valsalva maneuver or other means of decreasing venous return shows characteristic enlargement of the engorged varix. Phleboliths can sometimes be seen on plain-film radiographs. Patients may exhibit enophthalmos at rest, when the varix is not engorged. Treatment of orbital varices is usually conservative. Surgery is reserved for cases in which the varix threatens vision because of optic nerve or globe damage. Complete surgical excision is difficult because the varix is

CHAPTER 5: Orbital Neoplasms • 71

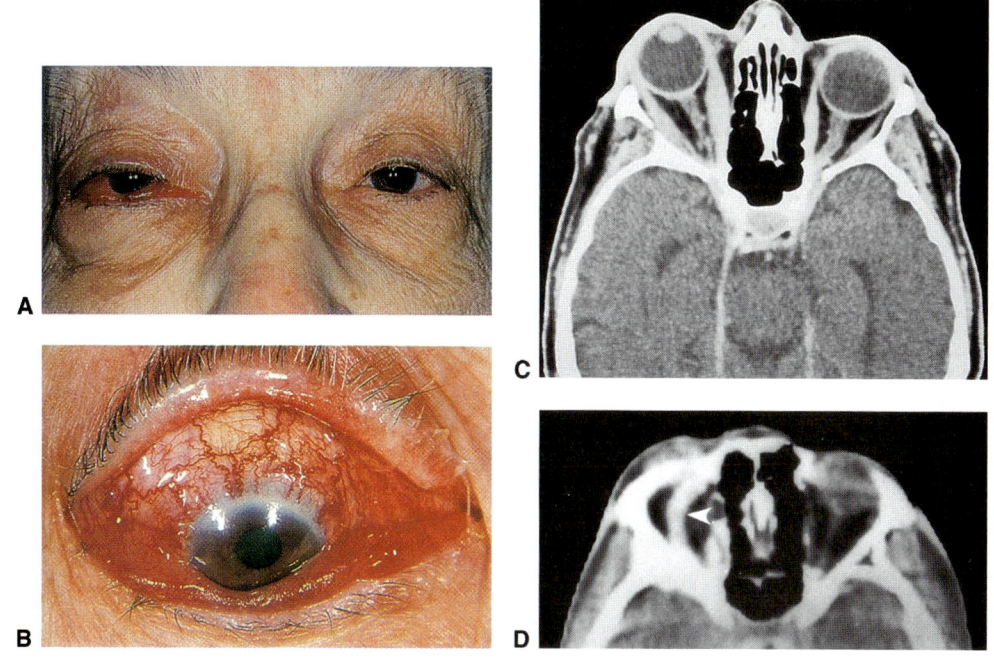

Figure 5-5 A, Carotid cavernous fistula, right eye, in elderly woman. **B,** Arterialization of episcleral and conjunctival vessels and chemosis of conjunctiva. **C,** CT scan demonstrating proptosis of right eye secondary to congested orbital tissues. Note enlarged medial rectus and lateral rectus muscles. *(Parts A–C courtesy of Jeffrey A. Nerad, MD.)* **D,** Axial CT scan showing dilated superior ophthalmic vein *(arrow)*, typical of carotid cavernous fistula.

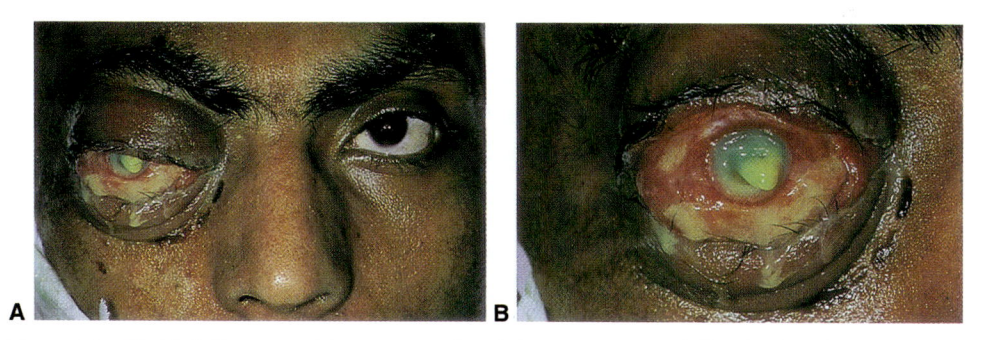

Figure 5-6 A, High-flow carotid cavernous fistula in a young man following head trauma. Note marked proptosis and exposure of eye. **B,** Corneal perforation resulting from exposure. *(Photographs courtesy of Robert C. Kersten, MD.)*

intertwined with normal orbital structures and directly communicates with the abundant venous reservoir in the cavernous sinus. Partial excision sometimes provides an adequate surgical result, and embolization using coils inserted through a distal venous cutdown has also been reported to diminish symptoms.

72 • Orbit, Eyelids, and Lacrimal System

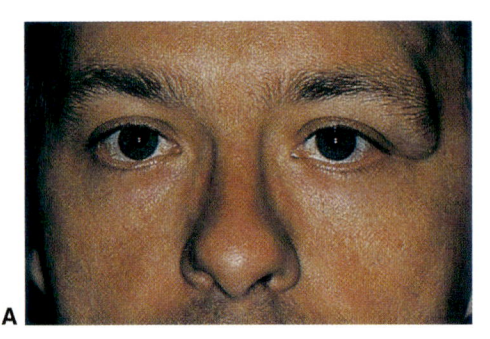

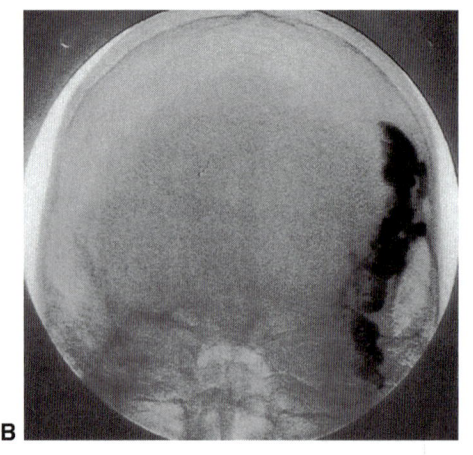

Figure 5-7 A, Congenital varix of left upper eyelid and temple. **B,** Venogram demonstrating large venous channels in periorbital area. *(Photographs courtesy of Jeffrey A. Nerad, MD.)*

Orbital hemorrhages

Orbital hemorrhages may result from trauma or spontaneous bleeding from vascular malformations. Rarely, spontaneous hemorrhage may be caused by a sudden increase in venous pressure (eg, a Valsalva maneuver). They almost always occur superiorly and should be allowed to spontaneously resorb unless there is associated visual compromise.

Atalla ML, McNab AA, Sullivan TJ, et al. Nontraumatic subperiosteal orbital hemorrhage. *Ophthalmology.* 2001;108:183–189.

Neural Tumors

Neural tumors include optic nerve gliomas, neurofibromas, meningiomas, and schwannomas.

Optic Nerve Gliomas

Optic nerve gliomas (Fig 5-8) are uncommon, usually benign tumors that occur predominantly in children in the first decade of life. *Malignant* optic nerve gliomas (glioblastomas) are very rare. They tend to affect middle-aged males, and initial signs and symptoms may resemble optic neuritis. However, they progress rapidly to blindness and death.

Approximately 25%–50% of optic nerve gliomas are associated with neurofibromatosis. The chief clinical feature is gradual, painless, unilateral, axial proptosis associated with loss of vision and an afferent pupillary defect. Other ocular findings may include optic atrophy, optic disc swelling, and strabismus. The chiasm is involved in roughly half of cases of optic nerve glioma. Intracranial involvement may be associated with decreased function of the hypothalamus and pituitary gland.

In the majority of cases, optic nerve gliomas are self-limited and show minimal growth. These characteristics have led some authors to consider them benign hamarto-

CHAPTER 5: Orbital Neoplasms • 73

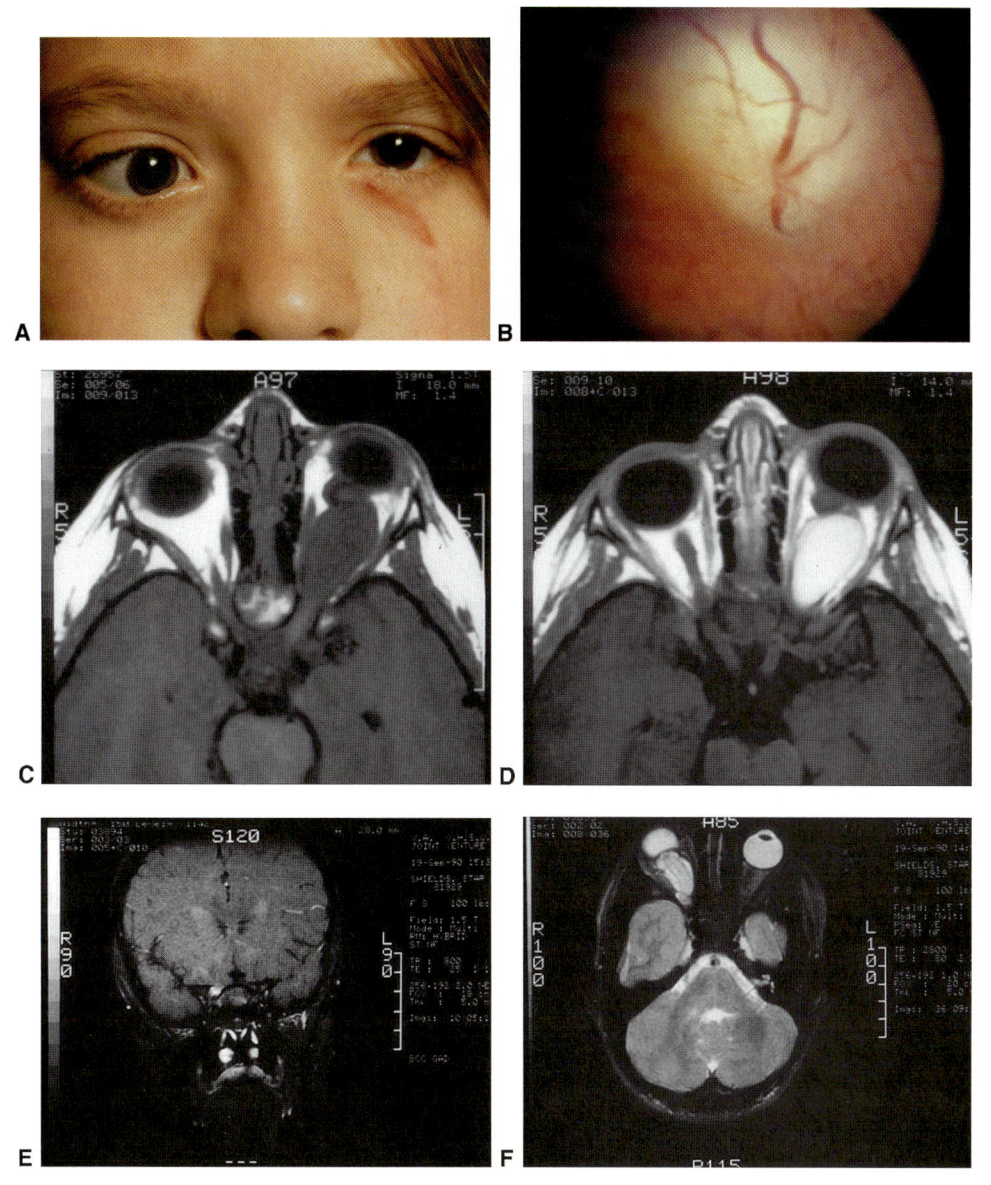

Figure 5-8 A, Clinical photograph of a child with right optic nerve glioma displaying proptosis with esotropia. **B,** Funduscopic view of same patient. Note swollen disc with obscured disc margins. **C,** T1-weighted axial MRI scan of optic nerve glioma demonstrating the so-called kink of the optic nerve. **D,** T2-weighted image of the same patient. **E,** Coronal MRI scan demonstrates involvement of the optic nerve near the chiasm. **F,** T2-weighted axial MRI scan demonstrating enlargement of the right optic nerve with apparent kink. Note that the central enlarged optic nerve is surrounded by tumor in the perineural space. *(Photographs courtesy of Roger A. Dailey, MD.)*

mas. However, cystic enlargement of the lesions can occur even without true cellular growth. Long-term follow-up of gliomas has shown that some tumors progress, especially when they present with midbrain involvement. Such involvement may prove fatal.

Gross pathology of resected tumors usually reveals a smooth, fusiform intradural lesion. Microscopically, the benign tumors in children are considered to be juvenile pilocytic (hairlike) astrocytomas. Other histopathologic findings include arachnoid hyperplasia, mucosubstance, and Rosenthal fibers. Optic gliomas arising in patients with neurofibromatosis often proliferate in the subarachnoid space; those occurring in patients without neurofibromatosis usually expand within the optic nerve without invasion of the dura mater.

Optic nerve gliomas can usually be diagnosed by means of orbital imaging. CT and MRI usually show fusiform enlargement of the optic nerve. MRI may be more accurate in defining the extent of optic canal lesions and intracranial disease.

It is usually unnecessary to perform a biopsy of a suspected optic nerve glioma, although a diagnosis can never be definitive without histologic examination. If a biopsy sample is obtained from the peripheral portion of the nerve, the presence of reactive meningeal hyperplasia occurring adjacent to the optic nerve glioma may cause the lesion to be misinterpreted as a fibrous meningioma.

Management

The treatment of optic nerve gliomas is controversial. Although most cases remain stable or progress very slowly, the occasional case behaves aggressively. A treatment plan must be carefully individualized for each patient. The following options may be considered.

Observation only Presumed optic nerve glioma, particularly with good vision on the involved side, may be carefully followed if the radiographic evidence is characteristic of this type of tumor and if the glioma is unequivocally confined to the orbit. Periodic follow-up examinations and appropriate radiographic studies (MRI, CT, or both) must be performed at regular intervals. Many patients maintain good vision for years and never require surgery.

Surgical excision When the tumor grows rapidly, the goal is to isolate the tumor from the optic chiasm to prevent the rare possibility of chiasmal invasion. An intracranial approach should be used so that a free surgical margin can be obtained. However, even if the tumor enlarges slowly and remains confined to the orbit, corneal exposure and cosmesis may also become indications for surgical excision. Removal through an intracranial approach may also be indicated at the time of initial diagnosis or after a short period of observation if the tumor involves the intracranial portion of the optic nerve between the bony optic canal and the optic chiasm. Complete excision is possible if the tumor ends 2–3 mm anterior to the chiasm. Excision may also be required if the glioma causes an increase in intracranial pressure.

Radiation therapy Initial radiation therapy is considered if the tumor cannot be resected (usually chiasm or tract lesions) and if symptoms (particularly neurologic) progress. Postoperative radiation of the chiasm and optic tract may also be considered if good radiographic studies document subsequent growth of the tumor within the chiasm or if chiasmal and optic tract involvement is extensive. Radiation is generally held as a last resort for children with incomplete orbital development.

Chemotherapy Combination chemotherapy using actinomycin D and vincristine has also been reported to be effective in patients with progressive chiasmatic/hypothalamic gliomas. Chemotherapy may delay the need for radiation therapy and thus enhance long-term intellectual development and preservation of endocrinologic function in children.

In summary, any treatment plan must be carefully individualized. Therapeutic decisions must be based on the tumor growth characteristics, the extent of optic nerve and chiasm involvement as determined by clinical and radiographic evaluation, the visual acuity of the involved and uninvolved eye, the presence or absence of concomitant neurologic or systemic disease, and the history of previous treatment.

> Dutton JJ. Gliomas of the anterior visual pathway. *Surv Ophthalmol.* 1994;38:427–452.
> Jenkin D, Angyalfi S, Becker L, et al. Optic glioma in children: surveillance, resection, or irradiation? *Int J Radiat Oncol Biol Phys.* 1993;25:215–225.
> Listernick R, Charrow J, Greenwald M, et al. Natural history of optic pathway tumors in children with neurofibromatosis type 1: a longitudinal study. *J Pediatr.* 1994;125:63–66.
> Massry GG, Morgan CF, Chung SM. Evidence of optic pathway gliomas after previously negative neuroimaging. *Ophthalmology.* 1997;104:930–935.

Neurofibromas

Neurofibromas, shown in Figures 5-9 and 5-10, are tumors composed chiefly of proliferating Schwann cells within the nerve sheaths. Axons, endoneural fibroblasts, and mucin are also visible. *Plexiform neurofibromas* are infiltrative tumors that usually occur in neurofibromatosis type 1. They are well-vascularized and can seldom be completely removed by surgical excision. *Discrete neurofibromas* are less common but can usually be excised surgically without recurrence.

Neurofibromatosis Type 1

Also known as *von Recklinghausen disease*, neurofibromatosis type 1 is inherited through an autosomal dominant gene with irregular penetrance. Because it is characterized by the presence of hamartomas involving the skin, eye, central nervous system, and viscera, it is classified as a phakomatosis. Neurofibromatosis type 1 is the most common phakomatous disorder involving the orbit. Among the disorders associated with this syndrome are

- Café-au-lait spots, which are areas of increased epidermal melanin caused by distinctive giant melanosomes (the number of café-au-lait spots generally increases in late childhood)
- Axillary freckling
- Fibroma molluscum (pedunculated skin nodules composed of connective tissue and other elements)
- Plexiform neurofibromas (diffuse proliferations of Schwann cells within nerve sheaths), which frequently involve the lateral area of the upper eyelid and cause

76 • Orbit, Eyelids, and Lacrimal System

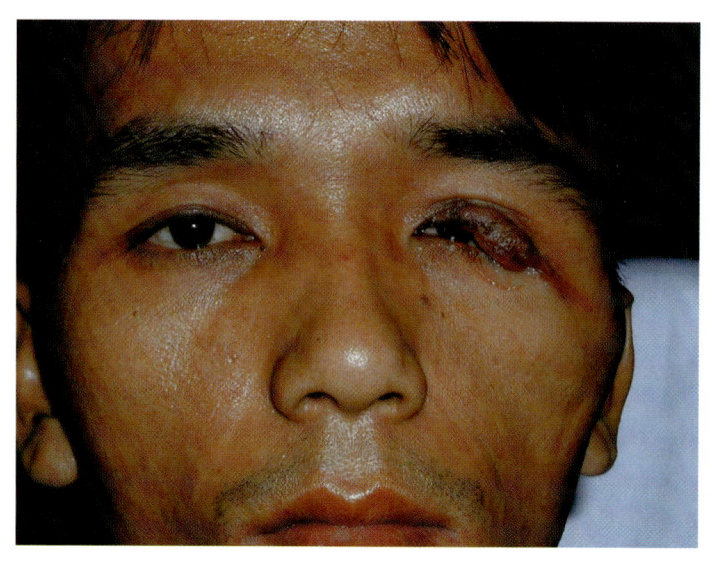

Figure 5-9 Ptosis of left upper eyelid, especially laterally, characteristic of plexiform neurofibroma infiltration. *(Photograph courtesy of Jerry Popham, MD.)*

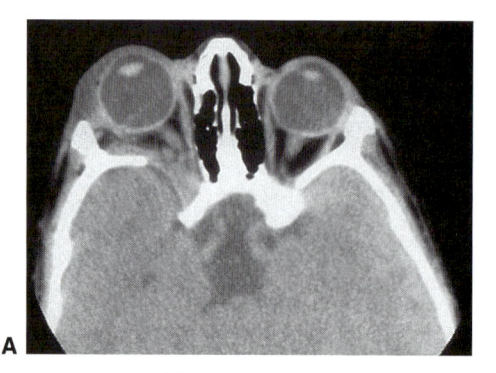

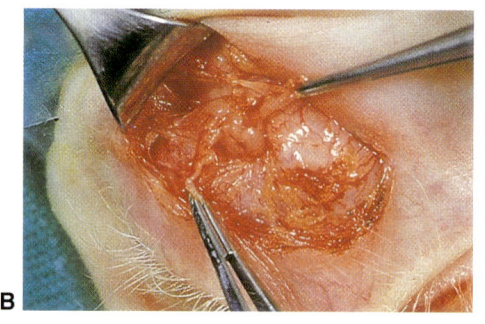

Figure 5-10 A, CT scan of patient with neurofibromatosis demonstrating slight proptosis, plexiform neurofibromas, and sphenoid wing dysplasia. **B,** Plexiform neurofibroma excision during ptosis surgery. Percutaneous palpation of the subcutaneous fibrous neoplastic cords visible here produces a "bag-of-worms" consistency. *(Photographs courtesy of Jeffrey A. Nerad, MD.)*

an S-shaped contour of the eyelid margin (on dissection, these tumors appear as tortuous, fibrous cords that infiltrate normal tissues)
- Dysplasia of orbital walls (pulsating proptosis may be produced by sphenoid bone dysplasia)
- Congenital glaucoma and pigmented iris nodules
- Optic nerve gliomas (approximately 25%–50% of all patients with optic nerve gliomas have neurofibromatosis)

See BCSC Section 6, *Pediatric Ophthalmology and Strabismus*, for further discussion of neurofibromatosis and other phakomatoses.

Farris SR, Grove AS. Orbital and eyelid manifestations of neurofibromatosis: a clinical study and literature review. *Ophthal Plast Reconstr Surg.* 1996;12:245–259.

Meningiomas

Meningiomas are invasive tumors that arise from arachnoid villi and usually originate intracranially along the sphenoid wing with secondary extension into the orbit through the bone, the superior orbital fissure, or the optic canal (Figs 5-11 and 5-12). Ophthalmic manifestations are related to the location of the primary tumor. Meningiomas arising near the sella and optic nerves cause early visual defects and papilledema or optic atrophy. Tumors arising near the pterion (posterior end of the parietosphenoid fissure, at the lateral portion of the sphenoid bone) often produce a temporal fossa mass and proptosis. Eyelid edema (especially of the lower eyelid) and chemosis are common.

CT commonly shows localized bone thickening (hyperostosis) associated with abnormal calcifications in the tumor. Sometimes bone absorption and destruction are apparent. MRI helps to outline the extent of meningiomas adjacent to the bone (especially when contrast enhancement is used).

Primary orbital meningiomas are much less common than those that arise intracranially and secondarily invade the orbit. Primary orbital meningiomas usually originate from the arachnoid of the optic nerve sheath. These optic nerve sheath meningiomas occur most commonly in women in their third and fourth decades of life. Symptoms usually include a gradual, painless, unilateral loss of vision. Examination typically shows decreased visual acuity and a relative afferent pupillary defect. Proptosis and ophthalmoplegia may also be present. At presentation, the optic nerve head may appear normal, atrophic, or swollen, and optociliary shunt vessels may be visible. Occasionally, optic nerve sheath meningiomas occur bilaterally, in which case they are associated with neurofibromatosis.

Imaging characteristics are usually sufficient to allow diagnosis of optic nerve sheath meningiomas. Both CT and MRI show diffuse tubular enlargement of the optic nerve with contrast enhancement. MRI has the additional benefit of identifying optic canal and intracranial tumor extension. Thus, MRI with gadolinium administration is the imaging modality of choice to diagnose and fully delineate the condition.

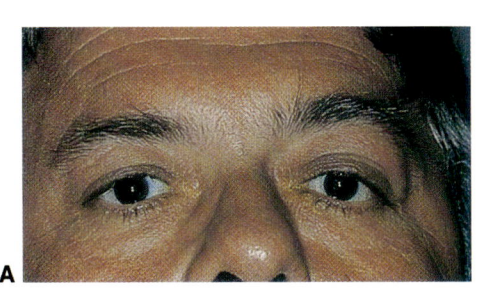

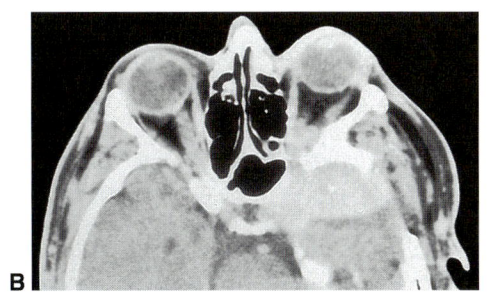

Figure 5-11 A, Left proptosis and fullness of left temple secondary to sphenoid wing meningioma. **B,** CT scan showing orbital and intracranial meningioma arising from sphenoid wing. Note hyperostosis of sphenoid bone. *(Photographs courtesy of Jeffrey A. Nerad, MD.)*

78 • Orbit, Eyelids, and Lacrimal System

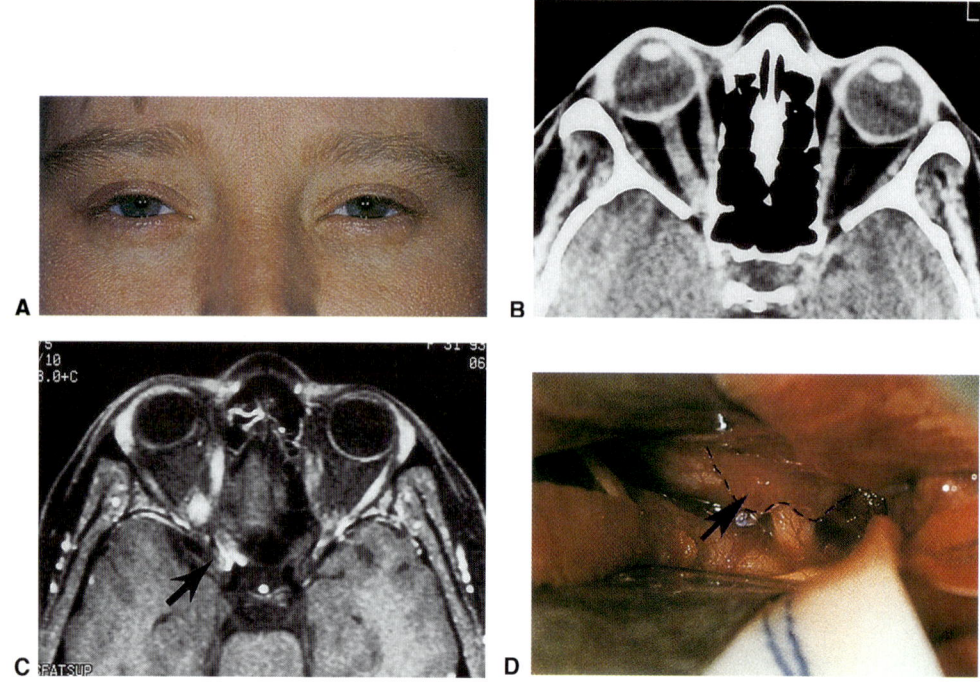

Figure 5-12 A, Primary optic nerve meningioma of right optic nerve, with minimal proptosis. **B,** CT scan showing thickened right optic nerve with calcification. **C,** MRI showing orbital apex mass with intracranial spread through optic canal. Note bright signal adjacent to flow void of right carotid artery (*arrow*). **D,** The meningioma is exposed through a craniotomy and superior orbitotomy. Intraoperative view shows intracranial prechiasmal optic nerve. Note cuff (*arrow, dashes*) of meningioma wrapping around optic nerve extending out from optic canal. *(Photographs courtesy of Jeffrey A. Nerad, MD.)*

Management

Treatment of optic nerve sheath meningioma must be individualized. Both the extent of visual loss and the presence of intracranial extension are important factors in treatment planning. Observation is indicated if vision is minimally affected and no intracranial extension is present. If the tumor is confined to the orbit and visual loss is significant or progressive, radiation therapy should be considered. Radiotherapy often results in stabilization or improvement of visual function. If the patient is observed or treated with radiation, periodic MRI is necessary to identify possible intracranial extension. With rare exceptions, attempts to surgically excise optic nerve sheath meningiomas results in visual loss. Thus, surgery is reserved for patients with intracranial extension or severe visual loss with severe proptosis. In such cases, the optic nerve is excised with the tumor from the back of the globe to the chiasm.

Dutton JJ. Optic nerve sheath meningiomas. *Surv Ophthalmol.* 1992;37:167–183.

Eng TY, Albright NW, Kuwahara G, et al. Precision radiation therapy for optic nerve sheath meningiomas. *Int J Radiat Oncol Biol Phys.* 1992;22:1093–1098.

Wright JE, McNab AA, McDonald WI. Primary optic sheath meningioma. *Br J Ophthalmol.* 1989;73:960–966.

Schwannomas

Schwannomas, sometimes known as *neurilemomas,* are proliferations of Schwann cells that are encapsulated by perineurium. These tumors have a characteristic biphasic pattern of solid areas with nuclear palisading *(Antoni A pattern)* and myxoid areas *(Antoni B pattern).* Hypercellular schwannomas sometimes recur even after what is thought to be complete removal, but they seldom undergo malignant transformation. These tumors are usually well encapsulated and can be excised with relative ease.

Mesenchymal Tumors

Rhabdomyosarcomas

Rhabdomyosarcoma (Fig 5-13) is the most common primary orbital malignancy of childhood. The average age of onset is 8–10 years. Although the classic clinical picture is one of a child with sudden onset and rapid evolution of unilateral proptosis, many rhabdomyosarcomas have a less dramatic course lasting from weeks to over a month of gradual progressive proptosis. There is often a marked adnexal response with edema and discoloration of the eyelids. Ptosis and strabismus may also be present. A mass may be palpable, particularly in the superonasal quadrant of the eyelid. However, the tumor may be retrobulbar or involve any other portion of the orbit and may rarely arise from the conjunctiva. The patient sometimes has a history of trauma to the orbital area. Although the history is purely coincidental, it can lead to a delay in diagnosis and treatment.

If a rhabdomyosarcoma is suspected, the workup should proceed on an urgent basis. CT, MRI, and ultrasonography can be used to define the location and extent of the tumor. CT is particularly helpful if the tumor has caused bony destruction, although the orbital walls remain intact in most orbital rhabdomyosarcomas.

A biopsy should be undertaken urgently, usually through an anterior orbitotomy. It is often possible to completely remove a rhabdomyosarcoma if it has a pseudocapsule; in any case, the smaller the volume of residual tumor, the more effective the combination of radiation and chemotherapy will be in causing its regression. In diffusely infiltrating

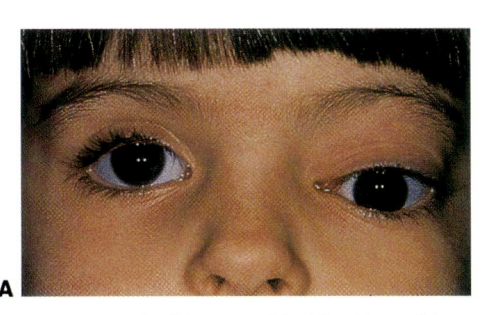

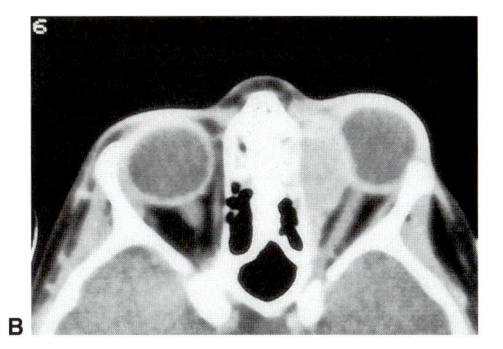

Figure 5-13 A, Six-year-old girl with rapid onset of axial proptosis, lateral and downward displacement of left eye. **B,** CT scan demonstrating a medial orbital mass proven by biopsy to be rhabdomyosarcoma. *(Photographs courtesy of Jeffrey A. Nerad, MD.)*

tumors, a large biopsy should be obtained so that adequate material is available for frozen sections, permanent light-microscopy sections, electron microscopy, and immunohistochemistry. Cross-striations are often not visible on light microscopy and may be more readily apparent on electron microscopy.

The physician should palpate the cervical and preauricular lymph nodes of patients with orbital rhabdomyosarcoma to rule out regional metastases. A chest radiograph, bone marrow aspirate and biopsy, and lumbar puncture should be obtained to search for more distant metastases. Sampling of the bone marrow and the cerebrospinal fluid is best performed under anesthesia. If a rhabdomyosarcoma is suspected, arrangements should be made to perform these studies while the patient is under anesthesia for the orbital biopsy.

Rhabdomyosarcomas arise from undifferentiated pluripotential mesenchymal elements in the orbital soft tissues and not from the extraocular muscles. They may be grouped into four categories:

- *Embryonal.* This is by far the most common type found in the orbits of infants and children, accounting for over 80% of cases. The embryonal form has a predilection for the superonasal quadrant of the orbit. The tumor is composed of loose fascicles of undifferentiated spindle cells, only a minority of which show cross-striations in immature rhabdomyosarcomas on trichrome staining. Embryonal rhabdomyosarcomas are associated with a good (94%) survival rate.
- *Alveolar.* This form has a predilection for the inferior orbit and accounts for 9% of orbital rhabdomyosarcomas. The tumor displays regular compartments composed of fibrovascular strands in which rounded rhabdomyoblasts either line up along the connective tissue strands or float freely in the alveolar spaces. This is the most malignant form of rhabdomyosarcoma.
- *Pleomorphic.* Pleomorphic rhabdomyosarcoma is the least common and the most differentiated form. In this type, many of the cells are straplike or rounded with cross-striations easily discovered with trichrome stain. The pleomorphic variety tends to occur in older persons and has the best prognosis (97% survival rate).
- *Botryoid.* This rare variant of embryonal rhabdomyosarcoma appears grapelike. It is not found in the orbit as a primary tumor; rather, the botryoid variant occurs as a secondary invader from the paranasal sinuses or from the conjunctiva.

Management

Before 1965, the standard treatment for orbital rhabdomyosarcoma was exenteration and the survival rate was poor. After 1965, this mutilating procedure was abandoned as primary management; radiation therapy and systemic chemotherapy have become the mainstays of treatment, based on the guidelines set forth by the Intergroup Rhabdomyosarcoma Studies I–IV. The total dose of local radiation varies from 4500 to 6000 cGy, given over a period of 6 weeks. The goal of systemic chemotherapy is to eliminate microscopic cellular metastases. Survival rates with radiation and chemotherapy are better than 90% if the orbital tumor has not invaded or extended beyond the bony orbital walls. Side effects of radiation in this young age group are common and include cataract, radiation dermatitis, and bony hypoplasia.

Kodet R, Newton WA Jr, Hamoudi AB, et al. Orbital rhabdomyosarcomas and related tumors in childhood: relationship of morphology to prognosis—an Intergroup Rhabdomyosarcoma Study. *Med Pediatr Oncol.* 1997;29:51–60.

Mannor GE, Rose GE, Plowman PN, et al. Multidisciplinary management of refractory orbital rhabdomyosarcoma. *Ophthalmology.* 1997;104:1198–1201.

Shields CL, Shields JA, Honavar SG, et al. Clinical spectrum of primary ophthalmic rhabdomyosarcoma. *Ophthalmology.* 2001;108:2284–2292.

Miscellaneous Mesenchymal Tumors

Tumors of fibrous connective tissue, cartilage, and bone are uncommon lesions that may involve the orbit. Among the miscellaneous mesenchymal tumors, *fibrous histiocytoma* is the most common orbital neoplasm. It is characteristically very firm and displaces normal structures. Both fibroblastic and histiocytic cells in a storiform (matlike) pattern are found in these locally aggressive tumors. Fewer than 10% have metastatic potential. This tumor is sometimes difficult to distinguish clinically and histologically from hemangiopericytoma. A new entity, *solitary fibrous tumor,* has been described. These tumors are composed of spindle-shaped cells that are strongly CD34-positive on immunohistochemical studies. They can occur anywhere in the orbit and may recur and undergo malignant degeneration if incompletely excised. A number of these mesenchymal tumors were probably misclassified (eg, as fibrous histiocytoma, hemangiopericytoma, schwannoma) before their typical immunochemistry was described.

Fibrous dysplasia (Fig 5-14) is a benign developmental disorder of bone that may involve a single region or be polyostotic. When associated with cutaneous pigmentation and endocrine disorders, the condition is known as *Albright syndrome.*

Katz BJ, Nerad JA. Ophthalmic manifestations of fibrous dysplasia—a disease of children and adults. *Ophthalmology.* 1998;105:2207–2215.

Osteomas are benign tumors that usually involve the frontal sinuses and can be completely excised in most patients.

Malignant mesenchymal tumors such as *liposarcoma, fibrosarcoma, chondrosarcoma,* and *osteosarcoma* rarely appear in the orbit. When chondrosarcomas and osteosarcomas are present, they usually destroy normal bone and have characteristic calcifications visible in radiographs and CT scans. Children with a history of bilateral retinoblastoma are at higher risk for osteosarcoma, chondrosarcoma, or fibrosarcoma, even if they have not been treated with therapeutic radiation.

Lymphoproliferative Disorders

Lymphoid Hyperplasias and Lymphomas

Lymphoproliferative lesions of the ocular adnexa constitute a fascinating and confusing disease complex about which our understanding continues to evolve. This heterogeneous group of neoplasms of the lymphoid system comprises distinct entities that are defined by clinical, histologic, immunologic, molecular, and genetic characteristics.

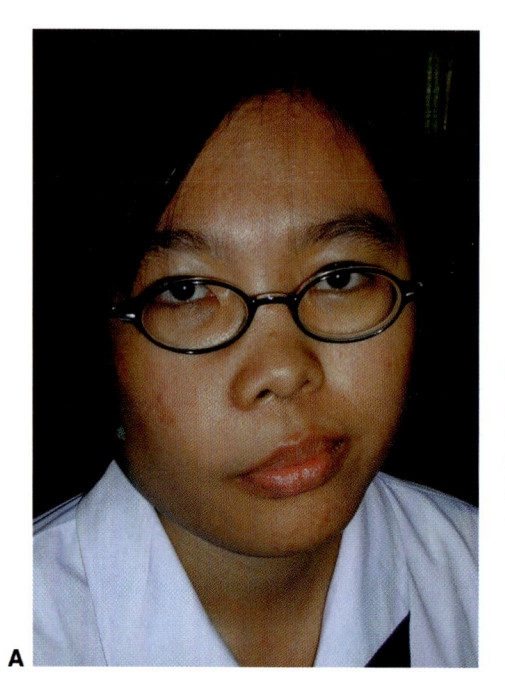

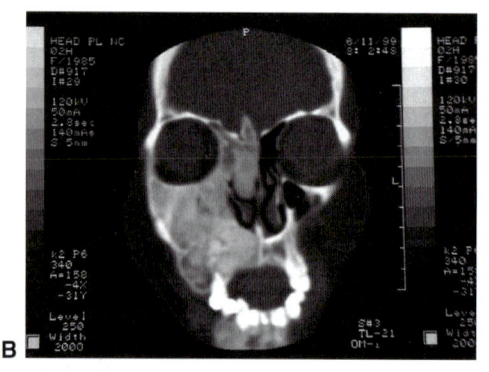

Figure 5-14 Fibrous dysplasia. **A,** This young woman manifests facial asymmetry due to fibrous dysplasia. **B,** CT scan shows characteristic hyperostosis of involved facial bones. *(Photographs courtesy of Jerry Popham, MD.)*

Lymphoproliferative neoplasms account for greater than 20% of all orbital mass lesions. The incidence of non–Hodgkin lymphoma of all anatomic sites has been increasing at a rate of 3%–4% per year (representing a 50% increase over the last 15 years), and this entity is now the fourth most common malignancy among men and women. Orbital lymphomas have been increasing at an even greater rate, although the factors responsible for this rise are poorly understood. Workers in occupations such as farming, paper processing, and others that all involve long-term exposure to bioactive solvents and reagents are at increased risk for non–Hodgkin lymphoma, as are patients with chronic autoimmune diseases.

Identification and classification of lymphoproliferative disorders

Historically, lymphoid tumors were classified as either *reactive lymphoid hyperplasias* (thought to be localized benign diseases of unknown cause) or *malignant lymphomas* (Figs 5-15, 5-16). More recently, it has been recognized that lymphoproliferative lesions represent a continuum and that ultimate behavior is difficult to predict. A considerable number of patients with histologically benign-appearing orbital lymphoid infiltrates eventually develop extraorbital lymphoma, while the malignant lymphoma of the ocular adnexa may be well-demarcated and may respond satisfactorily to local therapy without subsequent systemic involvement. Currently, 70%–80% of orbital lymphoproliferative lesions are designated as malignant lymphomas on the basis of monoclonal cell surface markers, whereas 90% are found to be malignant on the basis of molecular genetic studies. With further advances in evaluation of these lesions, the number designated as benign reactive hyperplasias is likely to continue to shrink.

CHAPTER 5: Orbital Neoplasms • 83

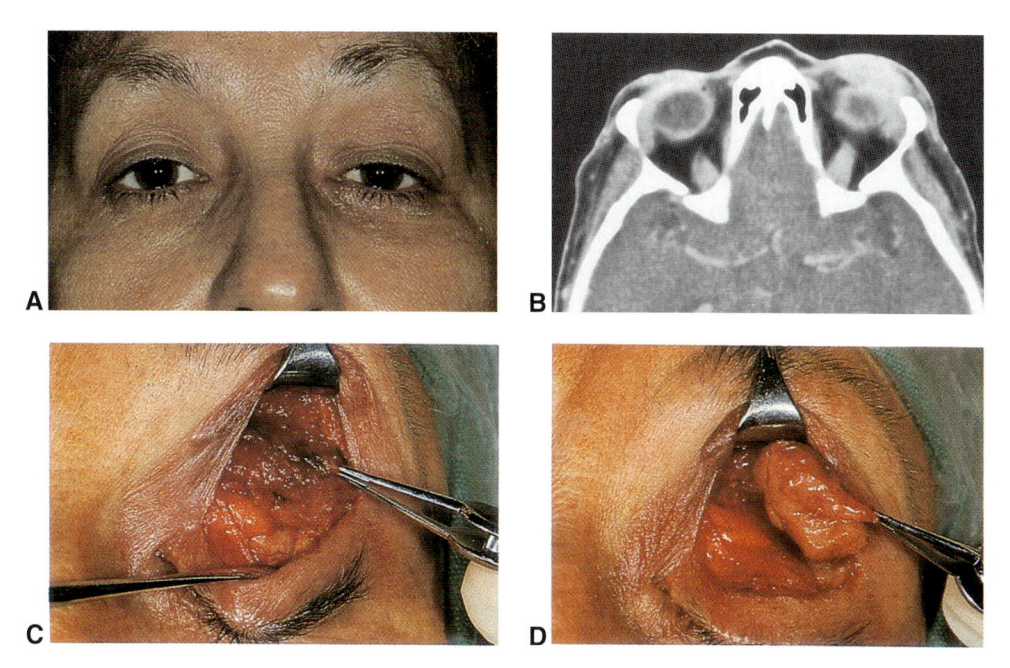

Figure 5-15 A, Bilateral upper eyelid ptosis and fullness. Bilateral upper eyelid masses can be palpated under orbital rim. **B,** CT scan demonstrating bilateral lacrimal gland enlargement with infiltration of anterior orbital tissues consistent with orbital lymphoma. **C,** Anterior orbitotomy is performed for biopsy of the mass. Note large mass *(grasped in forceps)* positioned between preaponeurotic fat and superior orbital rim. **D,** Incisional biopsy of mass is performed, confirming diagnosis of lymphoma. *(Photographs courtesy of Jeffrey A. Nerad, MD.)*

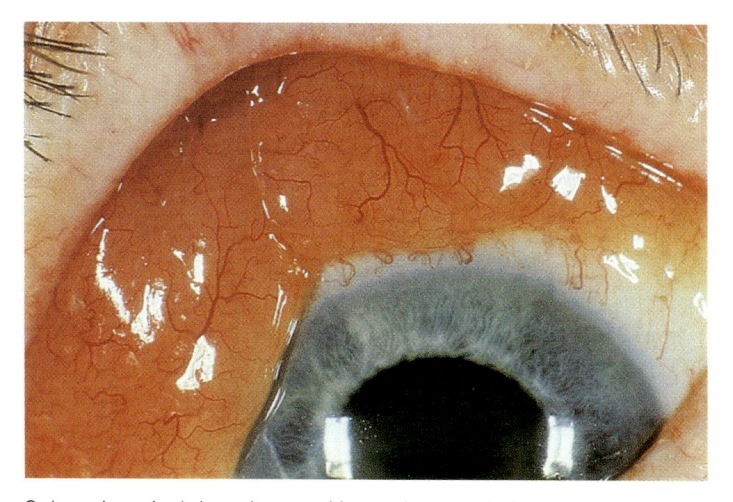

Figure 5-16 Subconjunctival lymphoma. Note characteristic salmon-patch appearance of lesion. *(Photograph courtesy of Jeffrey A. Nerad, MD.)*

The typical lymphoproliferative lesion presents as a gradually progressive painless mass. These tumors are often located anteriorly in the orbit or beneath the conjunctiva and may present as a palpable or visible mass (subconjunctival salmon-patch appearance). Lymphoproliferative lesions, whether considered benign or malignant, usually mold themselves around existing orbital structures rather than invading them; consequently, disturbances of extraocular motility or visual function are unusual. Reactive lymphoid hyperplasias and low-grade lymphomas often have a history of slow expansion over a period of months to years. Orbital imaging reveals a characteristic puttylike molding of the tumor around normal structures, and bone erosion or infiltration is usually not seen except with high-grade malignant lymphomas. Up to 50% of orbital lymphoproliferative lesions arise in the lacrimal fossa. Lymphomas in the retrobulbar fat may appear more infiltrative. Approximately 17% of lymphoid lesions occur bilaterally in the orbits, but this does not necessarily indicate systemic disease.

For all lymphoproliferative lesions, an open biopsy is recommended when possible to obtain an adequate tissue specimen for attempting to establish a diagnosis and to characterize the lesions to reflect distinct morphologic, immunologic, cytogenetic, and molecular properties under the Revised European American Lymphoma (REAL) classification. A portion of the tissue should be placed in a suitable fixative for light-microscopic studies. The majority of the specimen should be sent fresh to a molecular diagnostics laboratory for possible flow cytometry and polymerase chain reaction (PCR) analysis.

Both reactive hyperplasia and malignant lymphoma are hypercellular proliferations with sparse or absent stromal components. Histopathologically, light microscopy may reveal a continuum from benign reactive hyperplasia, to atypical lymphoid hyperplasia, to low-grade lymphoma, to more highly malignant lymphoma. Within this spectrum, it may be difficult to characterize a given lesion by light microscopy alone. In such cases, immunopathology and molecular diagnostic studies have been proposed as aids to further categorization.

Malignant lymphomas are thought to represent clonal expansions of abnormal precursor cells. Immunologic identification of cell-surface markers on lymphocytes can be used to classify tumors as containing B cells or T cells and as being either monoclonal or polyclonal in origin. Cells in smears, histologic sections, or cell suspensions can be studied using specific monoclonal antibodies directed against surface light-chain (κ or λ) immunoglobulins in order to determine whether they represent monoclonal (ie, malignant) proliferations.

Newer techniques of molecular analysis allow more precise identification of tumor clonality by extracting, amplifying, and hybridizing tumor DNA with radioactively labeled nucleotide probes. DNA hybridization is more sensitive than cell-surface marker typing in detecting clonality, but this technique is also more time-consuming and expensive. DNA genetic studies have demonstrated that most lymphoproliferative lesions that appear to be immunologically polyclonal actually harbor small monoclonal proliferations of B lymphocytes. Interestingly, the finding of monoclonality on either an immunophenotypic or a molecular genetic basis does not predict which tumors will go on to cause nonocular disease.

CHAPTER 5: Orbital Neoplasms • 85

Approximately 90% of orbital lymphoproliferations prove monoclonal and 10% polyclonal by molecular genetic studies, but both types of lesions may have prior, concurrent, or future systemic spread. This occurs in greater than half of periocular lymphomas, with 20%–30% of periocular lymphoproliferative lesions having a history of previous or concomitant systemic disease and an additional 30% developing it over 5 years. The anatomic site of origin offers some prediction of the risk of having or developing systemic non–Hodgkin lymphoma, with the risk being lowest for conjunctival lesions, greater for orbital lesions, and highest for lesions arising in the eyelid. Lymphoid lesions developing in the lacrimal fossa may carry a greater risk of systemic disease than those occurring elsewhere in the orbit. Bilateral periocular involvement markedly increases the risk of systemic disease, but such involvement is not, as one might suspect, definitive of systemic disease. It is also clear that the risk of systemic disease increases for decades after the original lesion is diagnosed, regardless of the initial lesion's location in the orbit or its clonality.

The REAL system has been shown to predict differences in the clinical behavior of ocular adnexal lymphomas. The REAL classification allocates adnexal lymphomas to one of five categories: marginal zone lymphoma, diffuse lymphoplasmacytoid/lymphoplasmacytic lymphoma, follicle center lymphoma, diffuse large B-cell lymphoma, and other rare lymphomas. Marginal zone lymphoma is also known as mucosa-associated lymphoid tumor (discussed next) and represents the largest group of orbital lymphomas, accounting for 40%–60%.

MALT-type tumors

Mucosa-associated lymphoid tumors (MALTs) were originally described as occurring in the gastrointestinal tract; approximately 50% of MALT-type lymphomas arise there. Recent studies have suggested that proliferation of early MALT-type tumors may be antigen-driven. Therapy directed at the antigen (eg, against *Helicobacter pylori* in gastric lymphomas) may result in regression of early lesions. Extranodal MALT-type lymphomas in other parts of the body usually arise in association with mucosa or other epithelial structures. In contrast, MALT-type lymphomas of the ocular adnexa do not appear to be preferentially associated with conjunctival or lacrimal gland involvement. Therefore, the MALT designation in the ocular adnexal marginal zone lymphomas refers merely to similar histologic and ultrastructural appearance and not to a predilection for mucosal or epithelial sites of origin.

It used to be thought that low-grade MALT-type lymphomas that originate as primary neoplasms in the orbit rarely undergo systemic dissemination. However, recent studies with long-term follow-up have demonstrated that at least 50% of patients will have developed systemic disease at 10 years and that the 5-year tumor-associated mortality rate for marginal zone lymphomas of the ocular adnexa is higher than previously thought, with progressively increasing mortality for higher-grade orbital lymphomas (Table 5-1). MALT lymphomas may temporarily regress, and spontaneous remission occurs in 5%–15% of cases. MALT lymphomas, however, may undergo histologic transformation to a more aggressive lymphoma, usually of a large-cell type. Such transformation occurs in 15%–20% of cases, usually after several years, and is not related to therapy. In

Table 5-1 Characteristics and Outcome for Patients Presenting With Ocular Adnexal Lymphoma Classified by Histologic Type (REAL Classification)

Characteristics		MZL	LPL	FCL	DLCL	H5	All
Number	All patients	82/192 (43%)	44/192 (23%)	26/192 (14%)	19/192 (10%)	21/192 (11%)	192
	Solely adnexal disease	67/123 (54%)	29/123 (24%)	14/123 (11%)	10/123 (8%)	3/123 (2%)	123/192 (64%)
Age at diagnosis (mean and range)	All patients	68 (18–87)	63 (31–86)	65 (18–86)	73 (35–90)	60 (3–81)	66 (3–90)
	Solely adnexal disease	68 (18–87)	62 (31–86)	61 (18–86)	74 (39–85)	58 (3–80)	66 (3–87)
Sex (proportion men)	All patients	35/82 (43%)	21/44 (48%)	12/26 (46%)	10/19 (53%)	16/21 (76%)	94/192 (49%)
	Solely adnexal disease	29/67 (43%)	15/29 (52%)	6/14 (43%)	5/10 (50%)	2/3 (67%)	57/123 (46%)
Clinical outcome characteristics in all patients							
Systemic spread at diagnosis	Proportion	15/82 (18%)	15/44 (34%)	11/26 (42%)	5/19 (26%)	16/21 (76%)	62/192 (32%)
	Odds ratio	[1.0]	2.3 (1.0, 5.3)	3.3 (1.3, 8.5)	1.6 (0.5, 5.1)	14.3 (4.5, 45.1)	
Extraorbital spread at diagnosis	Proportion	15/82 (18%)	15/44 (34%)	12/26 (46%)	9/19 (47%)	18/21 (86%)	69/192 (36%)
	Odds ratio	[1.0]	2.3 (1.0, 5.3)	3.8 (1.5, 9.9)	4.0 (1.4, 11.6)	26.8 (6.9, 102.7)	
Systemic spread at any time	Proportion	33/82 (40%)	25/44 (57%)	14/26 (54%)	9/19 (47%)	21/21 (100%)	102/192 (53%)
	Hazard ratio	[1.0]	1.0 (0.5, 2.0)	1.7 (0.7, 3.9)	2.0 (0.8, 5.1)	4.1 (1.9, 8.9)	
Extraorbital spread at any time	Proportion	33/82 (40%)	25/44 (57%)	16/26 (62%)	13/19 (68%)	21/21 (100%)	108/192 (56%)
	Hazard ratio	[1.0]	1.0 (0.5, 2.0)	1.9 (0.8, 4.3)	2.4 (1.0, 5.6)	4.1 (1.9, 8.9)	
All deaths	Proportion	24/82 (29%)	18/44 (41%)	10/26 (39%)	10/19 (53%)	14/21 (67%)	76/192 (40%)
Lymphoma related death	Proportion	11/82 (13%)	12/44 (27%)	8/26 (31%)	7/19 (37%)	11/21 (52%)	49/192 (26%)
	Hazard ratio	[1.0]	1.1 (0.5, 2.6)	2.0 (0.8, 5.0)	2.9 (1.1, 7.6)	3.9 (1.7, 9.2)	
Clinical outcome characteristics in patients with solely adnexal disease at diagnosis*							
Future extra	Proportion	18/67 (27%)	10/29 (35%)	4/14 (29%)	4/10 (40%)	3/3 (100%)	39/123 (32%)
	Hazard ratio	[1.0]	0.9 (0.4, 1.9)	1.3 (0.5, 4.0)	1.9 (0.7, 5.8)	3.1 (0.9, 10.5)	
All deaths	Proportion	19/67 (28%)	10/29 (35%)	4/14 (29%)	5/10 (50%)	1/3 (33%)	39/123 (32%)
Lymphoma related deaths	Proportion	6/67 (9%)	4/29 (14%)	3/14 (21%)	3/10 (30%)	1/3 (33%)	17/123 (14%)
	Hazard ratio	[1.0]	0.5 (0.1, 2.3)	2.1 (0.5, 8.7)	2.5 (0.6, 11.2)	3.2 (0.4, 26.9)	

Lymphoma types: MZL = marginal zone lymphoma, LPL = diffuse lymphoplasmacytoid/lymphoplasmacytic lymphoma, FCL = follicle center lymphoma, DLCL = diffuse large B-cell lymphoma, H5 = rare histologic variants.

Lower and upper 95% confidence limits are given in parentheses after odds and hazard ratios. [1.0] is the reference datum.

Systemic spread refers to remote noncontiguous disease. *Extraorbital spread* refers to both remote disease and local extraorbital extension.

* These data refer to patients presenting without a previous history of lymphoma or without extraorbital lymphoma diagnosed (usually as a result of staging) within 3 mo of biopsy.

(From Jenkins C, Rose GE, Bunce C, et al. Histological features of ocular adnexal lymphoma [REAL classification] and their association with patient morbidity and survival. *Br J Ophthalmol.* 2000;84:908.)

contrast, intermediate- and high-grade lymphomas grow rapidly and may be fatal within months if not treated.

Management

Because the various lymphoproliferative lesions show great overlap in terms of clinical behavior, all patients with hypercellular lymphoid lesions (whether monoclonal or polyclonal) should be examined by an oncologist. The examination usually includes a general physical examination, a complete blood count, a bone marrow biopsy, a liver and spleen scan, a bone scan, a chest radiograph, and serum immunoprotein electrophoresis for the detection of abnormal immunoglobulin production. The oncologist may also recommend CT of the thorax and abdomen to check for mediastinal and retroperitoneal lymph node involvement. The patient should be reexamined periodically because systemic lymphoma may occur many years after the presentation of an isolated orbital lymphoid neoplasm.

Although systemic corticosteroids are useful in idiopathic orbital inflammation (pseudotumor), they are not recommended in the treatment of lymphoproliferative lesions. Radiotherapy is the therapy of choice for patients with localized ocular adnexal lymphoproliferative disease. The eye should be protected with a metallic contact lens, and a dose of 2000–2500 cGy is administered. This regimen achieves local control in virtually all cases and, if the lesion is isolated, may prevent systemic spread, although such spread eventually occurs in at least 50% of lesions despite local irradiation. A surgical cure usually cannot be attained because of the infiltrative nature of lymphoid tumors.

Patients must be monitored indefinitely for the development of additional lymphoid neoplasms. The treatment for low-grade lymphoid lesions that have already undergone systemic dissemination is somewhat controversial because indolent lymphomas are generally refractory to chemotherapy and are associated with long-term survival, even if untreated. Many oncologists take a watchful waiting approach and treat only symptomatic disease. More aggressive lymphomas require radiation, aggressive chemotherapy, or both; up to one third of these lesions can be completely cured.

Coupland SE, Krause L, Delecluse H-J, et al. Lymphoproliferative lesions of the ocular adnexa: analysis of 112 cases. *Ophthalmology*. 1998;105:1430–1441.

Jenkins C, Rose GE, Bunce C, et al. Histological features of ocular adnexal lymphoma (REAL classification) and their association with patient morbidity and survival. *Br J Ophthalmol*. 2000;84:907–913.

Johnson TE, Tse DT, Byrne GE Jr, et al. Ocular-adnexal lymphoid tumors: a clinicopathologic and molecular genetic study of 77 patients. *Ophthal Plast Reconstr Surg*. 1999;15:171–179.

Kennerdell JS, Flores NE, Hartsock RJ. Low-dose radiotherapy for lymphoid lesions of the orbit and ocular adnexa. *Ophthal Plast Reconstr Surg*. 1999;15:129–133.

Margo CE, Mulla ZD. Malignant tumors of the orbit: analysis of the Florida Cancer Registry. *Ophthalmology*. 1998;105:185–190.

White WL, Ferry JA. Ocular adnexal lymphoma: a clinicopathologic study with identification of lymphomas of mucosa-associated lymphoid tissue type. *Ophthalmology*. 1995;102:1994–2006.

Plasma Cell Tumors

Lesions composed predominantly of mature plasma cells may be plasmacytomas or localized plasma cell–rich pseudotumors. However, multiple myeloma should be ruled out, particularly if there is bone destruction or any immaturity or mitotic activity among the plasmacytic elements. Some lesions are composed of lymphocytes and lymphoplasmacytoid cells that combine properties of both lymphocytes and plasma cells. Plasma cell tumors display the same spectrum of clinical involvement as do lymphoproliferative lesions but are much less common.

Histiocytic Disorders

Langerhans cell histiocytosis, formerly known as *histiocytosis X,* is a rare collection of disorders of the mononuclear phagocytic system. These disorders are now thought to result from abnormal immune regulation, and the basic disease in all subtypes is characterized by an accumulation of proliferating dendritic histiocytes in various tissues. The disease occurs most commonly in children, with a peak incidence between 5 and 10 years of age, and runs a gamut of severity from benign lesions with spontaneous resolution to chronic dissemination resulting in death. The older names representing the various manifestations of histiocytic disorders (*eosinophilic granuloma of bone, Hand-Schüller-Christian syndrome,* and *Letterer-Siwe disease*) are being displaced by the terms *unifocal* and *multifocal eosinophilic granuloma of bone,* and *diffuse soft tissue histiocytosis.*

The most frequent presentation in the orbit is a lytic defect usually affecting the orbital roof or sphenoid wing and causing progressive proptosis. Younger children more often present with significant overlying soft tissue inflammation; they are also more likely to have evidence of multifocal or systemic involvement. Even if the initial workup shows no evidence of systemic dissemination, younger patients require regular observation to detect subsequent multiorgan involvement.

Histiocytic disorders have a reported survival rate of only 50% in patients presenting under 2 years of age; if the disease develops after age 2, the survival rate rises to 87%. Treatment of localized orbital disease consists of confirmatory biopsy with debulking, which may be followed by intralesional steroid injection or low-dose radiation therapy. Spontaneous remission has also been reported. Although destruction of the orbital bone may be extensive at the time of presentation, the bone usually reossifies completely.

> Goodman DF, Gottsch JD, Whitmore SE. Eyelid manifestations of metabolic and storage diseases. *Ophthalmol Clin North Am.* 1992;5:361–371.
> Kramer TR, Noecker RJ, Miller JM, et al. Langerhans cell histiocytosis with orbital involvement. *Am J Ophthalmol.* 1997;124:814–824.
> Trocme SD, Baker RH, Bartley GB, et al. Extracellular deposition of eosinophil major basic protein in orbital histiocytosis X. *Ophthalmology.* 1991;98:353–356.

Juvenile Xanthogranuloma

Juvenile xanthogranuloma (or nevoxanthoendothelioma) is a benign condition that rarely involves the orbit. This disease, which develops in infants under the age of 2 years, is characterized by a histiocytic proliferation that is usually found in the skin and may involve the iris. Juvenile xanthogranuloma may cause spontaneous anterior chamber hemorrhages and secondary glaucoma with acute pain and photophobia. The condition usually regresses spontaneously by the age of 5; however, if ocular involvement warrants treatment, topical corticosteroids and IOP-lowering agents are generally sufficient.

Lacrimal Gland Tumors

Clinically, a significant number of lacrimal gland masses represent idiopathic inflammation (dacryoadenitis variant of orbital pseudotumor). They present with acute inflammatory signs and usually respond to anti-inflammatory medication and thus do not require surgical intervention and biopsy (see Chapter 4 under the heading of Idiopathic Orbital Inflammation [Orbital Inflammatory Syndrome, Orbital Pseudotumor]). Of those lacrimal gland tumefactions not presenting with inflammatory signs and symptoms, the majority represent lymphoproliferative disorders (discussed above): fully 50% of orbital lymphomas develop in the lacrimal fossa. Only a minority of lacrimal fossa lesions are epithelial neoplasms of the lacrimal gland. CT is helpful in evaluating lesions in the lacrimal gland region. CT contour analysis can be used to differentiate inflammatory conditions and lymphoid proliferations from frank lacrimal gland neoplasms. Inflammatory and lymphoid proliferations within the lacrimal gland tend to cause it to expand diffusely and appear elongated, whereas epithelial neoplasms appear as isolated globular masses. Inflammatory and lymphoproliferative lesions usually contour around the globe, whereas epithelial neoplasms tend to displace and indent it.

Epithelial Tumors of the Lacrimal Gland

Approximately 50% of epithelial tumors are benign mixed tumors (pleomorphic adenomas) and about 50% are carcinomas. Approximately half of the carcinomas are adenoid cystic tumors, and the remainder are composed of malignant mixed tumors, primary adenocarcinomas, mucoepidermoid carcinomas, and squamous carcinomas.

Pleomorphic adenoma (benign mixed tumor)

Shown in Figure 5-17, pleomorphic adenoma is the most common epithelial tumor of the lacrimal gland. This tumor usually occurs in adults during the fourth and fifth decades of life and affects slightly more males than females. Patients present with a progressive painless downward and inward displacement of the globe with axial proptosis. Symptoms are usually present for more than 12 months.

A firm lobular mass may be palpated near the superior lateral orbital rim, and orbital imaging often reveals enlargement or expansion of the lacrimal fossa. On CT, the lesion appears well-circumscribed but may have a slightly nodular configuration.

Microscopically, benign mixed tumors have a varied cellular structure consisting primarily of a proliferation of benign epithelial cells and a stroma composed of spindle-shaped cells with occasional cartilaginous, mucinous, or even osteoid degeneration or metaplasia. This variability accounts for the designation *mixed tumor*. The lesion is circumscribed by a pseudocapsule.

90 • Orbit, Eyelids, and Lacrimal System

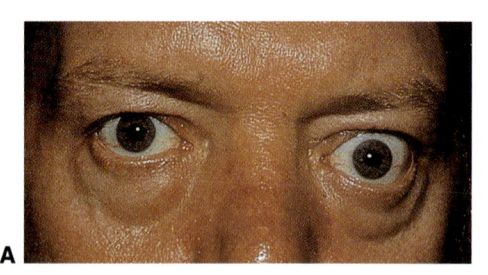

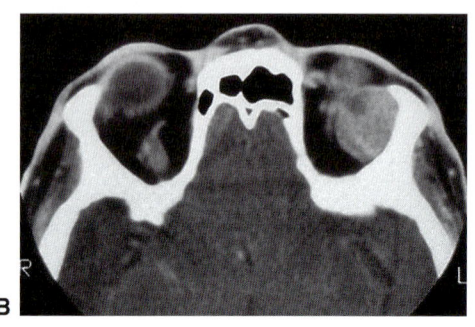

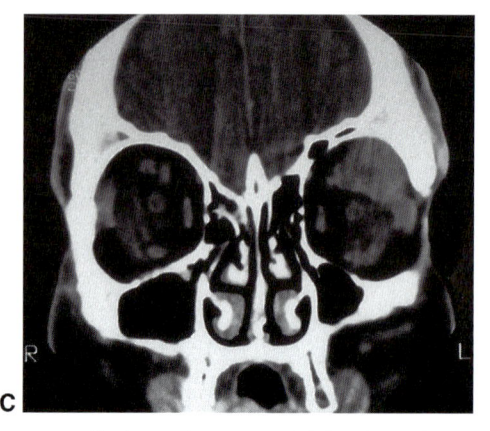

Figure 5-17 A, Proptosis and downward displacement of left eye in a man with benign mixed tumor of lacrimal gland. **B,** Axial CT scan showing rounded tumor in lacrimal fossa. No bony molding is present in this case. **C,** Coronal CT scan showing rounded mass in lacrimal gland consistent with benign mixed tumor. *(Photographs courtesy of Robert C. Kersten, MD.)*

Management Treatment should consist of complete removal of the tumor with its pseudocapsule and a surrounding margin of orbital tissue. Because of microscopic nodular extensions into the pseudocapsule, the lesion tends to recur if an insufficient margin of orbital tissue is removed. Surgery should be performed without a preliminary biopsy: when the capsule of the pleomorphic adenoma is incised for direct biopsy, the recurrence rate is 32%. These recurrences carry a significant risk of malignant degeneration. Analysis of the clinical presentation of the lesion and its CT contour helps the surgeon determine whether the lesion is likely to be a benign mixed tumor, in which case lateral orbitotomy is required for complete excision as the initial approach.

> Rose GE, Wright JE. Pleomorphic adenoma of the lacrimal gland. *Br J Ophthalmol.* 1992; 76:395–400.

Malignant mixed tumors

These lesions are histologically similar to benign mixed tumors but have areas of malignant change, usually poorly differentiated adenocarcinomas. They typically arise from long-standing primary benign mixed tumors or from a benign mixed tumor that has recurred following initial incomplete excision or violation of the pseudocapsule (see above). Radical orbitectomy with bone removal and exenteration has been performed, but long-term survival is poor.

Adenoid cystic carcinoma

Also known as *cylindroma*, adenoid cystic carcinoma is the most common malignant tumor of the lacrimal gland. This highly malignant tumor may cause pain because of perineural invasion and bone destruction. The relatively rapid course, with a history of generally less than 1 year, and early onset of pain help to differentiate this malignant tumor from benign mixed tumor, which tends to show progressive proptosis for more than a year and is painless. The tumor usually extends into the posterior orbit because of its capacity to infiltrate and its lack of true encapsulation.

Microscopically, this tumor is composed of disarmingly benign-appearing cells that grow in tubules, solid nests, or a cribriform Swiss-cheese pattern. The basaloid morphology is associated with worse survival than the cribriform variant. Infiltration of the orbital tissues, including perineural invasion, is common in microscopic sections.

Management of malignant lacrimal gland tumors

Suspicion of a malignant lacrimal gland tumor warrants percutaneous biopsy with permanent section confirmation. Exenteration and radical orbitectomy with removal of the roof, lateral wall, and floor along with the overlying soft tissues and anterior portion of the temporalis muscle has failed to demonstrate convincing improvement in long-term survival rates. High-dose radiation therapy in conjunction with surgical debulking may be offered as an alternative. Intracarotid chemotherapy has also been advocated, as has brachytherapy to the lacrimal fossa. Despite these measures, perineural extension into the cavernous sinus often occurs, and the typical clinical course is that of multiple painful recurrences with ultimate mortality from intracranial extension or systemic metastases, usually occurring a decade or more after the initial presentation.

> Bartley GB, Harris GJ. Adenoid cystic carcinoma of the lacrimal gland: is there a cure . . . yet? *Ophthal Plast Reconstr Surg.* 2002;18:315–318.
> Font RF, Smith SL, Bryan RG. Malignant epithelial tumors of the lacrimal gland. *Arch Ophthalmol.* 1998;116:613–616.
> Tellado MV, McLean IW, Specht CS, et al. Adenoid cystic carcinomas of the lacrimal gland in childhood and adolescence. *Ophthalmology.* 1997;104:1622–1625.
> Wright JE, Rose GE, Garner A. Primary malignant neoplasms of the lacrimal gland. *Br J Ophthalmol.* 1992;76:401–407.

Nonepithelial Tumors of the Lacrimal Gland

Most of the nonepithelial lesions of the lacrimal gland represent lymphoid proliferation or inflammations. Fully 50% of orbital lymphoproliferative lesions occur in the lacrimal gland. Inflammatory conditions such as idiopathic orbital inflammatory syndrome and sarcoidosis are covered in Chapter 4. Lymphoepithelial lesions may also occur either in Sjögren syndrome or as a localized lacrimal gland and salivary gland lesion (the so-called *Mikulicz syndrome*).

Lymphocytic infiltrates may be seen in middle-aged patients, particularly females, who develop bilateral swellings of the lacrimal gland, producing a dry eye syndrome. This condition can occur insidiously or following a symptomatic episode of lacrimal gland inflammation. The enlargement of the lacrimal glands may not be clinically apparent. Biopsy specimens of the affected glands show a spectrum of lymphocytic infiltrates, from scattered patches of lymphocytes to lymphocytic replacement of the lacrimal gland parenchyma with the survival of the inner duct cells surrounded by proliferating myoepithelial cells *(epimyoepithelial islands)*. This latter combination of lymphocytes and epimyoepithelial islands has led some authors to designate this manifestation as a lymphoepithelial lesion. Some patients with lymphocytic infiltrates may also have systemic rheumatoid arthritis and, therefore, have classic Sjögren syndrome. These lesions may develop into low-grade B-cell lymphoma (see earlier discussion of lymphoproliferative disorders).

Secondary Orbital Tumors

Secondary orbital tumors are those that extend into the orbit from contiguous structures, such as globe, eyelids, sinuses, or brain.

Globe and Eyelid Origin

Tumors and inflammations can spread into the orbit from within the eye (especially from choroidal melanomas and retinoblastomas) or from the eyelid (eg, sebaceous gland carcinoma, squamous cell carcinoma, and basal cell carcinoma). Primary eyelid tumors are discussed in Chapter 11. Retinoblastoma, choroidal melanoma, and other ocular neoplasms are covered in BCSC Section 4, *Ophthalmic Pathology and Intraocular Tumors;* and Section 6, *Pediatric Ophthalmology and Strabismus.*

Sinus Origin

Most tumors that secondarily involve the orbit arise from the nose or the paranasal sinuses (Fig 5-18). Proptosis and globe displacement are common, and the diagnosis is usually readily apparent on orbital CT or MRI. Imaging must be carried to the base of the sinuses for the proper evaluation of these lesions.

The sinuses are the most common sites of extraorbital disease that extends to displace the eye and cause proptosis. *Mucoceles* and *mucopyoceles* of the sinuses (Fig 5-19) are

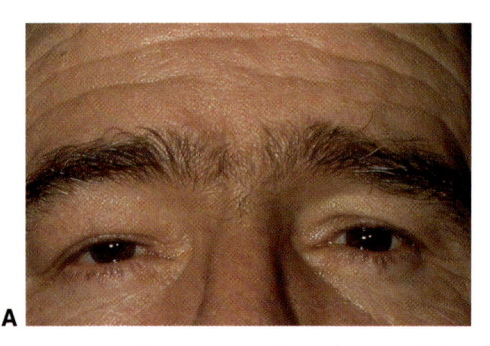

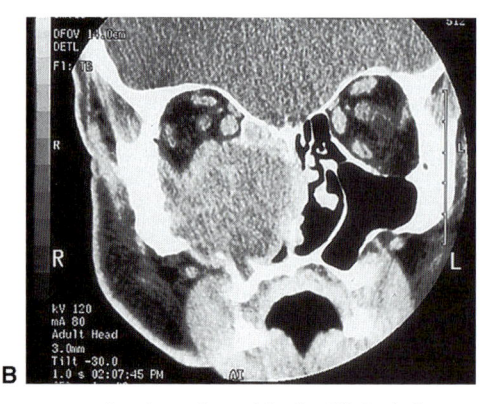

Figure 5-18 Squamous cell carcinoma of the sinus extending into the orbit. **A,** Clinical photo; note minimal proptosis despite large tumor of the sinus extending into the orbit. **B,** CT scan; sinus cancers typically do not show early clinical signs, usually presenting after the tumor has grown to a large size. *(Photographs courtesy of Jeffrey Nerad, MD.)*

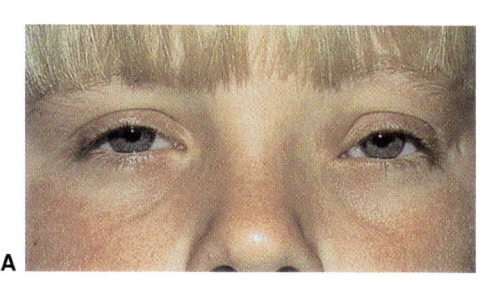

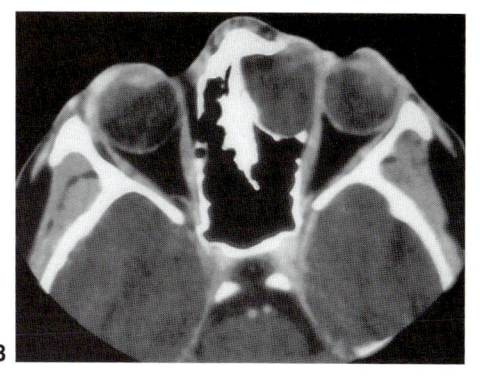

Figure 5-19 A, Fullness of superonasal left upper eyelid and lateral displacement of left medial canthal tendon in a boy with ethmoidal mucocele. **B,** CT scan demonstrating anterior ethmoidal mucocele pushing eye and medial canthal tendon laterally. *(Photographs courtesy of Robert C. Kersten, MD.)*

cystic structures with pseudostratified ciliated columnar (respiratory) epithelium. Resulting from obstruction of the sinus excretory ducts, they frequently invade the orbit by expansion and erosion of the bones of the orbital walls. The cysts are usually filled with thick mucoid secretions. If infected and filled with pus, the lesion is called a *pyocele*. Most mucoceles arise from the frontal or ethmoid sinuses. Preoperative diagnosis can usually be established by characteristic findings on orbital imaging. Surgical treatment includes evacuation of the mucocele and reestablishment of drainage of the affected sinus or obliteration of the sinus by mucosal stripping and packing with bone or fat.

Squamous cell carcinoma is the most common epithelial tumor secondarily invading the orbit. Malignancies usually arise within the maxillary sinuses, followed by the nasopharynx or the oropharynx. Nasal obstruction, epistaxis, or epiphora may be associated with the growth of such tumors. Treatment is usually a combination of surgical excision and radiation therapy and often includes exenteration if the periorbita is involved by tumor.

Nonepithelial tumors that can invade the orbit from the sinuses, nose, and facial bones include a wide variety of benign and malignant lesions. Among the most common of these are *osteomas, fibrous dysplasia,* and miscellaneous *sarcomas*.

Johnson LN, Krohel GB, Yeon EB, et al. Sinus tumors invading the orbit. *Ophthalmology.* 1984;91:209–217.

Brain Origin

Meningiomas may extend from within the intracranial cavity to the orbit (see the discussion of neural tumors earlier in this chapter). They often arise from the sphenoid wing and may compress the optic nerve or supraorbital fissure. They occur more often in women. Presentation is usually with chronic proptosis, motility disturbance, and visual loss; rarely, eyelid edema or erythema may be present. Treatment consists of neurosurgical and orbital excision or debulking in combination with postoperative radiation therapy.

Metastatic Tumors

Metastatic Tumors in Children

In children, distant tumors metastasize to the orbit more frequently than to the globe (in contrast to adults, who more frequently have metastases to the choroid).

Neuroblastoma

Metastatic orbital neuroblastoma typically produces an abrupt ecchymotic proptosis that may be bilateral. A deposition of blood in the lower eyelid may lead to the mistaken impression of injury. Commonly, bone destruction is apparent, particularly in the lateral orbital wall. Metastases typically occur late in the course of the disease, when the primary tumor can be detected readily in the abdomen, mediastinum, or neck. Congenital neuroblastoma of the cervical ganglia may produce an ipsilateral Horner syndrome with heterochromia (Fig 5-20).

> Miller NR, ed. *Walsh and Hoyt's Neuro-Ophthalmology.* 4th ed. Baltimore: Williams & Wilkins; 1988;3:1296–1300.

Leukemia

In advanced stages, leukemia may produce unilateral or bilateral proptosis. *Acute lymphoblastic leukemia* is the type of leukemia most likely to metastasize to the orbit. A primary leukemic orbital mass, called *granulocytic sarcoma*, or *chloroma*, is a rare variant of myelogenous leukemia. Typically, orbital lesions present in advance of blood or bone

Figure 5-20 A, Infant with left ptosis and miotic left pupil. **B,** Neck CT of infant showing neck mass causing Horner syndrome. At surgery, the mass was found to be a neuroblastoma. *(Photographs courtesy of John B. Holds, MD.)*

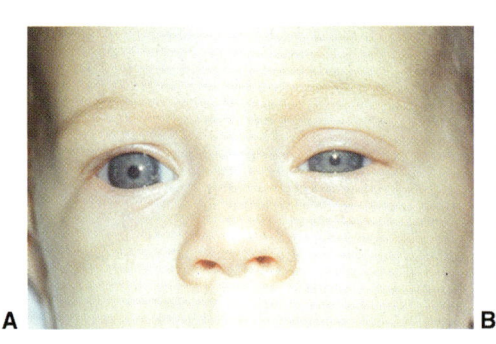

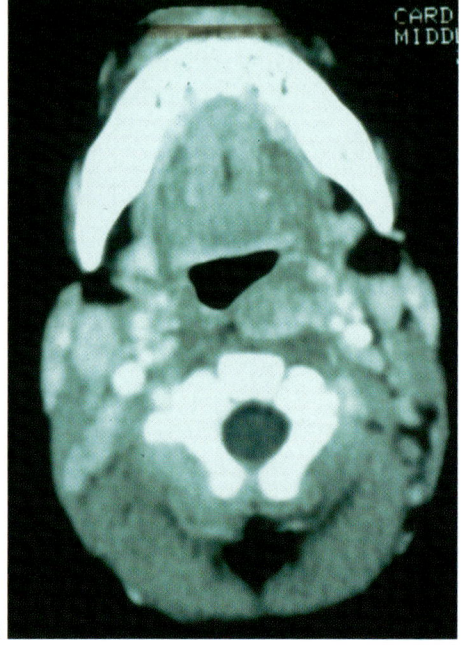

marrow signs of leukemia, which almost invariably follow within several months. Special stains for cytoplasmic esterase in the cells (Leder stain) indicate that these are granulocytic precursor cells. Chances for survival are enhanced if chemotherapy is instituted prior to the discovery of leukemic involvement in bone marrow or peripheral blood.

Stockl FA, Dolmetsch AM, Saornil MA, et al. Orbital granulocytic sarcoma. *Br J Ophthalmol.* 1997;81:1084–1088.

Metastatic Tumors in Adults

Although virtually any carcinoma of the internal organs and cutaneous malignant melanoma can metastasize to the orbit (Figs 5-21, 5-22), breast and lung tumors account for the majority of orbital metastases. The occurrence of pain, proptosis, inflammation, bone destruction, and early ophthalmoplegia suggests the possibility of metastatic carcinoma.

Some 75% of patients have a history of a known primary tumor, but in 25% the orbital metastasis may be the presenting sign. The extraocular muscles are frequently involved because of their abundant blood supply. Elevation of serum carcinoembryonic

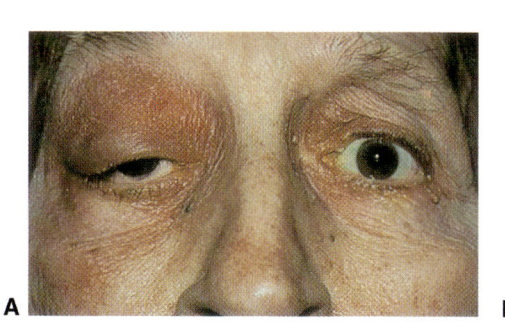

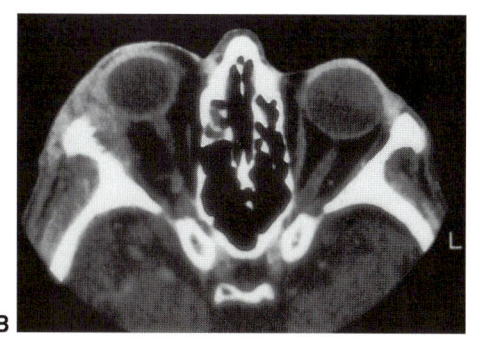

Figure 5-21 A, Right upper eyelid ptosis, superior orbital mass, and eyelid inflammation in an elderly man with prostate carcinoma. **B,** CT scan showing superotemporal orbital mass with adjacent bony changes proven by biopsy to be metastatic prostate cancer. *(Photographs courtesy of Robert C. Kersten, MD.)*

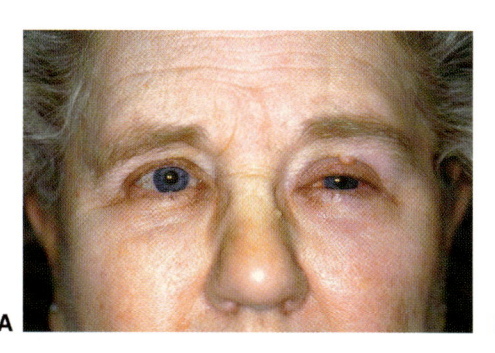

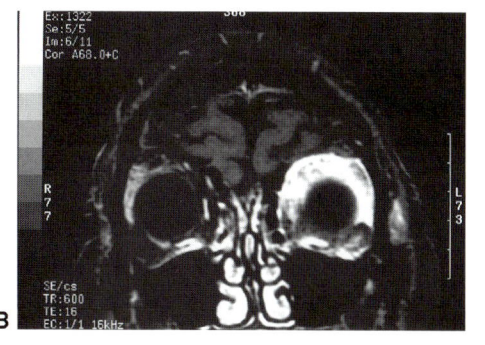

Figure 5-22 A, Woman with enophthalmos and motility restriction secondary to metastatic breast carcinoma to the orbit. **B,** CT scan. *(Photographs courtesy of John B. Holds, MD.)*

antigen levels may suggest a metastatic process. Fine-needle aspiration biopsy can be performed in the office and may obviate the need for orbitotomy and open biopsy.

Breast carcinoma

The most common primary source of orbital metastases in women is breast cancer. Metastases may occur many years after the breast has been removed; thus, a history should always include inquiries about previous cancer surgery. Rarely, breast metastases to the orbit may elicit a fibrous response that causes enophthalmos and possibly restriction of ocular motility (see Fig 5-22).

Some patients with breast cancer respond favorably to hormonal therapy. This response usually correlates with the presence of estrogen and other hormone receptors found in the tumor tissue. If metastatic breast cancer is found at the time of orbital exploration, fresh tissue should be submitted for estrogen-receptor assay even if this test was previously performed because estrogen-receptor content may vary between the primary and the metastatic lesion. Hormone therapy is most likely to help patients whose tumors are receptor-positive.

Bronchogenic carcinoma

The most frequent source of orbital metastasis in men is bronchogenic carcinoma. The primary lesion may be quite small, and CT of suspicious lung lesions may be performed in patients suspected of having orbital metastases.

Prostatic carcinoma

Metastatic prostatic carcinoma can produce a clinical picture resembling that of acute pseudotumor.

Management of Orbital Metastases

The treatment of metastatic tumors of the orbit is usually palliative, consisting of local radiation therapy. Some metastatic tumors, such as carcinoids and renal cell carcinomas, may be candidates for wide excision of the orbital lesion because some patients may survive for many years following resection of isolated metastases from these primary tumors. Consultation with the patient's oncologist should identify candidates who might benefit from wide excision.

> Char DH, Miller T, Kroll S. Orbital metastases: diagnosis and course. *Br J Ophthalmol.* 1997;81:386–390.
>
> Henderson JW, Campbell RJ, Farrow GM, et al. *Orbital Tumors.* 3rd ed. New York: Raven; 1994.
>
> Rootman J, ed. *Diseases of the Orbit: a Multidisciplinary Approach.* Philadelphia: Lippincott; 1988.

CHAPTER 6

Orbital Trauma

Orbital trauma can damage both the facial bones and adjacent soft tissues. Fractures may be associated with injuries to orbital contents, intracranial structures, and paranasal sinuses. Orbital hemorrhage and embedded foreign bodies may also be present and have secondary effects upon the orbital soft tissues. Decreased visual acuity, intraocular injuries, strabismus, and ptosis may occur.

Because of the high incidence of concomitant intraocular injury, an ocular examination must always be performed on patients who have sustained orbital trauma. Ocular damage accompanying orbital trauma may include hyphema, angle recession, corneoscleral laceration, retinal tear, retinal dialysis, and vitreous hemorrhage.

Midfacial (Le Fort) Fractures

Le Fort fractures involve the maxilla and are often complex and asymmetric (Figs 6-1, 6-2). By definition, Le Fort fractures must extend posteriorly through the pterygoid plates. Treatment may include dental stabilization with arch bars and open reduction with rigid fixation using mini- and microplating systems. These fractures may be divided into three categories, although clinically they often do not conform precisely to these groupings.

- *Le Fort I* is a low transverse maxillary fracture above the teeth with no orbital involvement.
- *Le Fort II* fractures generally have a pyramidal configuration and involve the nasal, lacrimal, and maxillary bones as well as the medial orbital floor.
- *Le Fort III* fractures cause craniofacial disjunction in which the entire facial skeleton may be completely detached from the base of the skull and suspended only by soft tissues. The orbital floor and medial and lateral orbital walls are involved.

Orbital Fractures

Zygomatic Fractures

Zygomatic-maxillary complex fractures are called *tripod fractures* (Fig 6-3), although the zygoma is usually fractured at four of its articulations with the adjacent bones (lateral orbital rim, inferior orbital rim, zygomatic arch, and lateral wall of the maxillary sinus).

98 • Orbit, Eyelids, and Lacrimal System

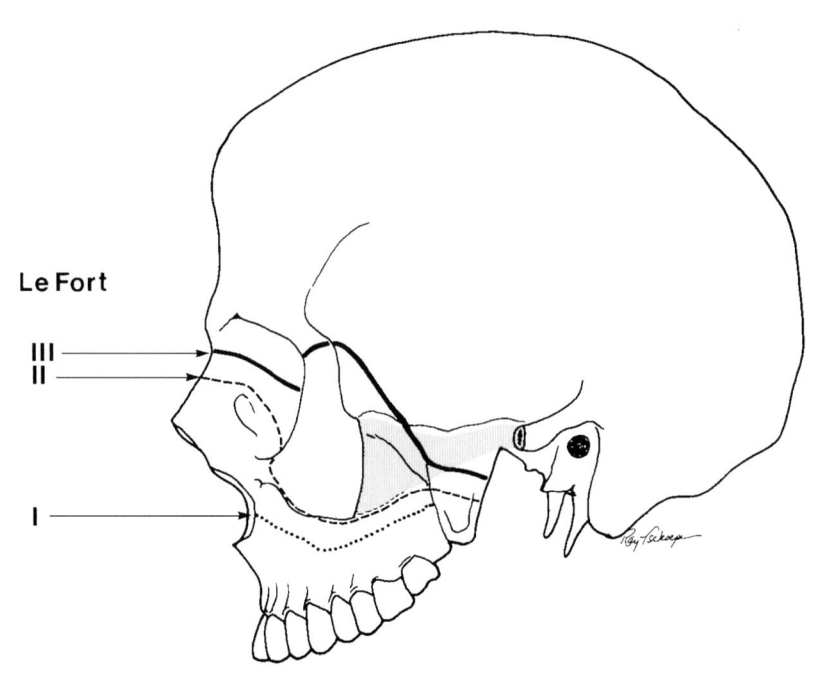

Figure 6-1 Le Fort fractures (lateral view). Note that all the fractures extend posteriorly through the pterygoid plates. *(After Converse JM, ed.* Reconstructive Plastic Surgery. *Philadelphia: Saunders; 1977:2.)*

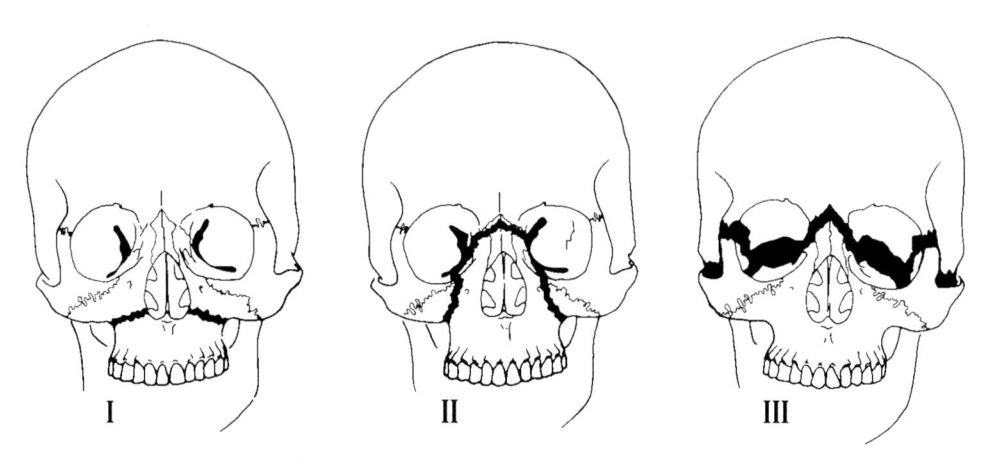

Figure 6-2 Le Fort's classification of midfacial fractures. Le Fort I, horizontal fracture of the maxilla, also known as Guerin fracture. Le Fort II, pyramidal fracture of the maxilla. Le Fort III, craniofacial disjunction. *(After Converse JM, ed.* Reconstructive Plastic Surgery. *Philadelphia: Saunders; 1977:2.)*

The zygomatic-maxillary complex fracture involves the orbital floor to varying degrees, but fractures of the zygomatic arch can occur without causing orbital damage. If the zygoma is not significantly displaced, no treatment is necessary. Displacement of the zygoma can cause cosmetic deformity, and impingement on the coronoid process of the mandible can cause pain and difficulty in opening the mouth.

CHAPTER 6: Orbital Trauma • 99

Figure 6-3 A, Zygomatic fracture (anterior view). Downward displacement of the globe and lateral canthus as a result of frontozygomatic separation and downward displacement of the zygoma and the floor of the orbit. **B,** Globe ptosis and lateral canthal dystopia due to widely displaced zygomaticomaxillary complex (ZMC) fracture. **C,** Three-dimensional CT scan of a ZMC fracture. Note the displaced zygoma and an additional fracture of the medial buttress. *(Part A after Converse JM, ed.* Reconstructive Plastic Surgery. *Philadelphia: Saunders; 1977:2; Parts B and C reproduced with permission from Nerad JA.* The Requisites in Ophthalmology: Oculoplastic Surgery. *Philadelphia: Mosby; 2001:340.)*

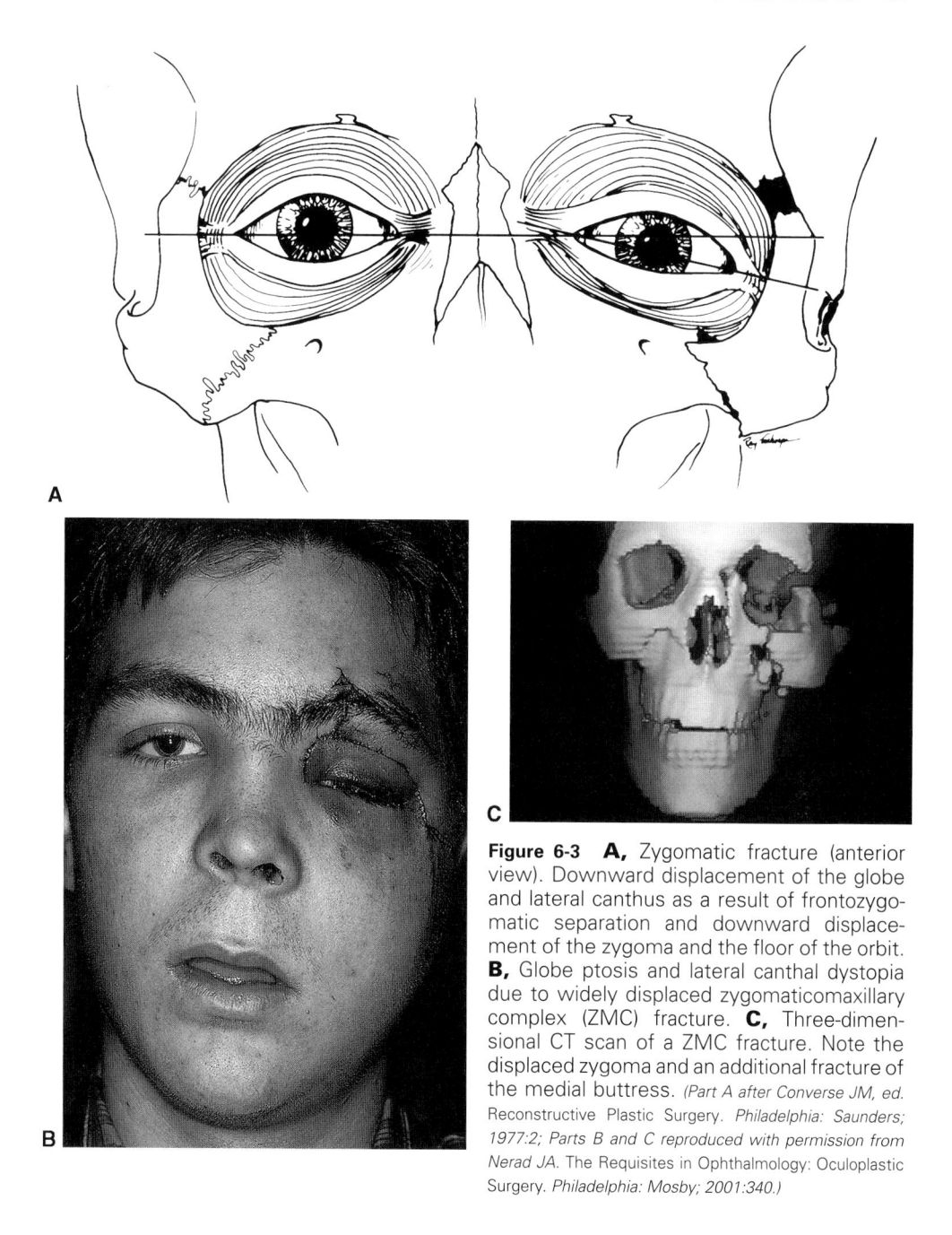

When treatment is indicated, the best results are obtained with open reduction of the fracture and fixation with miniature metal plates that are attached with bone screws. Exact realignment and stabilization of the maxillary buttress is key for accurate fracture reduction and can be achieved through a buccal sulcus incision. With this approach, it is not necessary to routinely explore the orbital floor unless it is significantly disrupted or the extraocular muscles are entrapped.

> Hartzell KN, Botek AA, Goldberg SH. Orbital fractures in women due to sexual assault and domestic violence. *Ophthalmology*. 1996;103:953–957.
>
> Iizuka T, Thoren H, Annino DJ, et al. Midfacial fractures in pediatric patients. *Arch Otolaryngol Head Neck Surg*. 1995;121:1366–1371.
>
> Shumrick KA, Kersten RC, Kulwin DR, et al. Criteria for selective management of the orbital rim and floor in zygomatic complex and midface fractures. *Arch Otolaryngol Head Neck Surg*. 1997;123:378–384.
>
> Shumrick KA, Kersten RC, Kulwin DR, et al. Extended access/internal approaches for the management of facial trauma. *Arch Otolaryngol Head Neck Surg*. 1992;118:1105–1112.

Orbital Apex Fractures

Orbital apex fractures usually occur in association with other fractures of the face, orbit, or skull and may involve the optic canal, superior orbital fissure, and structures that pass through them. Possible associated complications include damage to the optic nerves with decreased visual acuity, cerebrospinal fluid leaks, and carotid cavernous sinus fistulas. Indirect traumatic optic neuropathy usually results from stretching, tearing, twisting, or bruising of the fixed canalicular portion of the nerve as the cranial skeleton suffers sudden deceleration. Thin-section CT through the orbital apex and anterior clinoid processes demonstrates fractures at or adjacent to the optic canal in the large majority of patients. The management of neurogenic visual loss after blunt head trauma is discussed at the end of this chapter.

Orbital Roof Fractures

Orbital roof fractures are usually caused by blunt trauma or missile injuries and are more common in young children who have not yet pneumatized the frontal sinus. The brain and cribriform plate may be involved. Frontal trauma in older patients tends to be absorbed by the frontal sinus, which acts as a crumple zone, preventing extension along the orbital roof. Complications include intracranial injuries, cerebrospinal fluid rhinorrhea, pneumocephalus, subperiosteal hematoma, ptosis, and extraocular muscle imbalance. The entrapment of extraocular muscles is extremely rare, but development of a subperiosteal hematoma and secondary mass effect impinging on the superior rectus is not uncommon. In severely comminuted fractures, pulsating exophthalmos may occur as a delayed complication. Young children may develop nondisplaced linear roof fractures after fairly minor trauma, which may present with delayed ecchymosis of the upper eyelid. Most roof fractures do not require repair. Indications for surgery are generally neurosurgical, and treatment involves a team approach with a neurosurgeon and an orbital surgeon.

> Greenwald MJ, Boston D, Pensler JM, et al. Orbital roof fractures in childhood. *Ophthalmology*. 1989;96:491–496.

Medial Orbital Fractures

Direct (naso-orbital-ethmoidal) fractures (Fig 6-4) usually result from the face striking solid surfaces. These fractures commonly involve the frontal process of the maxilla, the lacrimal bone, and the ethmoid bones along the medial wall of the orbit. Patients characteristically have a depressed bridge of the nose and traumatic telecanthus. Complications include cerebral and ocular damage, severe epistaxis due to severance of the anterior ethmoidal artery by bone fragments, orbital hematoma, cerebrospinal fluid rhinorrhea, damage to the lacrimal drainage system, lateral displacement of the medial canthus, and associated fractures of the medial orbital wall and floor. Treatment includes repair of the nasal fracture and miniplate stabilization. Transnasal wiring of the medial canthus is less often required now that adequate bony reduction with miniplate fixation is often possible.

Indirect (blowout) fractures are frequently extensions of blowout fractures of the orbital floor. Isolated blowout fractures of the medial orbital wall also may occur. Surgical intervention is seldom necessary unless the medial rectus muscle or its associated tissues are entrapped. Significant enophthalmos is relatively rare after isolated medial wall blowouts. Emphysema of the eyelids and orbit is commonly associated with fractures of the medial orbital wall. (Fractures of the sinuses may allow air to enter the subcutaneous tissues, and this air may be seen on radiographs.)

Large, isolated medial wall fractures may result in cosmetically noticeable enophthalmos, but enophthalmos occurs less often in this setting than with isolated floor frac-

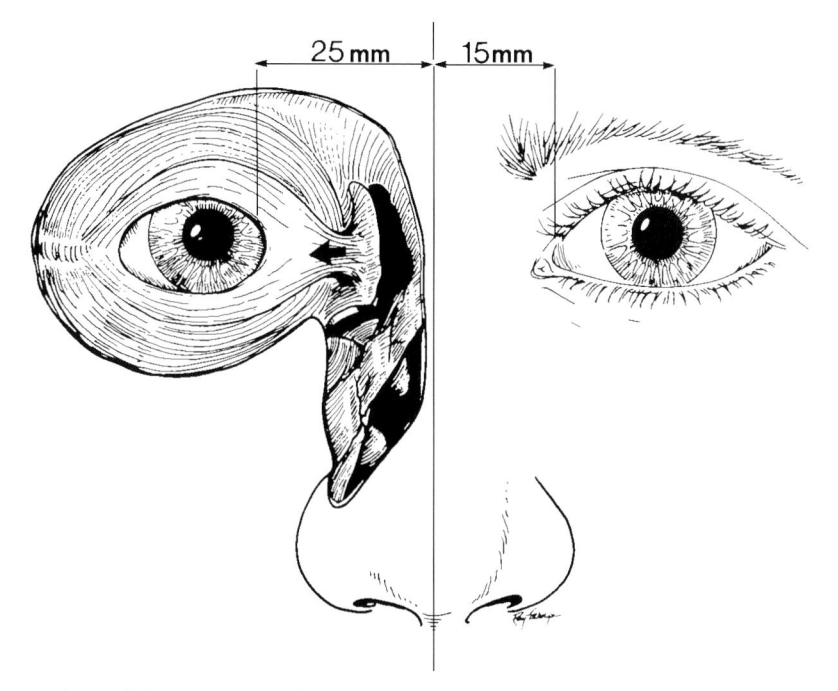

Figure 6-4 Lateral displacement of the medial orbital wall results in traumatic telecanthus and rounding of the medial canthus. *(After Beyer CK, Fabian FL, Smith B. Naso-orbital fractures, complications, and treatment.* Ophthalmology. *1982;89:458.)*

tures. The risk of enophthalmos is greatest when both the floor and the medial wall are fractured and displaced.

If surgery is required, the medial orbital wall may be approached by continuing the exploration of the floor up along the medial wall via the eyelid or transconjunctival approach. An alternative approach is a medial orbital incision through the skin or caruncle.

> Nolasco FP, Mathog RH. Medial orbital wall fractures: classification and clinical profile. *Otolaryngol Head Neck Surg.* 1995;112:49–56.

Orbital Floor Fractures

Direct fractures of the orbital floor can extend from fractures of the inferior orbital rim. Indications for repair of the orbital floor in these cases are the same as for indirect (blowout) fractures. Indirect fractures of the orbital floor are not associated with fracture of the inferior orbital rim.

Past theory held that blowout fractures resulted from a sudden increase in intraorbital pressure resulting from the application of force by a nonpenetrating object, usually smaller in diameter than the orbital entrance. According to this theory, the contents of the orbit are compressed posteriorly toward the apex of the orbit and the orbital bones break at their weakest point, usually the posterior medial part of the floor in the maxillary bone. The orbital contents may be entrapped or may prolapse through the fracture into the maxillary sinus. A more recent theory, however, is that the striking object causes a compressive force at the inferior rim, which leads directly to buckling of the orbital floor. The degree of increased orbital pressure determines whether or not orbital tissues are pushed down through the fracture into the maxillary antrum.

> Kersten RC. Blowout fracture of the orbital floor with entrapment caused by isolated trauma to the orbital rim. *Am J Ophthalmol.* 1987;103:215–219.
>
> Whitehouse RW, Batterbury M, Jackson A, et al. Prediction of enophthalmos by computed tomography after 'blow out' orbital fracture. *Br J Ophthalmol.* 1994;78:618–620.

Blowout fractures of the orbital floor are suggested by the patient's history, physical examination, and radiographs (Fig 6-5). There is a history of the orbital entrance being struck by an object, usually one larger than the diameter of the orbital opening (eg, a ball, an automobile dashboard, or a fist). An orbital blowout fracture should be suspected in any patient who has received a periorbital blow forceful enough to cause ecchymosis. Physical examination typically reveals the following:

- *Eyelid signs.* Ecchymosis and edema of the eyelids may be seen, but external signs of injury can be absent.
- *Diplopia with limitation on upgaze, downgaze, or both.* Limited vertical movement of the globe, vertical diplopia, and pain in the inferior orbit on attempted vertical movement of the globe are consistent with entrapment of the inferior rectus muscle or its adjacent septa in the fracture. Orbital edema and hemorrhage or damage to the extraocular muscles or their innervation can also limit movement of the globe. A significant limitation of both horizontal and vertical eye movements should alert the examiner to the likelihood of nerve damage or of generalized soft tissue injury. Limitations of globe movements caused by hemorrhage or edema generally im-

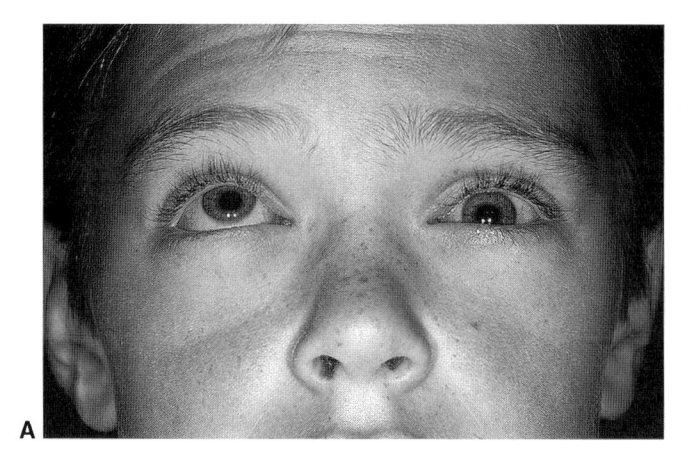

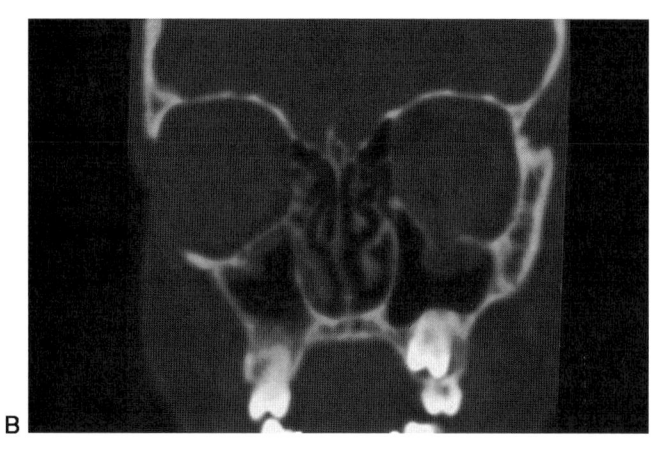

Figure 6-5 Decreased motility after a blowout fracture. **A,** Limited elevation of the eye after a blowout fracture. **B,** CT scan demonstrating an orbital floor fracture with prolapse of the intraorbital contents into the maxillary sinus, resulting in ocular restriction. *(Reproduced with permission from Nerad JA. The Requisites in Ophthalmology: Oculoplastic Surgery. Philadelphia: Mosby; 2001:333.)*

prove during the first 1–2 weeks after injury. If entrapment is present, a traction test should show restriction of passive movement of the eye; however, restriction can also result from edema and hemorrhage. A vertical traction test, sometimes called a *forced duction test*, is performed most easily by instilling anesthetic eyedrops followed by a cotton pledget containing 4% cocaine solution applied in the inferior cul-de-sac for several minutes. The insertion of the inferior rectus muscle is grasped through the conjunctiva with a toothed forceps, and an attempt is made to rotate the globe gently up and down. Comparing the intraocular pressure as measured in primary position and in upgaze usually shows a significant increase in upgaze if the inferior rectus is entrapped. Comparing ductions and versions also helps differentiate paretic from entrapped extraocular muscles.

- *Enophthalmos and ptosis of the globe.* These findings occur with large fractures in which the orbital soft tissues prolapse into the maxillary sinus. A medial wall fracture, if associated with the orbital floor fracture, may significantly contribute to enophthalmos because of prolapse of the orbital tissues into both the ethmoid and the maxillary sinuses. Enophthalmos may be masked by orbital edema immediately following the injury, but enophthalmos becomes more apparent as the orbital edema subsides and contracture pulls the soft tissues farther into the sinus.

- *Hypoesthesia in the distribution of the infraorbital nerve.*
- *Emphysema of the orbit and eyelids.* Any fracture that extends into a sinus may allow air to escape into the subcutaneous tissues, but this occurs most commonly with medial wall fractures.

In patients with orbital floor fractures, vision loss can result from injury to the optic nerve or increased orbital pressure causing a *compartment syndrome* (see below under "Traumatic Visual Loss With Clear Media"). An orbital hemorrhage should be suspected if loss of vision is associated with proptosis and increased intraocular pressure. Injuries to the globe and ocular adnexa may also be present.

CT scans with coronal or sagittal views are usually indicated to help guide treatment. They allow evaluation of extraocular muscle entrapment and fracture size to predict anticipated enophthalmos.

The majority of blowout or other orbital floor fractures do not require surgical intervention. Orbital blowout fractures are usually observed for 7–10 days to allow swelling and orbital hemorrhage to subside. Oral steroids (1 mg/kg per day for the first 7 days) decrease edema and may also limit the risk of long-term diplopia from inferior rectus contracture and fibrosis.

An exception to initial observation occurs in pediatric patients, in whom the inferior rectus muscle may become tightly trapped beneath a trapdoor fracture. In these patients, vertical globe excursion is significantly limited and CT reveals the inferior rectus muscle within the maxillary sinus. Attempted ocular excursions may result in bradycardia due to stimulation of the oculocardiac reflex. Urgent repair should be undertaken. Release of the entrapped muscle without delay may limit ultimate restriction and fibrosis.

Egbert JE, May K, Kersten RC, et al. Pediatric orbital floor fracture—direct extraocular muscle involvement. *Ophthalmology.* 2000;107:1875–1879.

Jordan DR, Allen LH, White J, et al. Intervention within days for some orbital floor fractures: the white-eyed blowout. *Ophthal Plast Reconstr Surg.* 1998;14:379–390.

Although the indications for surgery are controversial, certain guidelines are helpful in determining when surgery is advisable:

- *Diplopia with limitation of upgaze and/or downgaze within 30° of the primary position with a positive traction test result 7–10 days after injury and with radiologic confirmation of a fracture of the orbital floor.* These findings indicate functional entrapment of tissues affecting the inferior rectus muscle. Diplopia may improve significantly over the course of the first 2 weeks as orbital edema, hemorrhage, or both resolve and as some of the entrapped tissues stretch. However, if the findings are still present after 2 weeks and if the entrapped tissues are not freed, vertical diplopia is likely to persist. As mentioned above, tight entrapment of the inferior rectus muscle with a frozen globe is an indication for immediate repair.
- *Enophthalmos exceeding 2 mm that is cosmetically unacceptable to the patient.* Enophthalmos is usually masked by orbital edema immediately after the trauma, and several weeks may pass before the extent of this problem is fully appreciated. Appropriate measurements must be taken at the initial evaluation and at subsequent visits. If significant enophthalmos is present within the first 2 weeks and

associated with a large orbital floor fracture, even greater enophthalmos can be anticipated in the future.
- *Large fractures involving at least half of the orbital floor, particularly when associated with large medial wall fractures (determined by CT).* Orbital fractures of this size have a high incidence of subsequent significant enophthalmos.

Gilbard SM, Mafee MF, Lagouros PA, et al. Orbital blowout fractures: the prognostic significance of computed tomography. *Ophthalmology.* 1985;92:1523–1528.

Harris GJ, Garcia GH, Logani SC, et al. Correlation of preoperative computed tomography and postoperative ocular motility in orbital blowout fractures. *Ophthal Plast Reconstr Surg.* 2000;16:179–187.

Hawes MJ, Dortzbach RK. Surgery on orbital floor fractures: influence of time of repair and fracture size. *Ophthalmology.* 1983;90:1066–1070.

Putterman AM, Stevens T, Urist MJ. Nonsurgical management of blowout fractures of the orbital floor. *Am J Ophthalmol.* 1974;77:232–239.

Rubin PAD, Bilyk JR, Shore JW. Management of orbital trauma: fractures, hemorrhage, and traumatic optic neuropathy. In: *Focal Points: Clinical Modules for Ophthalmologists.* San Francisco: American Academy of Ophthalmology; 1994: vol 12, no 7.

Management

When surgery is indicated for blowout fractures of the orbital floor, it generally is preferable to proceed with the repair within 2 weeks of the initial trauma. Scar tissue formation and contracture of the prolapsed tissue make later correction of entrapment and diplopia difficult. Patients (usually children) with frank extraocular muscle entrapment on CT have profoundly limited vertical excursions and should undergo immediate repair. Although larger fractures in which eventual enophthalmos is anticipated are also easier to fix within the first 2 weeks of surgery, satisfactory correction of enophthalmos can usually be obtained even if surgery is delayed.

The surgical approach to blowout fractures of the orbital floor can be made through an infraciliary or lower eyelid crease incision. Currently popular approaches through the eyelid to the floor include a conjunctival (inferior fornix) incision combined with a lateral cantholysis. The approaches through the lower eyelid have the following steps in common: elevation of the periorbita from the orbital floor, release of the prolapsed tissues from the fracture, and usually the placement of an implant over the fracture to prevent recurrent adhesions and prolapse of the orbital tissues.

The development of mini- and microplating systems and their various metallic orbital implants has significantly improved the management of large unstable orbital floor fractures. A number of synthetic materials can be used for floor support. Bone grafts are rarely indicated except in large unstable fractures, where they may be directly fixated to the infraorbital rim with miniscrews or miniplates.

Delayed treatment for blowout fractures to correct debilitating strabismus and diplopia or cosmetically unacceptable enophthalmos may include exploration of the orbital floor in an attempt to free the scarred tissues entrapped or prolapsed through the fracture and to replace them in the orbit. Other measures are strabismus surgery and procedures to camouflage the enophthalmos with its associated narrowed palpebral fissure and deep superior sulcus.

Complications of blowout fracture surgery include decreased visual acuity or blindness, diplopia, undercorrection or overcorrection of enophthalmos, lower eyelid retraction, infraorbital nerve hypoesthesia, infection, extrusion of the implant, lymphedema, and damage to the lacrimal pump.

Intraorbital Foreign Bodies

If foreign bodies within the orbit are radiopaque, they can be localized by plain-film radiographs or by CT or MRI. (Some wooden foreign bodies may be missed on CT and are seen better on MRI. However, MRI should be avoided if there is a possibility that the foreign object is ferromagnetic.) If an embedded foreign body causes an orbital infection that drains to the skin surface, it is sometimes possible to locate the object by surgically following the fistulous tract posteriorly. Treatment of orbital foreign bodies initially involves culturing the wound (or the foreign body if it is removed) and administering antibiotics. Foreign bodies should be removed if they are composed of vegetable matter or if they are easily accessible in the anterior orbit. In many cases, objects can be safely observed without surgery if they are inert and have smooth edges or are located in the posterior orbit. Specifically, BBs are common intraorbital foreign bodies and are usually best left in situ. MRI can be safely performed with a BB in the orbit.

> Finkelstein M, Legmann A, Rubin PAD. Projectile metallic foreign bodies in the orbit. *Ophthalmology*. 1997;104:96–103.
>
> McGuckin JF Jr, Akhtar N, Ho VT, et al. CT and MR evaluation of a wooden foreign body in an in vitro model of the orbit. *Am J Neuroradiol*. 1996;17:129–133.

Orbital Hemorrhage

Hemorrhage into the orbit can arise spontaneously or result from accidental or surgical trauma in association with an underlying orbital lymphangioma or varix. Drainage or aspiration is seldom necessary unless visual function is compromised by (1) compression of the optic nerve or (2) increased orbital pressure that impedes arterial perfusion. Occasionally, a blood (hematic) cyst may form following accidental trauma, usually beneath the periosteum in the superior orbit. The cyst may become apparent well after the injury and progress slowly to displace the globe anteriorly and inferiorly and erode bone. The cyst can be evacuated through an anterior transcutaneous extraperiosteal route if it does not resolve spontaneously.

> Kersten RC, Kersten JL, Bloom HR, et al. Chronic hematic cysts of the orbit. *Ophthalmology*. 1988;95:1549–1553.

Traumatic Visual Loss With Clear Media

Many patients complain of decreased vision following periocular trauma. The decrease may be due to injuries of the cornea, lens, vitreous, or retina as previously discussed.

Patients without globe damage may also complain of decreased vision because of serosanguinous drainage obscuring incident light. In addition, swelling of the eyelids may cause difficulty in opening the eyes sufficiently to clear the visual axis. However, a small percentage of patients have true visual loss without any evidence of globe injury. Visual loss in this setting suggests traumatic dysfunction of the optic nerve. Such visual loss usually results from one of three mechanisms:

- Direct injury to the optic nerve from a penetrating wound
- Disruption of the blood supply to the optic nerve due to a compartment syndrome, in which posttraumatic orbital edema or hemorrhage causes orbital pressure to increase above arterial perfusion pressure
- Indirect injury caused by force from a frontal blow transmitted to the optic nerve in the orbital apex and optic canal

All patients with decreased visual acuity following periorbital trauma should be immediately examined for evidence of direct globe injury. Two key diagnostic questions should be answered when the patient has reduced vision with an apparently normal globe:

- Is an afferent pupillary defect present?
- Is there a "tight" orbit?

Detection of an afferent defect in the presence of an intact globe strongly suggests traumatic optic neuropathy; however, the examiner must remember that detection of an afferent defect may be difficult if the patient has received narcotics that can cause bilateral pupillary constriction. The second key diagnostic determination is that of intraorbital pressure. Periorbital trauma may cause significant retrobulbar hemorrhage or edema, which can lead to proptosis, ptosis, and limitation of extraocular motility. A Schiøtz tonometer or Tono-Pen may be used in the emergency room to measure intraocular pressure, which is increased in the tight orbit in response to the underlying increased orbital pressure. Although fundus examination may reveal a central retinal artery occlusion, visual loss is more often caused by occlusion of the posterior ciliary arteries, which have a lower perfusion pressure than the central retinal artery.

Patients with a tight orbit, increased intraocular pressure, and decreased visual acuity with afferent pupillary defect should undergo emergent decompression of the orbit. This is most easily achieved in the emergency room under local anesthesia by disinsertion of the lids from the lateral canthus, allowing the orbital volume to expand anteriorly. Lateral canthotomy alone does not sufficiently increase the orbital volume; inferior cantholysis and sometimes superior cantholysis are also required. Surgical relief of the increased orbital pressure is a priority. Although intraocular pressure is elevated in the setting of traumatic orbital hemorrhage, the elevation reflects the increased orbital pressure and is not indicative of glaucoma (although angle-closure glaucoma can rarely occur following retrobulbar hemorrhages).

If a tight orbit has been ruled out, then a mechanism other than an ischemic compartment syndrome should be sought to explain the visual loss. The circumstances suggest indirect trauma to the optic nerve. Patients with this disorder usually have a history of blunt trauma to the frontal region or rapid deceleration of the cranium and often have experienced loss of consciousness associated with head trauma. Thin-section CT scans of the orbital apex and anterior clinoid process demonstrate fractures adjacent to the optic canal through or adjacent to the optic canal in the large majority of cases.

Management

The proper management of neurogenic visual loss after blunt head trauma is controversial. No treatment, high-dose corticosteroids, and surgical decompression of the optic canal are all currently considered to be reasonable options. Interest in high-dose methylprednisolone (30 mg/kg loading dose and 15 mg/kg every 6 hours) was prompted by its success in the National Acute Spinal Cord Injury Study II, wherein the regimen was found to produce significant improvement in patients treated within 8 hours of injury. In such megadoses, the therapeutic effect appears to be based on the steroid's antioxidant, rather than anti-inflammatory, properties. The success seen with methylprednisolone for spinal cord injuries may not be applicable to the treatment of traumatic optic neuropathy, however, and no randomized trials have been conducted for optic nerve injuries.

For a time, interest focused on surgical decompression of the optic canal in patients in whom high-dose steroids failed. Decompression of the medial wall of the bony optic canal through a transethmoidal sphenoidal route undertaken within 5 days of injury was purported to return vision to patients with indirect traumatic optic neuropathy. However, the optimal management of traumatic optic neuropathy remains unresolved because no large randomized studies have been carried out. A recent multicenter, prospective, nonrandomized study failed to demonstrate clear benefit for either corticosteroid therapy or optic canal decompression. Successful results with steroid therapy or surgical treatment remain anecdotal, and a number of traumatic optic neuropathy cases have documented significant visual improvement without therapy.

Joseph MP, Lessell S, Rizzo J, et al. Extracranial optic nerve decompression for traumatic optic neuropathy. *Arch Ophthalmol.* 1990;108:1091–1093.

Levin LA, Beck RW, Joseph MP, et al. The treatment of traumatic optic neuropathy: the International Optic Nerve Trauma Study. *Ophthalmology.* 1999;106:1268–1277.

Levin LA, Joseph MP, Rizzo JF III, et al. Optic canal decompression in indirect optic nerve trauma. *Ophthalmology.* 1994;101:566–569.

Steinsapir KD, Goldberg RA. Traumatic optic neuropathy. *Surv Ophthalmol.* 1994;38:487–518.

CHAPTER 7

Orbital Surgery

Surgical Spaces

There are four surgical spaces within the orbit (Fig 7-1):
- The *subperiorbital surgical space*, which is the potential space between the bone and the periorbita
- The *extraconal surgical space* (peripheral surgical space), which lies between the periorbita and the muscle cone with its fascia
- The *intraconal surgical space* (central surgical space), which lies within the muscle cone
- The *episcleral surgical space*, which lies between Tenon's capsule and the globe

Orbital lesions may involve more than one space, and an orbital pathologic process may require a combination of approaches. Incisions to reach these surgical spaces via anterior or lateral orbitotomies are shown in Figure 7-2.

Anterior Orbitotomy

Superior Approach

More orbital lesions are located in the superoanterior part of the orbit than in any other location. Lesions in this area can usually be reached through a transcutaneous or transconjunctival route. Care must be taken to avoid damaging the levator and superior oblique muscles, trochlea, lacrimal gland, and sensory nerves and vessels leaving or entering the orbit along the superior orbital rim.

Transcutaneous routes

The *transseptal route* provides entry into the peripheral surgical space. The upper eyelid crease is an excellent skin incision location for this route because this crease provides good surgical exposure and the scar is hidden.

For the *extraperiosteal route*, skin incisions in the upper eyelid crease offer good exposure to the superior orbital rim, where the periosteum can be incised, and are generally preferable to incisions adjacent to the eyebrow. Access to the supraorbital rim can be readily obtained by dissecting superiorly in the postorbicular fascial plane, and cosmesis is superior. Exposure of the orbital rim allows entry into the subperiosteal space while the periorbita protects the orbital structures from the plane of dissection. Exposure

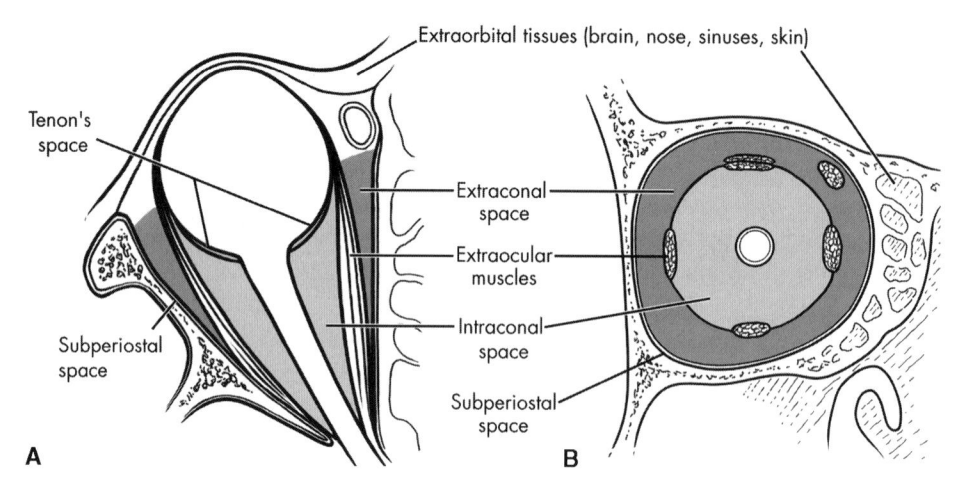

Figure 7-1 Surgical spaces of the orbit. **A,** Axial view. **B,** Coronal view. *(Reproduced with permission from Nerad JA. The Requisites in Ophthalmology: Oculoplastic Surgery. Philadelphia: Mosby; 2001:350.)*

of the orbital rim also allows much of the dissection to be performed without orbital fat in the surgical field.

Occasionally, a coronal scalp flap is used to expose superior orbital lesions. The purpose of this route is to avoid visible scars on the face; however, alopecia often occurs along the incision, and balding in men may expose the scar later. This route is most helpful for extensive lesions that require bone removal. Although coronal incisions have been used to gain access for lateral orbitotomy, extensive elevation of the temporalis muscle is required, which may result in cosmetically significant temporal wasting postoperatively.

Transconjunctival route

Incisions in the superior conjunctiva can be used to reach the episcleral, central, or peripheral surgical spaces.

Vertical eyelid splitting

Vertical splitting of the upper eyelid at the junction of the medial and central thirds allows extended transconjunctival exposure for the removal of superior medial intraconal tumors.

Inferior Approach

The inferior approach is suitable for masses that are visible or palpable in the inferior conjunctival fornix of the lower eyelid, as well as for deeper inferior extraconal orbital masses. This route is also used to approach the orbital floor for fracture repair or decompression.

Transcutaneous routes

An infraciliary blepharoplasty incision in the lower eyelid and dissection beneath the orbicularis muscle to expose the inferior orbital septum and inferior orbital rim mini-

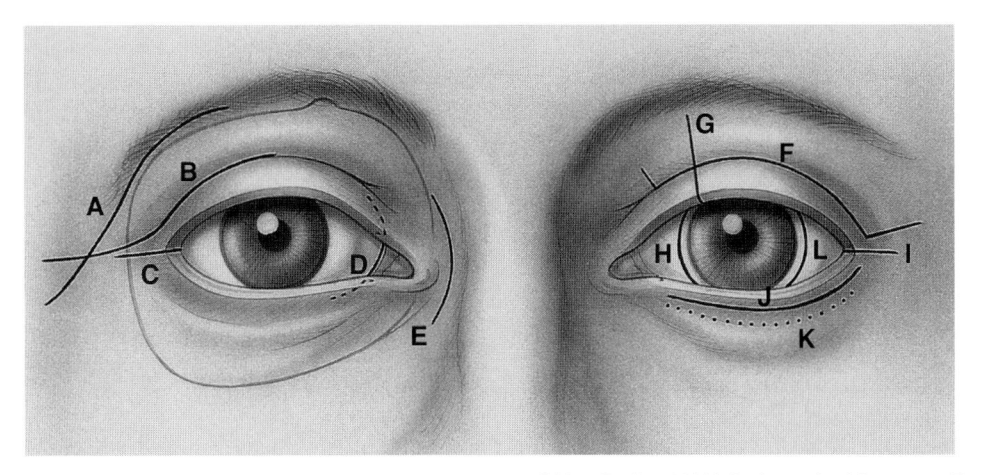

Figure 7-2 Sites of surgical entry into the orbit. *A*, Older Stallard-Wright lateral orbitotomy. *B*, Newer eyelid crease lateral orbitotomy. *C*, Canthotomy lateral orbitotomy. *D*, Transcaruncular medial orbitotomy. *E*, Frontoethmoidal (Lynch) medial orbitotomy. *F*, Upper eyelid crease anterior orbitotomy. *G*, Vertical eyelid split superomedial orbitotomy. *H*, Medial bulbar conjunctival orbitotomy. *I*, Lateral canthotomy anterior orbitotomy. *J*, Subciliary inferior orbitotomy. *K*, Transconjunctival inferior orbitotomy. *L*, Lateral bulbar conjunctival orbitotomy. *(Illustration by Christine Gralapp after a drawing by Jennifer Clemens.)*

mizes visible scarring. An incision in the lower eyelid crease can provide the same exposure but leaves a slightly more obvious scar. However, placement of the incision in the eyelid crease reduces the risk of scar contracture and ectropion. The septum can then be incised to expose the peripheral surgical space. Care should be taken to avoid cutting lower eyelid tissue perpendicular to normal skin lines, as this disrupts lymphatic drainage and may cause persistent postoperative lymphedema.

For the *extraperiosteal route*, a skin incision beneath the eyelashes or in the lower eyelid crease allows exposure of the rim where the periosteum can be incised to expose the floor of the orbit. Fractures of the orbital floor are reached by the extraperiosteal route. Incisions directly over the orbital rim cause a more objectionable scar.

Transconjunctival route

The transconjunctival approach (Fig 7-3) has largely replaced the transcutaneous route for exposure of tumors in the inferior orbit and for management of fractures of the orbital floor and medial wall (Fig 7-4). An incision may be made through the inferior conjunctiva and lower eyelid retractors to reach the peripheral surgical space and orbital floor. Exposure of the floor is optimized when this incision is combined with a lateral canthotomy and cantholysis. Incision of the bulbar conjunctiva and Tenon's capsule allows entry to the episcleral surgical space, and if the inferior rectus is retracted, the intraconal surgical space can be accessed.

Medial Approach

When dissecting in the medial orbit, the surgeon should be careful to avoid damaging the medial canthal tendon, lacrimal canaliculi and sac, trochlea, superior oblique tendon

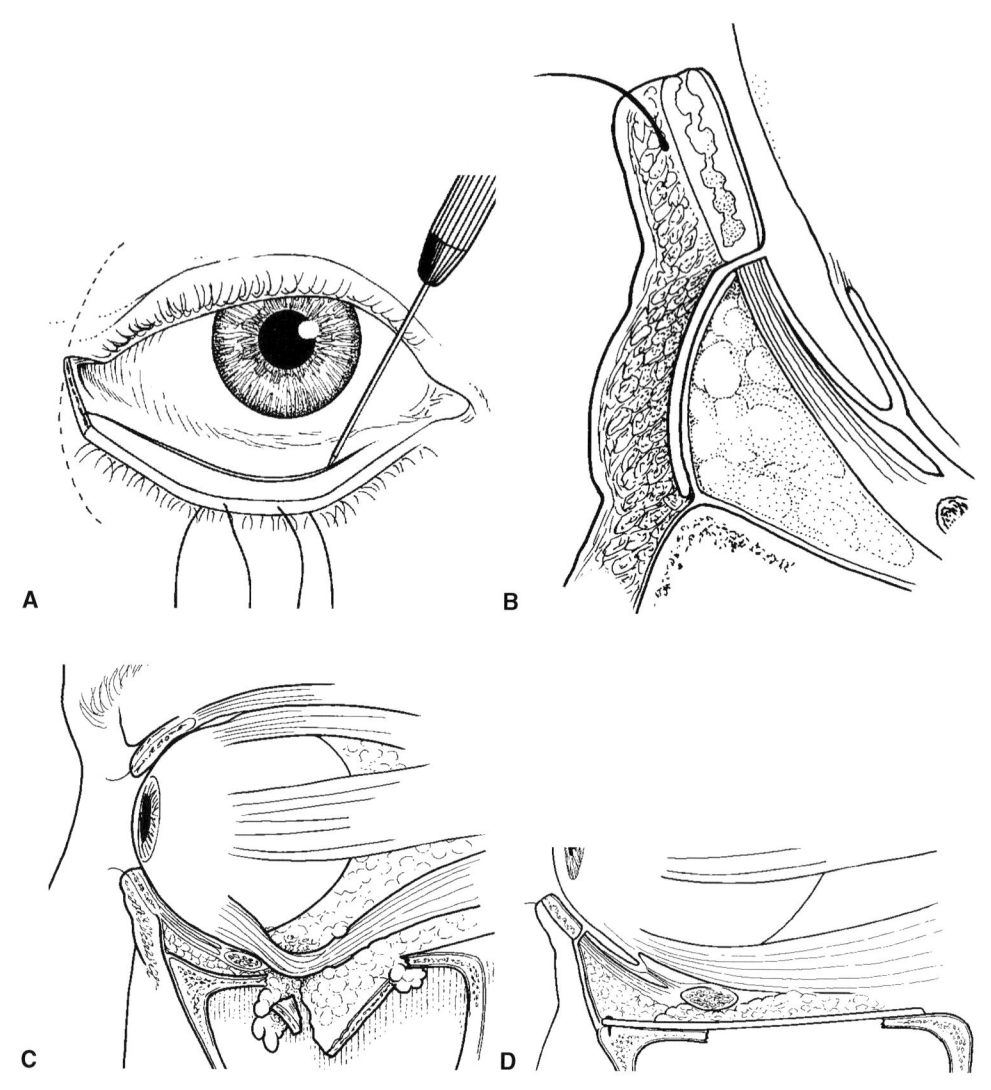

Figure 7-3 Inferior transconjunctival approach to the orbital floor. **A,** Canthotomy, cantholysis, and conjunctival incision. **B,** Plane of dissection anterior to the orbital septum. **C,** Tissue trapped in fracture. **D,** Reconstruction of orbital floor with implant after freeing entrapped tissue. *(Reproduced with permission from Nerad JA.* The Requisites in Ophthalmology: Oculoplastic Surgery. *Philadelphia: Mosby; 2001:335–336.)*

and muscle, inferior oblique muscle, and sensory nerves and vessels along the medial aspect of the superior orbital rim.

Transcutaneous route

Tumors within or near the lacrimal sac, frontal or ethmoidal sinuses, and medial rectus can be approached through a skin incision (Lynch or frontoethmoidal incision) placed vertically just medial to the insertion of the medial canthal tendon (approximately 9–10 mm medial to the medial canthal angle). This route usually is used to enter the sub-

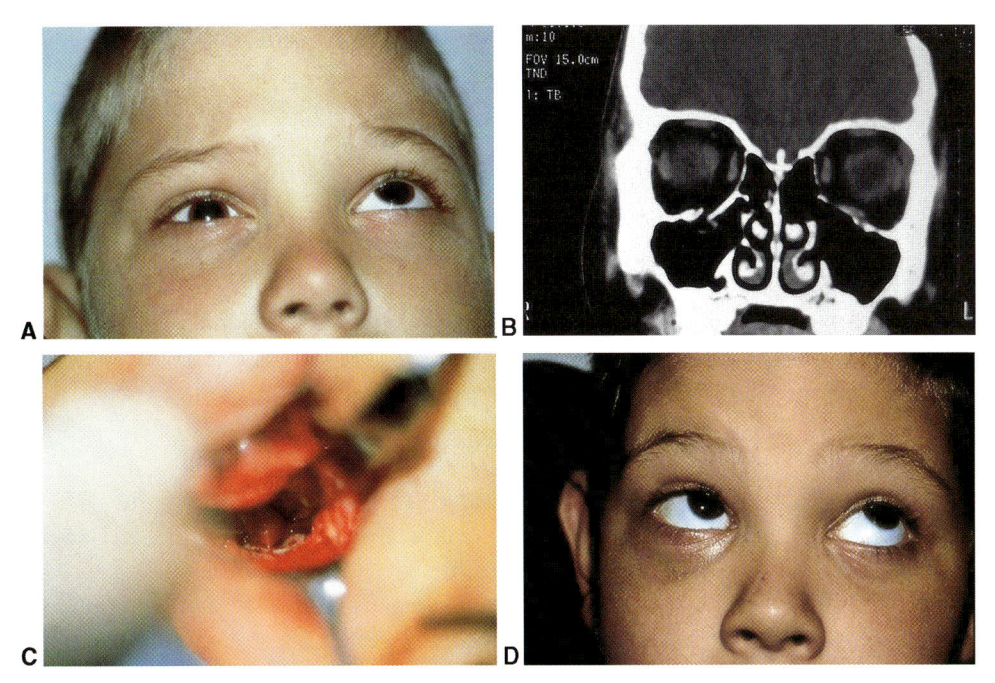

Figure 7-4 A, Marked restriction of elevation of the right eye in a young child with white-eyed blowout fracture. **B,** Coronal CT demonstrates right orbital floor trapdoor fracture. The inferior rectus muscle is displaced beneath the fracture into the maxillary sinus. **C,** Transconjunctival exploration of the orbital floor. The inferior rectus muscle can be seen entrapped in the fracture line. **D,** Restoration of elevation following release of the entrapped muscle. *(Photographs courtesy of Robert C. Kersten, MD.)*

periosteal space. The medial canthal tendon can be reflected with the periosteum and, therefore, does not need to be incised.

Transconjunctival route

An incision in the bulbar conjunctiva allows entry into the peripheral surgical space. If the medial rectus is detached, the central surgical space can be entered to expose the region of the anterior optic nerve for examination, biopsy, or decompression. If the posterior optic nerve or muscle cone needs to be visualized well, a combined medial/lateral orbitotomy can be performed. A lateral orbitotomy with removal of the lateral orbital wall to allow the globe to be displaced temporally is followed by a medial orbitotomy with detachment of the medial rectus muscle to provide good exposure of the posterior central surgical space. A canthotomy incision combined with elevation of overlying soft tissue provides good exposure of the rim.

Transcaruncular route

An incision through the caruncle with dissection posterior to the lacrimal sac allows access to the subperiosteal space along the medial wall. Dissection can be carried medially to the periosteum, allowing it to be elevated along the medial wall. This incision has the advantage of providing better cosmetic results than the traditional frontoethmoidal or Lynch incision, but the surgeon must be careful to protect the lacrimal canaliculi and to remain posterior to the lacrimal apparatus. The combination of the transcaruncular route with an inferior transconjunctival incision allows extensive exposure of the inferior and medial orbit. This approach provides excellent access for repair of medial wall fractures, for medial orbital bone decompression, and for drainage of medial subperiosteal abscesses.

Lateral Orbitotomy

A lateral orbitotomy is usually indicated when a lesion is located within the muscle cone, behind the equator of the globe, or in the lacrimal gland fossa, particularly when a benign mixed tumor of the lacrimal gland is suspected. In children, the more shallow orbit usually allows extensive exposure without the need for bone removal. The traditional S-shaped Stallard-Wright skin incision, extending from beneath the eyebrow laterally and curving down along the zygomatic arch, allowed good exposure of the lateral rim but left a more noticeable scar. It has largely been replaced for lateral orbital exposure by newer approaches, either through an upper eyelid crease incision or a lateral canthotomy incision. Both of these approaches allow subcutaneous undermining and exposure of the lateral orbital rim and anterior portion of the zygomatic arch with reflection of the temporalis muscle.

An oscillating saw is used to remove the bone of the lateral rim to expose the underlying periorbita, which is then opened. An operating microscope is often useful during intraorbital surgery, especially if dissection proceeds inside the muscle cone. Good exposure of the central surgical space can be achieved with retraction of the lateral rectus muscle. Tumors can occasionally be prolapsed into the incision by gentle pressure over the eyelids. A cryosurgical probe or Allis forceps can be useful in providing firm traction on encapsulated tumors. In the case of cavernous hemangiomas, a suture through the lesion allows not only traction but also slow decompression of the tumor to facilitate its removal.

Complete hemostasis should be accomplished prior to closure. A drain may be placed through the skin to reach the deep orbital tissues. The periosteum is loosely closed to allow postoperative hemorrhage to decompress. The lateral orbital rim is usually replaced and may either be sutured in place or plated or fixated by firmly suturing the investing periosteum. The overlying tissues are then returned to their normal positions and sutured. Steel wire is avoided because it can cause artifacts on follow-up CT scans.

Radical surgery, such as exenteration or extensive resection with potential for significant functional morbidity, should not be performed on the basis of a frozen-section biopsy report. The surgeon should await the permanent-section histopathology report and discuss the matter further with the patient before proceeding with disfiguring or disabling surgery. Lacrimal lesions thought to be malignant are usually biopsied by an anterior approach through the orbital septum (see under Epithelial Tumors of the Lacrimal Gland in Chapter 5).

Corticosteroids may be administered intravenously at the start of the operation and continued for several days postoperatively to reduce orbital edema. Intravenous antibiotics may also be given preoperatively and continued for 48 hours postoperatively if the sinuses are entered during the orbital surgery. Otherwise, prophylactic systemic antibiotics are usually not necessary in orbital surgery.

> Harris GJ, Logani SC. Eyelid crease incision for lateral orbitotomy. *Ophthal Plast Reconstr Surg.* 1999;15:9–18.

Orbital Decompression

Historically, the primary indication for orbital decompression in thyroid ophthalmopathy was reduced vision caused by pressure of swollen extraocular muscles on the optic nerve. However, since surgical techniques have improved, the deformity of exophthalmos is now also considered an indication in many cases. The goal of orbital decompression is to allow the edematous muscles to expand into periorbital spaces, relieving pressure on the optic nerve (and its blood supply) and reducing proptosis.

Decompression historically involved removal of the medial orbital wall and much of the orbital floor to allow orbital tissues to expand into the ethmoid and maxillary sinuses. The approach was made through the maxillary sinus (Caldwell-Luc) or transcutaneous anterior orbitotomy incision. The approach currently favored by most orbital surgeons is a transconjunctival incision combined with a lateral cantholysis to disinsert and evert the lower eyelid. Extension of this incision superonasally with a transcaruncular approach allows excellent access to the medial orbital wall. A transnasal endoscopic approach to the medial orbit may also be useful. The lateral orbital wall may be removed or repositioned outward to allow further decompression into the infratemporal fossa. Additional decompression can be achieved by burring down the medial surface of the sphenoid wing. This procedure is usually combined with the medial orbital decompression.

In patients with large restricted inferior rectus muscles, orbital floor decompression may exacerbate globe ptosis, upper lid retraction, and vertical globe excursion because of prolapse of the enlarged inferior rectus into the maxillary sinus. Recently, surgeons have advocated a balanced decompression of the medial and lateral orbital walls (Fig 7-5), leaving the floor intact in these cases. Decompression through the orbital roof into the anterior cranial fossa is rarely advisable. Craniofacial surgical techniques used to move the orbital bones forward can increase the effectiveness of decompression in particularly severe cases. Recent years have seen increased interest in removing orbital fat to decrease orbital volume, with or without associated bony decompression.

> Garrity JA, Fatourechi V, Bergstralh EJ, et al. Results of transantral orbital decompression in 428 patients with severe Graves' ophthalmopathy. *Am J Ophthalmol.* 1993;116:533–547.
>
> Goldberg RA. The evolving paradigm of orbital decompression surgery [editorial]. *Arch Ophthalmol.* 1998;116:95–96.
>
> Goldberg RA, Hwang MM, Garbutt MV, et al. Orbital decompression for non-Graves' orbitopathy: a consideration of extended indications for decompression. *Ophthal Plast Reconstr Surg.* 1995;11:245–252.

116 • Orbit, Eyelids, and Lacrimal System

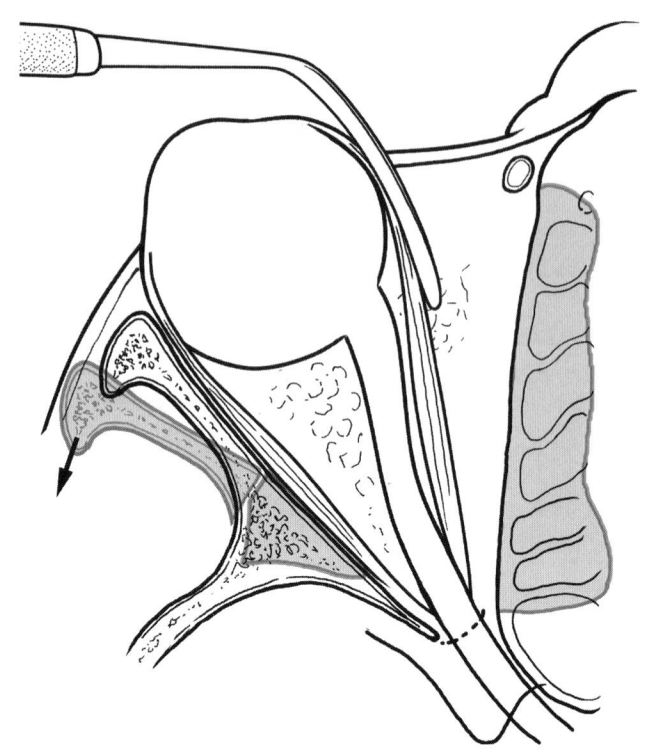

Figure 7-5 "Balanced" orbital decompression: medial and lateral *(shaded areas)*. *(After McCord CD Jr. Orbital decompression for Graves' disease: exposure through lateral canthal and inferior fornix incision. Ophthalmology. 1981;88:526.)*

Postoperative Care

Measures used to reduce postoperative edema are elevation of the head, iced compresses on the eyelids, a drain that is removed in 24–36 hours, and systemic steroids. Visual acuity should be checked frequently at routine intervals in the first 12 hours after surgery. Systemic antibiotics may be given. Patching of the operative site should be discouraged because it can delay diagnosis of a postoperative hemorrhage. Ice packs minimize swelling and still allow frequent observation of the operative site and vision monitoring.

Special Surgical Techniques in the Orbit

Fine-needle aspiration biopsy may have limited value in selected cases of lymphoid lesions, secondary tumors invading the orbit from the sinuses, suspected metastatic tumors, and blind eyes with optic nerve tumors. The technique is not very effective for obtaining tissue from fibrous lesions, from which it is difficult to aspirate cells. Although fine-needle aspiration biopsy has not been considered a good technique for biopsy of lymphoproliferative disorders, it may assist in the diagnosis of selected cases when used with flow cytometry with monoclonal antibodies or Southern blot analysis.

Fine-needle aspiration biopsy is performed with a 4 cm 22- or 23-gauge needle attached to a syringe with a pistol-grip holder. The needle is passed through the skin or conjunctiva. If necessary, the needle can be guided into the tumor by ultrasonography or CT. Cells (and occasionally a small block of tissue) are aspirated from the lesion. A skilled cytologist is required to study the specimen. See BCSC Section 4, *Ophthalmic Pathology and Intraocular Tumors,* for further discussion of fine-needle aspiration biopsy.

Masses or traumatic injuries may involve the skull base, including posterior and superior aspects of the orbit. Advanced surgical techniques provide access to these areas via a frontotemporal-orbitozygomatic approach. Such operations often require the combined efforts of the orbital surgeon, neurosurgeon, and otorhinolaryngologist. These techniques allow removal of tumors such as meningiomas, hemangiomas, hemangiopericytomas, schwannomas, and gliomas that might not otherwise be resectable. In addition, this approach may provide access to the optic canal for decompression.

McDermott MW, Durity FA, Rootman J, et al. Combined frontotemporal-orbitozygomatic approach for tumors of the sphenoid wing and orbit. *Neurosurgery.* 1990;26:107–116.

Complications of Orbital Surgery

Complications from orbital surgery can be reduced by a complete preoperative evaluation, choice of the appropriate approach, adequate exposure, careful manipulation of the tissues, good hemostasis, and consultations with a neurosurgeon or otorhinolaryngologist (or both) when appropriate.

The most serious complication is decreased or lost vision. This complication may be caused by excessive traction on the globe and optic nerve, contusion of the optic nerve, or hemorrhage. A patient who has severe orbital pain postoperatively should be evaluated immediately for possible orbital hemorrhage. If this pain is associated with decreased visual acuity, proptosis, ecchymosis, increased intraocular pressure, and an afferent pupillary defect, the surgeon should consider immediately opening the wound and evacuating the hematoma.

In cases of orbital decompression, removal of the orbital floor tends to cause downward displacement of the globe and may cause postoperative exacerbation of upper eyelid retraction. This effect may be minimized by balancing medial and lateral decompressions and avoiding or limiting removal of the orbital floor. Hypoesthesia over the distribution of the second division of cranial nerve V may also follow orbital floor decompression. Motility disorders are encountered in up to one third of patients after orbital decompression, but the vast majority of these patients had preexisting restrictive myopathy.

Other complications of orbital surgery include extraocular muscle damage, ptosis, neuroparalytic keratopathy, pupillary changes, vitreous hemorrhage, detached retina, hypoesthesia of the forehead, keratitis sicca, cerebrospinal fluid leak, and infection.

Kersten RC, Nerad JA. In: Tasman W, Jaeger EA, eds. *Duane's Clinical Ophthalmology.* Philadelphia: Lippincott-Raven; 1995;5:1–36.

CHAPTER 8

The Anophthalmic Socket

It is occasionally necessary to remove an eye or the contents of an orbit to enhance patient comfort and cosmesis, to protect the vision in the fellow eye, or to safeguard life. With loss of an eye, the patient can suffer depression or a degraded self-image. The ophthalmologist can assist the patient both before and after anophthalmic surgery by providing reassurance and psychological support. Discussions of the procedure, the rehabilitation process, and expected functional changes can help the patient with adjustment. With very few exceptions, the monocular patient may resume the full range of home, vocational, and athletic activities.

When resuming full activity, however, patients should take a cautious approach to allow adjustment to the changes in perception. The loss of depth perception and visual field may limit a patient's ability to perform as a commercial pilot or driver or to operate hazardous equipment safely. The ophthalmologist can also help safeguard the remaining eye through regular follow-up examinations and the prescription of polycarbonate safety glasses for full-time wear.

> Brady FB. *A Singular View: The Art of Seeing with One Eye.* Oradell, NJ: Medical Economics Co; 1972.
>
> Czeisler CA, Shanahan TL, Klerman EB, et al. Suppression of melatonin secretion in some blind patients by exposure to bright light. *N Engl J Med.* 1995;332:6–11.

The indications for anophthalmic surgery are diverse, and the procedure of choice varies. *Enucleation* involves removal of the entire globe while preserving other orbital tissues. *Evisceration* is the removal of the intraocular contents (lens, uvea, retina, vitreous, and sometimes cornea), leaving the sclera and extraocular muscles intact. *Exenteration* refers to the removal of all or parts of the orbital tissues including the globe. The cosmetic goals in anophthalmic surgery are to minimize any condition that draws attention to the anophthalmos. Surgical efforts to produce orbital and eyelid symmetry and to promote good prosthetic position and motility enhance cosmesis.

Enucleation

Enucleation allows for the complete histologic examination of the eye and optic nerve, possibly influencing subsequent treatment and contributing to medical knowledge. It also eliminates any concern that surgery might contribute to the risk of sympathetic ophthalmia in the fellow eye. Enucleation is always the procedure of choice if the nature of the intraocular pathology is unknown.

Enucleation is indicated for primary intraocular malignancies not amenable to alternative modes of therapy such as external- or proton-beam irradiation or episcleral plaque brachytherapy. Retinoblastoma and choroidal melanoma are the ocular tumors that most commonly require enucleation. Evisceration should not be performed in cases of suspected intraocular malignancy. When enucleation is performed for an intraocular tumor, care must be taken to avoid opening the globe during surgery, and the globe should be handled gently to minimize the risk of disseminating tumor cells. In cases of suspected retinoblastoma, the surgeon should obtain a long segment of optic nerve with the enucleation specimen to increase the chances of completely resecting the tumor. A lateral canthotomy during enucleation surgery may provide the desired surgical exposure.

Blind eyes with opaque media should be suspected of harboring an occult neoplasm unless another cause of ocular disease can be surmised. Although blind or phthisical eyes are not at increased risk for malignancy, a tumor can occasionally be the cause of globe degeneration. Ultrasonography is useful in evaluating these eyes and planning proper management.

In severely traumatized eyes, enucleation within the first 10–14 days may be considered if the risk of sympathetic ophthalmia and harm to the remaining eye is judged to be greater than the likelihood of recovering useful vision in the traumatized eye. Sympathetic ophthalmia is thought to be a delayed hypersensitivity immune response to the uveal antigens. The condition can occur from 9 days to 50 years after corneoscleral perforation. The incidence of sympathetic ophthalmia in fellow eyes following penetrating ocular trauma in eyes that were not enucleated has been estimated at 0.19%. Enucleation with complete removal of the uveal pigment may be beneficial in preventing a subsequent immune response. However, the infrequency of sympathetic ophthalmia coupled with improved medical therapy for uveitis has made early enucleation strictly for prophylaxis a debatable practice. Additionally, it has been demonstrated that the majority of severely injured eyes do not subsequently require removal for pain and thus can be treated by fitting a cosmetic scleral shell to provide excellent cosmesis and motility. Follow-up visits are required to examine the fellow eye for signs of inflammation, the presence of which requires prompt medical therapy. Although there is some conflicting evidence, removal of an eye that has already stimulated sympathetic ophthalmia is unlikely to prevent progression of the disease.

Painful eyes without useful vision can be managed with enucleation or evisceration. Patients with end-stage neovascular glaucoma, chronic uveitis, or previously traumatized blind eyes can obtain dramatic relief from discomfort and improved cosmesis with either procedure. For debilitated patients unable to undergo surgery and rehabilitation, retrobulbar injection of ethanol may provide adequate pain relief. In a disfigured eye without pain, however, it is generally advisable to initially consider a trial of a cosmetic scleral shell. If tolerated, scleral shells give superior cosmesis and motility.

Guidelines for Enucleation

A functionally and aesthetically acceptable anophthalmic socket must have the following components:

- An orbital implant of sufficient volume centered within the orbit
- A socket lined with conjunctiva or mucous membrane with fornices deep enough to hold a prosthesis
- Eyelids with normal appearance and adequate tone to support a prosthesis
- Good transmission of motility from the implant to the overlying prosthesis
- A comfortable ocular prosthesis that looks similar to the normal eye

Enucleation can be performed satisfactorily under local or general anesthesia; however, most patients prefer general anesthesia or sedation when an eye is removed.

Enucleation in Childhood

Enucleation in early childhood, as well as congenital anophthalmos or microphthalmos, may lead to underdevelopment of the involved bony orbit with secondary facial asymmetry. Orbital soft tissue volume is a critical determinant of orbital bone growth. When enucleation is necessary in childhood, a large implant should be used to replace orbital volume. An adult-sized implant should be placed as soon as possible to encourage symmetric orbital bone growth. Volume loss in the adult anophthalmic socket may be adequately replaced by a 20–22 mm sphere implant. Rarely should an implant smaller than 18 mm be used even in the very young.

Recently, surgeons have reported good success with autogenous dermis-fat grafts as anophthalmic implants in children. Reportedly, these grafts continue to grow along with the expanding orbit. The opposite effect has been observed in adults, in whom loss of volume generally occurs when dermis-fat grafts are used as primary anophthalmic implants.

> Heher KL, Katowitz JA, Low JE. Unilateral dermis-fat graft implantation in the pediatric orbit. *Ophthal Plast Reconstr Surg.* 1998;14:81–88.

Orbital Implants

The function of an implant is to replace lost orbital volume, to maintain the structure of the orbit, and to impart motility to the overlying ocular prosthesis.

Implants used today are usually either spheres or buried implants with front surface projections to which the extraocular muscles can be attached in various ways. Spherical implants may be grouped according to the materials from which they are manufactured: *inert materials,* such as glass, silicone, or methylmethacrylate; and *biointegrated materials,* such as porous polyethylene or hydroxyapatite. The latter are designed to be incorporated by soft tissue ingrowth into the socket.

Inert spherical implants provide comfort and low rates of extrusion, but they offer ocular motility only through passive movement of the socket. Buried motility implants with front surface projections push the overlying prosthesis with a direct force and probably improve prosthetic motility. The front surface projections, however, may pinch conjunctiva between the implant and prosthesis and lead to a painful socket or erosion over the implant.

Hydroxyapatite and porous polyethylene implants allow for drilling and placement of a peg to integrate the prosthesis directly with the moving implant. Drilling is usually carried out 6–12 months after enucleation. Although drilled porous implants offer excellent motility, they may also have a higher rate of postoperative exposure. Interestingly, the majority of surgeons who place porous implants do not subsequently drill a peg, reporting satisfactory motility even without pegging the prosthesis directly to the implant. In this case, their function is similar to that of any other spherical implant.

Locations for implants are either within Tenon's capsule or behind posterior Tenon's capsule in the muscle cone. Spheres may be covered with other materials such as homologous sclera or autogenous fascia, which serve as further barriers to migration and extrusion. Secure closure of Tenon's fascia over the anterior surface of an anophthalmic implant is an important barrier to later extrusion.

Extraocular muscles should not be crossed over the front surface of a sphere implant or purse-stringed anteriorly. These techniques allow the implant to migrate when the muscles slip off the anterior surface. Muscles sutured into the normal anatomic locations, either directly to the implant or to homologous sclera or autogenous fascia surrounding the implant, allow superior motility and prevent migration.

Prostheses

An ocular prosthesis is fitted within 4–8 weeks after enucleation. The ideal prosthesis is custom-fitted to the exact dimensions of the orbit after postoperative edema has subsided. Premade, or stock, eyes are less satisfactory cosmetically, limit prosthetic motility, and may trap secretions between the prosthesis and the socket.

Following enucleation surgery, an acrylic or silicone conformer is placed in the conjunctival fornices to maintain the conjunctival space that will eventually accommodate the prosthesis. An anophthalmic socket without a conformer or prosthesis in place can contract in a matter of days, preventing placement of the prosthesis.

> Custer PL, Trinkhaus KM, Fornoff J. Comparative motility of hydroxyapatite and alloplastic enucleation implants. *Ophthalmology.* 1999;106:513–516.
>
> Edelstein C, Shields CL, De Potter P, et al. Complications of motility peg placement for the hydroxyapatite orbital implant. *Ophthalmology.* 1997;104:1616–1621.
>
> Goldberg RA, Holds JB, Ebrahimpour J. Exposed hydroxyapatite orbital implants. *Ophthalmology.* 1992;99:831–836.
>
> Karesh JW, Dresner SC. High-density porous polyethylene (Medpor) as a successful anophthalmic socket implant. *Ophthalmology.* 1994;101:1688–1696.
>
> Kim YD, Goldberg RA, Shorr N, et al. Management of exposed hydroxyapatite orbital implants. *Ophthalmology.* 1994;101:1709–1715.
>
> Nerad JA, Carter KD. The anophthalmic socket. In: *Focal Points: Clinical Modules for Ophthalmologists.* San Francisco: American Academy of Ophthalmology; 1992: vol 10, no 9.
>
> Remulla HD, Ruben PAD, Shore JW, et al. Complications of porous spherical orbital implants. *Ophthalmology.* 1995;102:586–593.
>
> Rubin PAD, Popham JK, Bilyk JR, et al. Comparison of fibrovascular ingrowth into hydroxyapatite and porous polyethylene orbital implants. *Ophthal Plast Reconstr Surg.* 1994;10: 96–103.

Intraoperative Complications of Enucleation

Removal of the wrong eye

This is one of the most feared complications in ophthalmology. Always reexamine the chart, the operative permit, and the patient with ophthalmoscopy in the operating room immediately before enucleation. Marking the skin near the eye to be enucleated and having the patient point to the involved eye give further assurance.

Ptosis and extraocular muscle damage

Avoiding excessive dissection near the orbital roof and apex reduces the chance of damaging the extraocular muscles or their innervation.

Evisceration

Evisceration involves the removal of the contents of the globe, leaving the sclera, extraocular muscles, and optic nerve intact. Evisceration should be considered *only* if the presence of an intraocular malignancy has been ruled out.

Advantages of Evisceration

- *Less disruption of orbital anatomy.* Thus, the chance of injury to extraocular muscles and nerves and atrophy of fat is reduced with less dissection within the orbit. The relationships between the muscles, globe, eyelids, and fornices remain undisturbed.
- *Good motility of the prosthesis.* The extraocular muscles remain attached to the sclera. Motility of the prosthesis is generally better than that achieved following enucleation.
- *Better treatment of endophthalmitis.* Evisceration is preferred by some surgeons in cases of endophthalmitis, because extirpation and drainage of the ocular contents can occur without invasion of the orbit. The chance of contamination of the orbit with possible subsequent orbital cellulitis or intracranial extension is therefore theoretically reduced.
- *A technically simpler procedure.* Performing this less invasive procedure may be important when general anesthesia is contraindicated or when bleeding disorders increase the risk of orbital dissection.

Disadvantages of Evisceration

Although not all surgeons agree on the exact indications for enucleation and evisceration, it should be emphasized that evisceration should never be performed if a tumor is suspected. It has been suggested that sympathetic ophthalmia may rarely be caused by a reaction to residual uveal tissue in the eviscerated socket, although an initial report of four cases over 25 years ago has not been subsequently confirmed by additional case reports. Finally, evisceration affords a less complete specimen for pathologic examinations.

Levine MR, Pou CR, Lash RH. Evisceration: is sympathetic ophthalmia a concern in the new millennium? The 1998 Wendell Hughes Lecture. *Ophthal Plast Reconstr Surg.* 1999;15:4–8.

Massry GG, Holds JB. Evisceration with scleral modification. *Ophthal Plast Reconstr Surg.* 2001;17:42–47.

Techniques of Evisceration

Evisceration can be performed either with retention of the cornea or with excision of the cornea. The cornea can be retained if it is of normal thickness and shows no active corneal disease. The corneal epithelium and endothelium should be removed at the time of surgery. If there is mild thinning of the cornea, a bridge flap of conjunctiva and Tenon's capsule can be brought down from the bulbar area just above the cornea and sutured over the cornea. This technique has the advantage of allowing placement of a larger implant, thus enhancing orbital volume. The disadvantage is that the cornea may erode eventually, and extrusion of the implant can result. Regardless of the technique used for evisceration, all visible pigmented uvea should be removed before the implant is placed.

If there is active disease in the cornea, the cornea should be excised and the implant sutured within the sclera. Posterior relaxing incisions of the sclera (radially in each quadrant or concentric to optic nerve) may be utilized to allow placement of a larger implant.

Anophthalmic Socket Complications and Treatment

Deep Superior Sulcus

Deep superior sulcus deformity is caused by decreased orbital volume (Fig 8-1). This deformity can be corrected by increasing the orbital volume by placing a secondary implant subperiosteally on the orbital floor. This implant pushes the initial implant and superior orbital fat upward to fill out the superior sulcus. If a relaxed lower eyelid is present, it is tightened, usually with lid shortening at the lateral canthus. This procedure elevates the prosthesis and superior orbital fat to fill out the superior sulcus deformity. Dermis-fat grafts may be implanted in the upper eyelid to fill out the sulcus, but eyelid contour and function may be damaged and the graft may undergo resorption. Superior sulcus deformity may also be corrected by replacing the original implant with a larger secondary anophthalmic implant.

Figure 8-1 Superior sulcus deformity following enucleation of right eye.

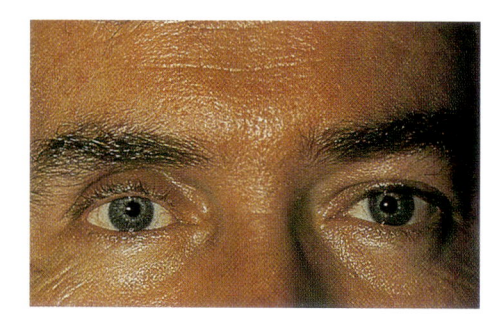

Contracture of Fornices

Preventing contracted fornices includes preserving as much conjunctiva as possible and limiting dissection in the fornices. Placing extraocular muscles in the normal anatomic positions also minimizes shortening of the fornices. The patient should wear a conformer as continuously as possible postoperatively to minimize conjunctival shortening. Conformers and prostheses should not be removed for periods greater than 24 hours. The prosthesis can be removed frequently and cleaned in the presence of infection but should be replaced promptly after irrigation of the socket.

Exposure and Extrusion of Implant

Implants may extrude if placed too far forward or if closure of anterior Tenon's fascia is not satisfactory. Postoperative infection, poor wound healing, poorly fitting prostheses or conformers, and pressure points between the implant and prosthesis may also contribute to extrusion of the implant. Exposed implants are subject to infection. Although small defects over porous implants may rarely close spontaneously, most exposures should be covered with scleral patch grafts or autogenous tissue grafts to promote conjunctival healing (Fig 8-2).

A dermis-fat graft may be used when a limited amount of conjunctiva remains in the socket. This graft increases the net amount of conjunctiva available as the conjunctiva reepithelializes over the front surface of the dermis. Unpredictable reabsorption of volume is a serious drawback to the dermis-fat graft technique in adults. In children, dermis-fat grafts appear to continue to grow along with the surrounding orbit and may help stimulate orbital development if enucleation is required during infancy or childhood.

Contracted Sockets

Causes of contracted sockets include

- Radiation treatment (usually as treatment of the tumor that necessitated removal of the eye)

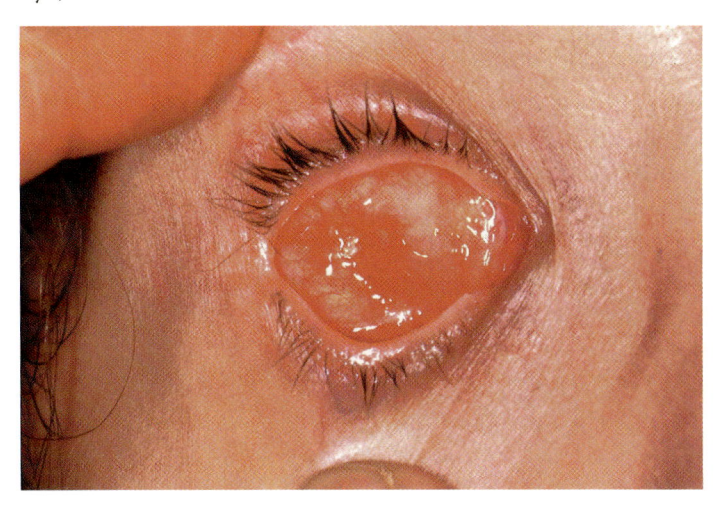

Figure 8-2 Exposure of the hydroxyapatite orbital implant in a patient who had undergone enucleation for trauma.

- Extrusion of an enucleation implant
- Severe initial injury (alkali burns or extensive lacerations)
- Poor surgical techniques (excessive sacrifice or destruction of conjunctiva and Tenon's capsule; traumatic dissection within the socket causing excessive scar tissue formation)
- Multiple socket operations
- Removal of the conformer or prosthesis for prolonged periods

Sockets are considered to be contracted when the fornices are too small to retain a prosthesis (Fig 8-3). Socket reconstruction procedures involve incision or excision of the scarred tissues and placement of a graft to enlarge the fornices. Full-thickness mucous membrane grafting is preferred because this allows the grafted tissue to match conjunctiva histologically. Buccal mucosal grafts may be taken from the cheeks (beware of damaging the duct to the parotid gland) or from the upper lip, lower lip, or hard palate. Goblet cells and mucus production are preserved.

Contracture of the fornices alone (more common with the inferior fornix) usually is associated with milder degrees of socket contracture. In these cases, the buccal mucosal graft is placed in the defect, and a silicone sheet is attached by sutures to the superior or inferior orbital rim, depending on which fornix is involved. In 2 weeks, the sheet may be removed and a prosthesis placed.

Anophthalmic Ectropion

Lower eyelid ectropion may result from the loosening of lower eyelid support under the weight of a prosthesis. Frequent removal of the prosthesis as well as a larger prosthesis accelerate the development of lid laxity. Tightening the lateral or medial canthal tendon may remedy the situation. Ectropion repair may also be combined with correction of

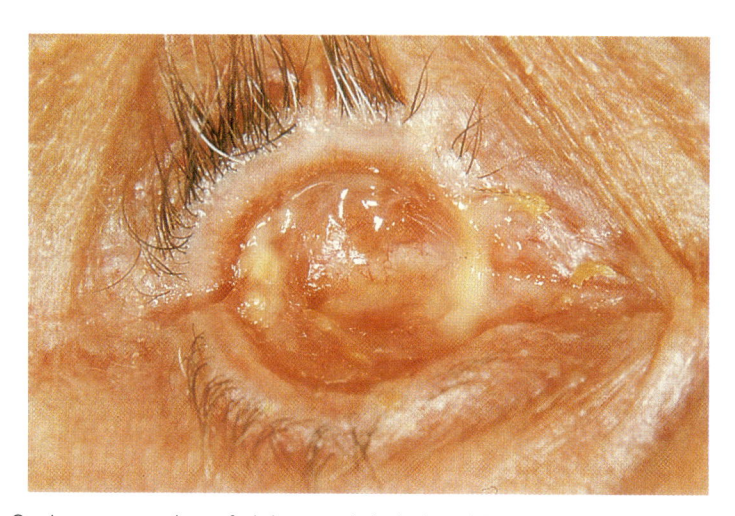

Figure 8-3 Socket contraction of right anophthalmic orbit. Note obliteration of conjunctival fornices. Patient is unable to wear an ocular prosthesis.

eyelid retraction by recessing the inferior retractor muscle layer and grafting mucous membrane tissue in the inferior fornix.

Anophthalmic Ptosis

Ptosis of the anophthalmic socket results from superotemporal migration of sphere implants, cicatricial tissue in the upper fornix, or damage to the levator muscle or nerve. Small amounts of ptosis may be managed by modification of the prosthesis. Greater amounts of ptosis require tightening of the levator aponeurosis; this procedure is best done under local anesthesia with intraoperative adjustment of eyelid height and contour, because mechanical forces may cause the surgeon to underestimate true levator function. Frontalis suspension is usually a less acceptable procedure because there is no visual drive to stimulate contracture of the frontalis muscle to elevate the eyelid.

Lash Margin Entropion

Lash margin entropion, trichiasis, and ptosis of the eyelashes are common in the anophthalmic socket. Contracture of fornices or cicatricial tissue near the lash margin contributes to these abnormalities. Horizontal tarsal incisions and rotation of the lash margin (such as the Wies procedure) may correct the problem. In more severe cases, splitting of the eyelid margins at the gray line with mucous membrane grafting to the eyelid margin may correct the entropic lash margin.

Cosmetic Optics

The style of frames and tinted lenses chosen for spectacles can help to camouflage residual defects in reconstructed sockets. Plus (convex) lenses or minus (concave) lenses may be placed in the glasses in front of the prosthesis to change its apparent size. Prisms in the glasses may be used to change the apparent vertical position of the prosthesis.

> Neuhaus R, Hawes MJ. Inadequate inferior cul-de-sac in the anophthalmic socket. *Ophthalmology*. 1992;99:153–157.
> Smit TJ, Koornneef L, Zonneveld FW, et al. Computed tomography in the assessment of the postenucleation socket syndrome. *Ophthalmology*. 1990;97:1347–1351.
> Smit TJ, Koornneef L, Zonneveld FW, et al. Primary and secondary implants in the anophthalmic orbit: preoperative and postoperative computed tomographic appearance. *Ophthalmology*. 1991;98:106–110.

Exenteration

Exenteration involves the removal of the soft tissues of the orbit, including the globe.

Considerations for Exenteration

Exenteration should be considered in the following circumstances:

- *Destructive tumors extending into the orbit from the sinuses, face, eyelids, conjunctiva, or intracranial space* (Fig 8-4). However, exenteration is not indicated for all such

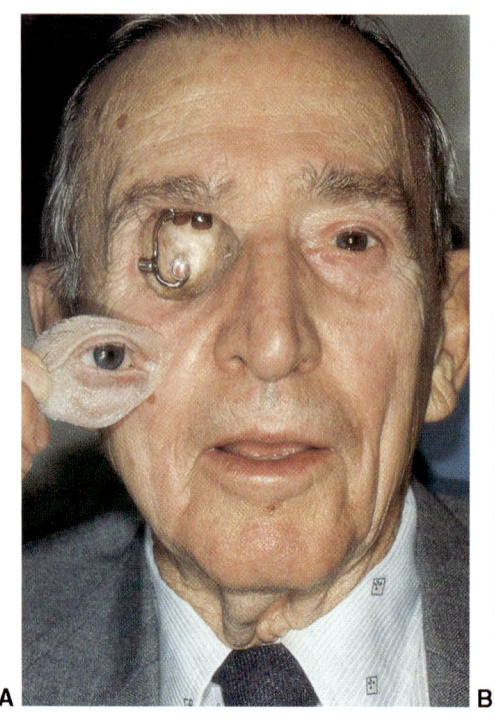

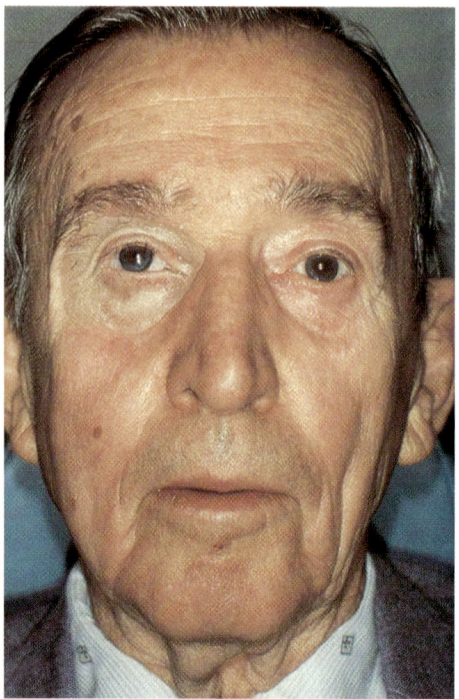

Figure 8-4 Orbital exenteration and osseointegrated prosthesis. **A,** Exenterated socket for sebaceous cell carcinoma. **B,** Prosthesis in place, retained with magnets attached to bone-anchored framework. *(Photographs courtesy of Jeffrey A. Nerad, MD.)*

tumors: some are responsive to radiation, and some have extended too far to be completely removed by surgical excision.

- *Intraocular malignant melanomas or retinoblastomas that have extended outside the globe (if evidence of distant metastases is excluded).* When local control of the tumor would benefit the nursing care of the patient, exenteration is indicated.
- *Malignant epithelial tumors of the lacrimal gland.* Although the procedure is somewhat controversial, these tumors usually require extended exenteration with radical bone removal of the roof, lateral wall, and floor.
- *Sarcomas and other primary orbital malignancies that do not respond to nonsurgical therapy.* Some tumors such as rhabdomyosarcomas that were previously treated by exenteration are now treated by radiation and chemotherapy.
- *Fungal infection.* Subtotal or total exenteration may be necessary for the management of orbital phycomycosis, which occurs most commonly in patients who are diabetic or immunosuppressed. However, attention is now being focused on achieving control through more limited debridement of involved orbital tissues.

Types of Exenteration

Exenterations vary in the amount of tissue that is removed. Following are the types of exenteration:

- *Subtotal.* The eye and adjacent intraorbital tissues are removed to locally excise the lesion (leaving periorbita and part or all of eyelids). This technique is used for some locally invasive tumors, for debulking of disseminated tumors, or for partial treatment in selected patients.
- *Total.* All intraorbital soft tissues, including periorbita, are removed, with or without the skin of the eyelids.
- *Extended.* All intraorbital soft tissues are removed, together with adjacent structures (usually bony walls and sinuses).

Following removal of the orbital contents, the bony socket may be allowed to spontaneously granulate and epithelialize or may be covered by a split-thickness skin graft, which may be placed onto bare bone or over a temporalis muscle or temporoparietal fascial flap.

The technique selected depends on the pathologic process. The goal is to remove all lesions along with appropriate margins of adjacent tissue while retaining as much healthy tissue as possible.

Bartley GB, Garrity JA, Waller RR, et al. Orbital exenteration at the Mayo Clinic: 1967–1986. *Ophthalmology.* 1989;96:468–474.

Günalp I, Gündüz K, Dürük K. Orbital exenteration: a review of 429 cases. *Int Ophthalmol.* 1996;19:177–184.

Johnson TE, Tabbara KF, Weatherhead RG, et al. Secondary squamous cell carcinoma of the orbit. *Arch Ophthalmol.* 1997;115:75–78.

Levin PS, Dutton JJ. A 20-year series of orbital exenteration. *Am J Ophthalmol.* 1991;112: 496–501.

Yeatts RP, Marion JR, Weaver RG, et al. Removal of the eye with socket ablation: a limited subtotal exenteration. *Arch Ophthalmol.* 1991;109:1306–1309.

PART II

Periocular Soft Tissues

Introduction

The eyelids and periocular structures exist in a continuum with the rest of the face. Ophthalmic plastic surgeons have long recognized the need to incorporate a variety of upper face, midface, and lower face and neck procedures for repair of involutional periocular problems, reconstruction, and cosmetic enhancement. It is not possible to safely and satisfactorily treat all periocular problems without thorough knowledge of the anatomy and procedures available for facial surgery. Although the surgeon should approach each operation with a basic surgical plan in mind, innovation and flexibility are essential in facial and eyelid surgery. Alternative scenarios should be mentally well rehearsed before surgery. Appropriate preoperative planning minimizes intraoperative indecision and ultimately enhances the final surgical result.

CHAPTER 9

Anatomy

Face

The surgeon who undertakes surgical manipulation of the face should clearly understand its anatomy and response to injury (ie, wound healing). The structural planes of the face include skin, subcutaneous tissue, the *superficial musculoaponeurotic system (SMAS)* and investing mimetic muscles, the deep facial fascia, and the plane containing the facial nerve, parotid duct, and buccal fat pad.

Subcutaneous fat lies beneath the dermis except in the eyelid. The thickness varies from person to person and from one area of the face to another. The cheeks, temples, and neck have the thickest subcutaneous fat pad. Connective tissue septa divide the subcutaneous fat into lobules.

Deep to orbicularis muscle overlying the maxillary and zygomatic periosteum is a plane of nonseptate fat called the *suborbicularis oculi fat (SOOF)*. This fat is continuous superiorly with the *retro-orbicularis oculi fat (ROOF)* situated deep to the eyebrow and extending in a varying amount as preaponeurotic fat into the upper eyelid.

The superficial facial fascia, an extension of the superficial cervical fascia in the neck, invests the facial mimetic muscles (platysma, zygomaticus major, zygomaticus minor, and orbicularis oculi), making up the SMAS (Fig 9-1). The SMAS distributes facial muscle contractions facilitating facial expression. These muscle actions are transmitted to the skin by ligamentous attachments located between the SMAS and the dermis. Relaxation of these supportive facial ligaments causes laxity and descent of facial soft tissue. Dissection and repositioning of the SMAS has important implications for facial cosmetic surgery.

The SMAS is connected to the underlying bone and overlying skin by a network of fibrous septa and ligaments. Thus, facial support is transmitted from the deep fixed structures of the face to the overlying dermis. Two major components of this system are the osteocutaneous ligaments (orbitomalar, zygomatic, and mandibular) and the ligaments formed by a condensation of superficial and deep facial fascias (parotidocutaneous and masseteric). As these ligaments become attenuated in conjunction with facial dermal elastosis, facial aging becomes apparent.

The mimetic muscles (Fig 9-2) can be grouped into superficial and deep categories. Superficial mimetic muscles that receive neurovascular supply to the posterior surface include the orbicularis oculi, platysma, zygomaticus major, zygomaticus minor, and risorius.

136 • Orbit, Eyelids, and Lacrimal System

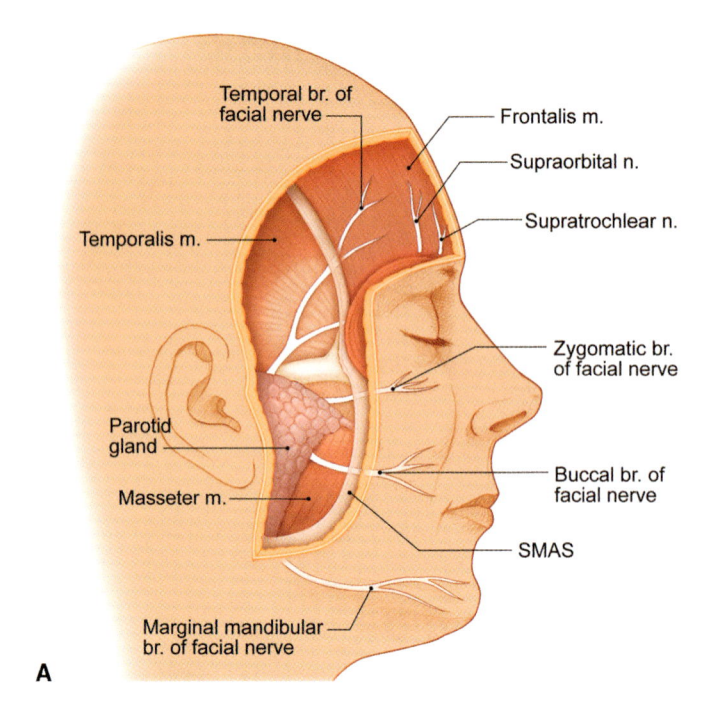

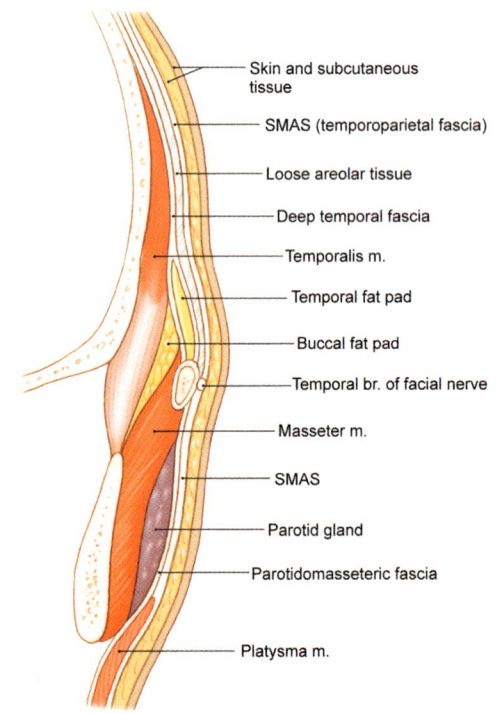

Figure 9-1 **A,** Superficial musculoaponeurotic system (SMAS). Note that the facial nerve branches inferior to the zygomatic arch are deep to the SMAS. **B,** Coronal section of face. The temporal branch of the facial nerve is found within the superficial portion of the temporal parietal fascia (extension of the SMAS). *(Illustrations by Christine Gralapp.)*

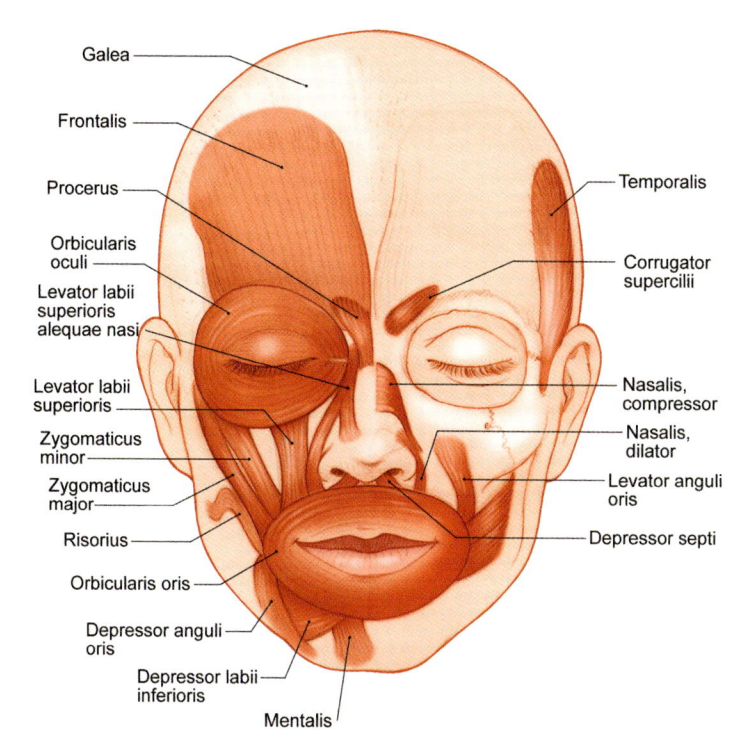

Figure 9-2 Facial mimetic muscles. *(Illustration by Christine Gralapp.)*

Deep mimetic muscles, which receive neurovascular supply to the anterior surface, include the buccinator, mentalis, and levator anguli oris. Other facial muscles include the orbicularis oris, masseter, temporalis, and multiple lip elevators and depressors.

The parotidomasseteric fascia is a continuation of the deep cervical fascia of the neck. It is important to remember that the facial nerve lies deep to this thin layer in the lower face. In the temporal region, above the zygomatic arch, this layer is continuous with the deep temporal fascia and the facial nerve (frontal branch) lies superficial to this fascial layer.

In the neck, the deep cervical fascia is found on the superficial surface of the strap muscles superior to the hyoid bone. It overlies the myelohyoid muscle and extends superiorly over the body of the mandible.

The facial nerve (CNVII), which innervates the mimetic muscles, divides into five major branches deep to the parotid gland (Fig 9-3): temporal (frontal), zygomatic, buccal, marginal mandibular, and cervical. Facial nerve injury creates regional paralysis leading to facial dysfunction and deformity. In general, dissection deep to the SMAS in the upper face and temporal region avoids the frontal nerve, whereas dissection superficial to the SMAS (especially anterior to the parotid gland) avoids the remaining facial nerve branches in the lower face. The face receives its sensory innervation from the three branches of the fifth cranial nerve: V_1, V_2, and V_3. Damage to these nerves causes numbness and paresthesia.

In the *upper face*, the frontal branch of the facial nerve pierces the frontalis muscle from its posterior surface. The supraorbital and supratrochlear neurovascular bundles

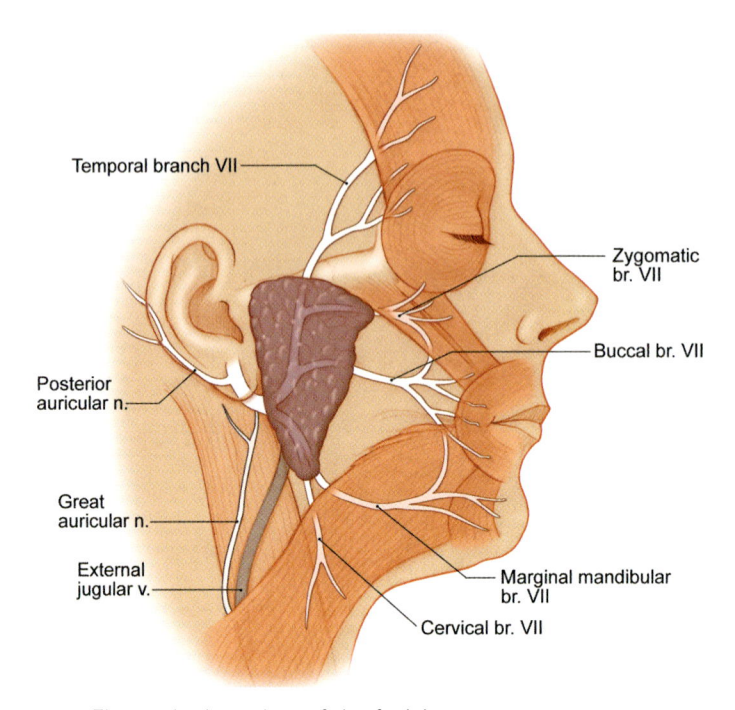

Figure 9-3 Five major branches of the facial nerve. *(Illustration by Christine Gralapp.)*

(branches of V_1) exit their respective foramina, coursing superiorly beneath the skin's surface and either within the superficial (superficial branch) or deep (deep branch) frontalis fascia. Dissection deep to the frontalis (ie, subgaleal or subperiosteal plane) avoids the frontal branch of the facial nerve and all sensory nerves. The frontalis, corrugator, and procerus muscles animate the forehead and glabella (see Fig 9-2). The frontalis elevates the eyebrows, causing transverse forehead rhytids. Chronic, static rhytidosis in the forehead results from chronic frontalis contracture related to brow ptosis and dermatochalasis. Chronic forehead rhytidosis may therefore be reduced with forehead lifting, brow lifting, blepharoplasty, or a combination thereof. Chronic contraction of the corrugator and procerus muscles leads to glabellar furrows that usually respond to botulinum toxin injections or direct muscle transection as part of a brow lift procedure.

In the *temporal area*, the frontal branch of the facial nerve (see Fig 9-3) crosses the zygomatic arch and courses superomedially in the deep layers of the temporoparietal fascia (SMAS). The temporoparietal fascia bridges the SMAS of the lower face to the galea aponeurosis of the upper face. Deep to the temporoparietal fascia, a dense, immobile fascia termed the *deep temporal fascia* overlies the temporalis muscle (see Fig 9-1B). Dissection along this fascia allows mobilization of the temporal forehead while avoiding the overlying frontal branch of the facial nerve. This is an important anatomic principle in brow and forehead lifting procedures.

In the *lower face*, the facial nerve branches, sensory nerves, vascular networks, and parotid gland and duct are deep to the SMAS (see Fig 9-1). The superficial mimetic muscles receive their neurovascular supply on their posterior surfaces; the deep mimetic muscles receive their neurovascular supply anteriorly. Dissection just superficial to the

SMAS, parotid gland, and parotidomasseteric fascia in the lower face avoids injury to all of these structures. In the neck, the deep cervical fascia is found on the superficial surface of the strap muscles superior to the hyoid bone.

Eyelids

For discussion purposes, the eyelids can be conveniently divided into the following seven structural layers:

- Skin and subcutaneous tissue
- Muscles of protraction
- Orbital septum
- Orbital fat
- Muscles of retraction
- Tarsus
- Conjunctiva

Figures 9-4, 9-5, and 9-6 detail the anatomy of the eyelids.

Skin and Subcutaneous Tissue

Eyelid skin is the thinnest of the body and unique in having no subcutaneous fat layer. Because the thin skin of the eyelids is subjected to constant movement with each blink, the laxity that often occurs with age is not unexpected. In both the upper and lower eyelids, the pretarsal tissues are normally firmly attached to the underlying tissues, whereas the preseptal tissues are more loosely attached, creating potential spaces for fluid accumulation. The upper eyelid crease approximates the attachments of the levator aponeurosis to the pretarsal orbicularis bundles and skin. This site is near or at the level of the superior border of the tarsus. The upper eyelid fold consists of the loose preseptal skin and subcutaneous tissues immediately superior to the tarsus. Asians normally have a relatively low upper eyelid crease because the orbital septum fuses with the levator aponeurosis between the eyelid margin and the superior border of the tarsus. This also allows preaponeurotic fat to occupy a position more inferior and anterior in the eyelid, creating a more pronounced upper eyelid fold. The crease in the lower eyelid is less well defined than that of the upper eyelid.

Protractors

The orbicularis oculi muscle is the main protractor of the eyelid. Contraction of this muscle, innervated by cranial nerve VII, narrows the palpebral fissure. Specific portions of this muscle also constitute the lacrimal pump.

The orbicularis muscle is divided into *pretarsal, preseptal,* and *orbital* parts (Fig 9-7). These divisions are both anatomic and physiologic. The palpebral (pretarsal and preseptal) parts are more involved in involuntary eyelid movements (blink), whereas the orbital portion is primarily involved in forced eyelid closure (winking and blepharospasm). The pretarsal parts of the upper and lower eyelid orbicularis arise from deep origins at the posterior lacrimal crest and superficial origins at the anterior limb of the medial canthal

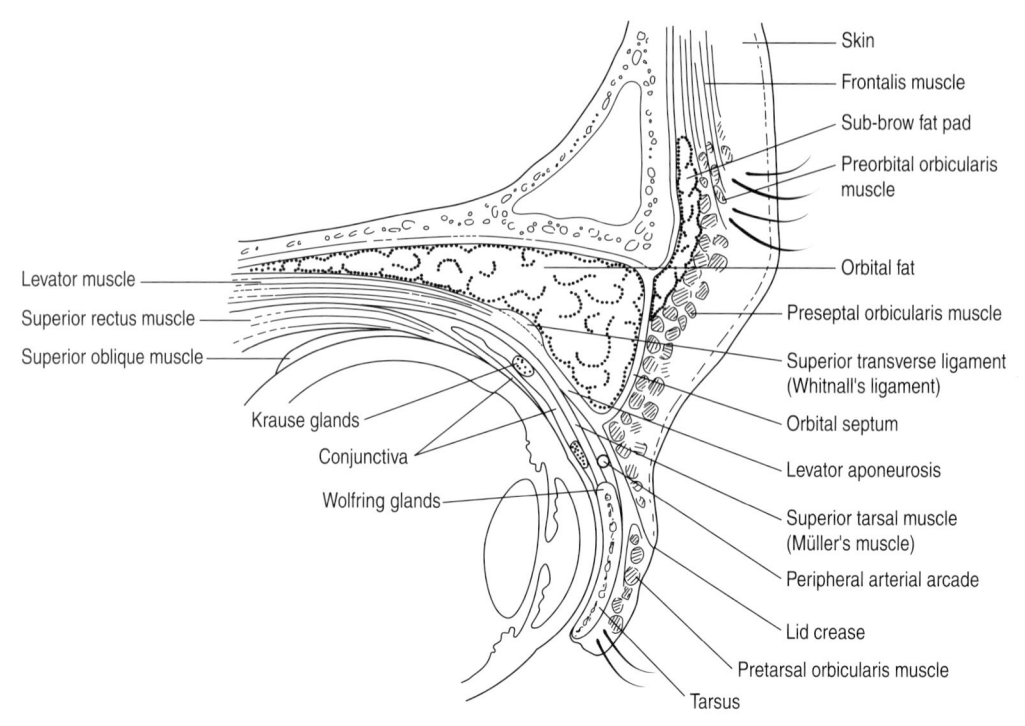

Figure 9-4 Upper eyelid anatomy. *(Modified from Stewart WB.* Surgery of the Eyelid, Orbit, and Lacrimal System. *Ophthalmology Monograph 8, vol 2. San Francisco: American Academy of Ophthalmology; 1994:85. Illustration by Jeanne C. Koelling.)*

tendon. The deep head of the pretarsal muscle (Horner's tensor tarsi), a localized bundle of pretarsal orbicularis, encircles both canaliculi to facilitate tear drainage. The upper and lower eyelid segments of the pretarsal orbicularis fuse in the lateral canthal area to become the lateral canthal tendon. The corrugator muscle draws the head of the eyebrows to the nose and is responsible for vertical furrows on the bridge of the nose. Contraction of the procerus muscle depresses the head of the eyebrow, resulting in horizontal furrows in the skin overlying the bridge of the nose.

The preseptal orbicularis muscles have deep origins from the fascia around the lacrimal sac and the posterior lacrimal crest. Superficial origins arise from the anterior limb of the medial canthal tendon. Laterally, the preseptal muscles form the lateral palpebral raphe overlying the lateral orbital rim. The orbital portions of the orbicularis muscle arise from the anterior limb of the medial canthal tendon and the surrounding periosteum. These fibers course over the zygoma, covering the elevator muscles of the lip.

Orbital Septum

The orbital septum, a thin multilayered sheet of fibrous tissue, arises from the periosteum over the superior and inferior orbital rims at the arcus marginalis. In the upper eyelid, the orbital septum fuses with the levator aponeurosis 2–5 mm above the superior tarsal border in non-Asians. In the lower eyelid, the orbital septum fuses with the capsulopalpebral fascia at or just below the inferior tarsal border. The fused capsulopalpebral orbital

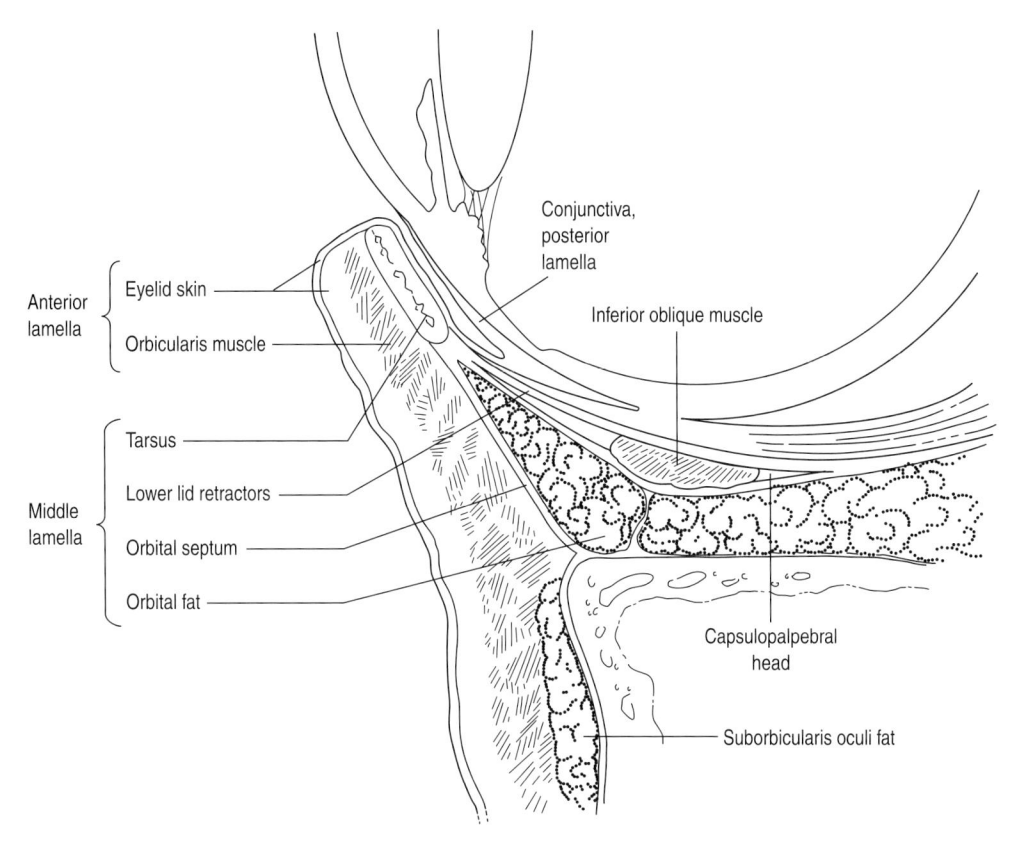

Figure 9-5 Lower eyelid anatomy. *(Modified from Stewart WB. Surgery of the Eyelid, Orbit, and Lacrimal System. Ophthalmology Monograph 8, vol 2. San Francisco: American Academy of Ophthalmology; 1994:23. Illustration by Jeanne C. Koelling.)*

septum complex, along with a small contribution from the inferior tarsal smooth muscle, inserts on both the posterior and the anterior tarsal surfaces as well as the tapered inferior border of the tarsus. In elderly patients, the septum in both the upper and the lower eyelids can become quite attenuated.

> Meyer DR, Linberg JV, Wobig JL, et al. Anatomy of the orbital septum and associated eyelid connective tissues. *Ophthal Plast Reconstr Surg.* 1991;7:104–113.

Orbital Fat

The orbital septum serves as a barrier between the orbit and the eyelid to limit the spread of infection and hemorrhage. The orbital fat normally lies posterior to the orbital septum and anterior to the levator aponeurosis. With age-related attenuation of the septum, orbital fat sometimes herniates anteriorly into the eyelids. The central orbital fat pad is an important landmark in both elective eyelid surgery and eyelid laceration repair because it lies directly behind the orbital septum and in front of the levator aponeurosis.

142 • Orbit, Eyelids, and Lacrimal System

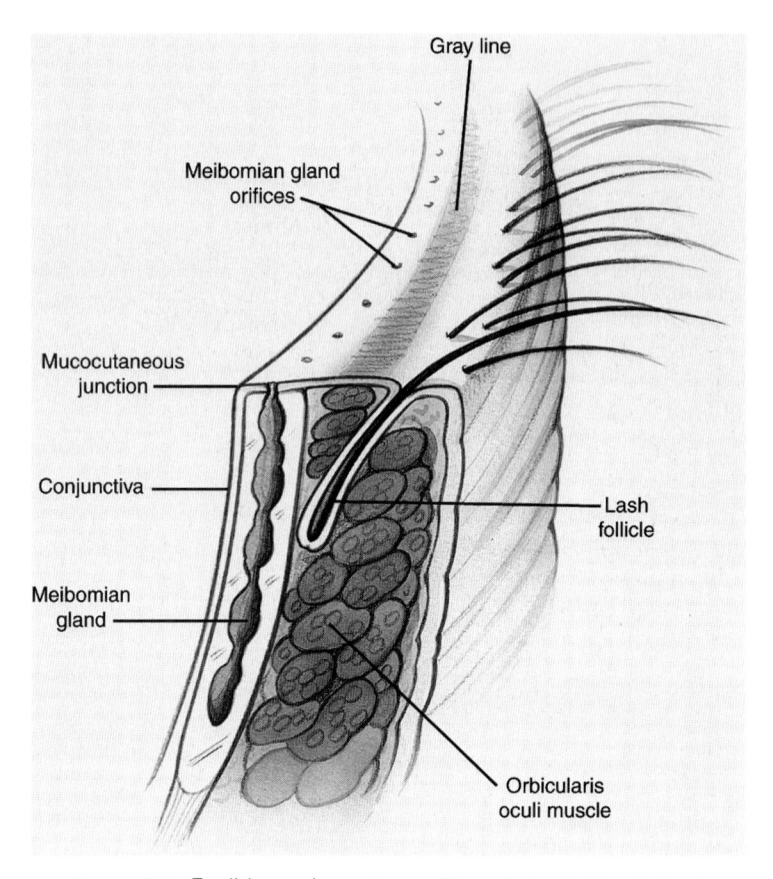

Figure 9-6 Eyelid margin anatomy. *(Illustration by Christine Gralapp.)*

Retractors

The retractors of the upper eyelid are the levator muscle with its aponeurosis and the sympathetically innervated superior tarsal muscle (Müller's muscle). In the lower eyelid, the retractors are the capsulopalpebral fascia and the inferior tarsal muscle.

Upper eyelid retractors

The levator muscle originates in the apex of the orbit from the periorbita of the lesser wing of the sphenoid, just above the annulus of Zinn. The muscular portion of the levator is approximately 40 mm long; the aponeurosis is 14–20 mm in length. The superior transverse ligament (Whitnall's ligament) is a condensation of elastic fibers of the anterior sheath of the levator muscle located in the area of transition from levator muscle to levator aponeurosis, which is composed of collagen and elastic fibers (Fig 9-8).

Whitnall's ligament functions primarily as a suspensory support for the upper eyelid and the superior orbital tissues. The ligament also acts as a fulcrum for the levator, transferring its vector force from an anterior–posterior to a superior–inferior direction. Its analogue in the lower eyelid is Lockwood's ligament. Medially, Whitnall's ligament attaches to connective tissue around the trochlea and superior oblique tendon. Laterally, it forms septa through the stroma of the lacrimal gland, then arches upward to attach to

CHAPTER 9: Anatomy • 143

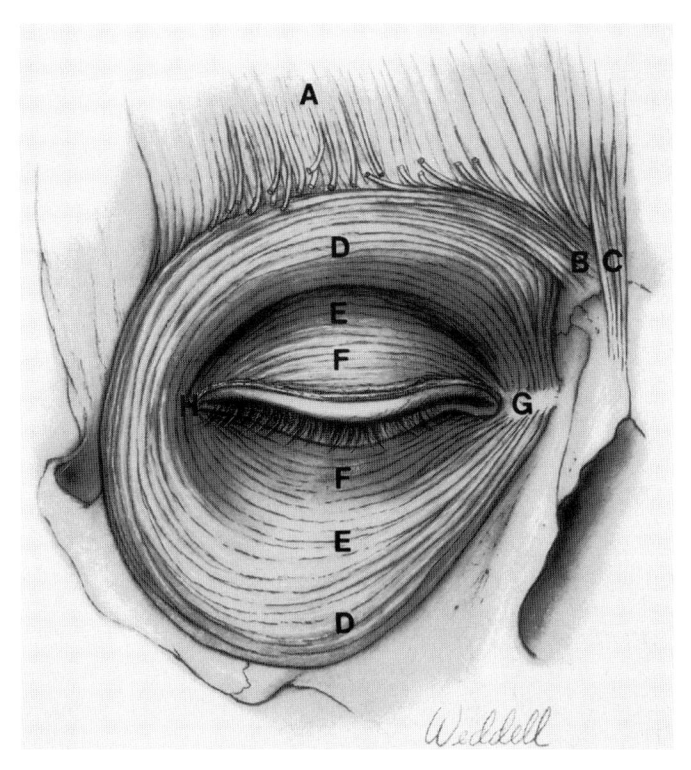

Figure 9-7 Orbicularis muscle and related musculature. *A,* Frontalis muscles; *B,* superciliary corrugator muscle; *C,* procerus muscle; *D,* orbicularis muscle (orbital portion); *E,* orbicularis muscle (preseptal portion); *F,* orbicularis muscle (pretarsal portion); *G,* medial canthal tendon; *H,* lateral canthal tendon. *(From Beard C.* Ptosis. *3rd ed. St. Louis: Mosby; 1981.)*

the inner aspect of the lateral orbital wall approximately 10 mm above the orbital tubercle. There are other attachments to the roof of the orbit. Whitnall's ligament has sometimes been confused with the horns of the levator aponeurosis and mistakenly illustrated as a structure to be cut during ptosis surgery. However, the horns of the levator aponeurosis lie more inferior and toward the canthi. The lateral horn inserts onto the lateral orbital tubercle; the medial horn inserts onto the posterior lacrimal crest.

As the levator aponeurosis continues toward the tarsus, it divides into an anterior and posterior portion a variable distance above the superior tarsal border. The anterior portion is composed of fine strands of aponeurosis that insert into the septa between the pretarsal orbicularis muscle bundles. These fine attachments are responsible for the close apposition of the pretarsal skin and orbicularis muscle to the underlying tarsus. The upper eyelid crease is formed by the most superior of these attachments and by contraction of the underlying levator complex. The upper eyelid fold is created by the overhanging skin and orbicularis muscle superior to the crease.

Codere F, Tucker NA, Renaldi B. The anatomy of Whitnall ligament. *Ophthalmology.* 1995; 102:2016–2019.

Doxanas MT, Anderson RL. Oriental eyelids. An anatomic study. *Arch Ophthalmol.* 1984; 102:1232–1235.

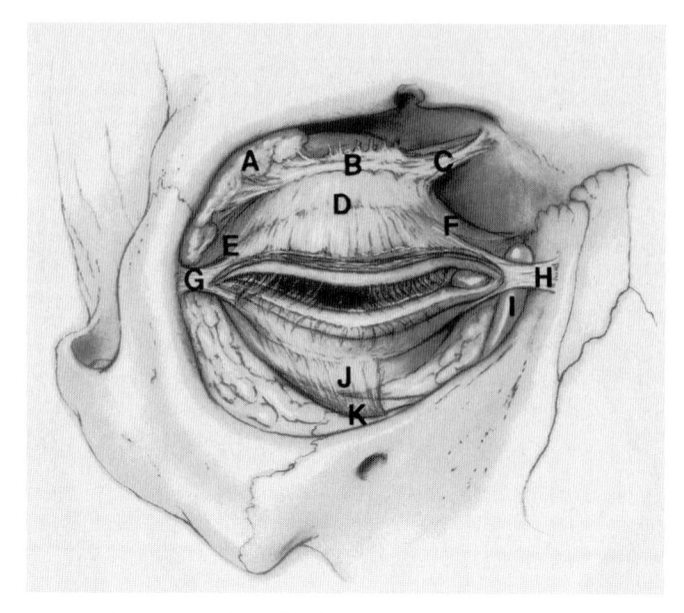

Figure 9-8 Deeper eyelid and anterior orbital structures from anterior view. *A,* Lacrimal gland; *B,* superior transverse ligament (Whitnall's ligament); *C,* superior oblique tendon sheath; *D,* levator aponeurosis; *E,* lateral horn; *F,* medial horn; *G,* lateral canthal tendon; *H,* medial canthal tendon; *I,* lacrimal sac; *J,* lower eyelid retractors; *K,* inferior oblique muscle. *(From Beard C.* Ptosis. *3rd ed. St. Louis: Mosby; 1981.)*

Stasior GO, Lemke BN, Wallow IH, et al. Levator aponeurosis elastic fiber network. *Ophthal Plast Reconstr Surg.* 1993;9:1–10.

The posterior portion of the levator aponeurosis inserts firmly onto the anterior surface of the lower half of the tarsus. It is most firmly attached approximately 3 mm above the eyelid margin and is only very loosely attached to the superior 2–3 mm of the tarsus. The lateral horn of the levator aponeurosis is strong, and it divides the lacrimal gland into orbital and palpebral lobes, attaching firmly to the orbital tubercle. The medial horn of the aponeurosis is more delicate and forms loose connective attachments to the posterior aspect of the medial canthal tendon and to the posterior lacrimal crest. Disinsertion, dehiscence, or rarefaction of the aponeurosis may give rise to ptosis following intraocular inflammation or intraocular surgery. In many cases of ptosis following intraocular surgery, a small amount of aponeurotic ptosis was already present.

Müller's muscle originates at the undersurface of the levator aponeurosis approximately at the level of Whitnall's ligament, 12–14 mm above the upper tarsal margin. This sympathetically innervated muscle extends inferiorly to insert along the upper eyelid superior tarsal margin. This muscle provides approximately 2 mm of elevation of the upper eyelid; if it is interrupted (as in Horner syndrome), mild ptosis results. Müller's muscle is firmly attached to the adjacent conjunctiva posteriorly, especially just above the superior tarsal border. The peripheral arterial arcade is found between the levator aponeurosis and Müller's muscle just above the superior tarsal border. This vascular arcade serves as a useful surgical landmark to identify Müller's muscle.

Lower eyelid retractors

The capsulopalpebral fascia in the lower eyelid is analogous to the levator aponeurosis in the upper eyelid. The fascia originates as the capsulopalpebral head from attachments to the terminal muscle fibers of the inferior rectus muscle. The capsulopalpebral head divides as it encircles the inferior oblique muscle and fuses with its sheath of the inferior oblique muscle. Anterior to the inferior oblique muscle, the two portions of the capsulopalpebral head join to form Lockwood's suspensory ligament. The capsulopalpebral fascia extends anteriorly from this point, sending strands to the inferior conjunctival fornix, the suspensory ligament of the fornix. The capsulopalpebral fascia inserts onto the inferior tarsal border, just after it fuses with the orbital septum.

The inferior tarsal muscle in the lower eyelid is analogous to Müller's muscle. The poorly developed inferior tarsal muscle runs posterior to the capsulopalpebral fascia. The smooth muscle fibers are most abundant in the area of the inferior fornix.

Tarsus

The tarsi are firm dense plates of connective tissue that serve as the skeleton of the eyelids. The upper eyelid tarsal plates measure 10–12 mm vertically in the center of the eyelid; the maximum lower eyelid tarsal plate measurement is 4 mm or less. The tarsal plates have rigid attachments to the periosteum medially and laterally. The upper eyelid tarsal plate often becomes laterally displaced with age as a result of stretching of the medial supporting tendons. Both tarsal plates are usually 1 mm thick and taper at the medial and lateral ends. In the upper eyelid, the marginal arterial arcade lies 2 mm superior to the margin near the follicles of the cilia and anterior to the tarsal plate. The marginal arterial arcade should not be confused with the peripheral arterial arcade, which lies superior to the tarsus between the levator aponeurosis and Müller's muscle. The lower eyelid often has only one arterial arcade located at the inferior tarsal border.

Conjunctiva

The conjunctiva is composed of nonkeratinizing squamous epithelium. It forms the posterior layer of the eyelids and contains the mucin-secreting goblet cells and the accessory lacrimal glands of Krause and Wolfring. The accessory lacrimal glands are found in the subconjunctival tissue mainly in the upper eyelid between the superior tarsal border and the fornix. A few accessory lacrimal glands are found in the lower eyelid in the area of the inferior fornix. Traditionally, secretions from these glands have been regarded as the major components of the basic lacrimal secretion in contrast with the reflex tear secretion from the parasympathetically innervated main lacrimal gland. Concepts regarding basic and reflex tearing are still evolving, however, and all tearing may be found to be caused by reflex.

Other Anatomical Considerations

Suborbicularis fat pads

The suborbicularis oculi fat (SOOF) consists of the deep subcutaneous fat and connective tissue lying beneath the orbicularis muscle in the lower eyelid and extending into the midfacial soft tissues. The SOOF plays an important role in the aging process of gradual gravitational descent of the midfacial soft tissues. Recent studies and surgical procedures suggest that elevation of the SOOF into its previous anatomic position restores the normal youthful contours in the lower eyelid and midfacial soft tissues.

Similarly, the sub-brow fat pad undergoes gravitational descent, compounding a redundant upper eyelid skin fold. The displaced sub-brow fat pad can easily be confused with a coexisting redundant upper eyelid fold and prominent prolapsed upper eyelid preaponeurotic fat pad. An adequate functional and aesthetic result requires that standard blepharoplasty surgery be used to surgically resect the redundant aspect of the sub-brow fat pad.

Canthal tendons

The configuration of the palpebral fissure is maintained by the medial and lateral canthal tendons in conjunction with the attached tarsal plates. The two origins of the medial canthal tendon from the anterior and posterior lacrimal crests fuse just temporal to the lacrimal sac and then again split into an upper limb and a lower limb that attach to the upper and lower tarsal plates. The attachment of the tendon to the periosteum overlying the anterior lacrimal crest is diffuse and strong; the attachment to the posterior lacrimal crest is more delicate but important in maintaining apposition of the eyelids to the globe, allowing the puncta to lie in the tear lake.

The lateral canthal tendon attaches at the lateral orbital tubercle on the inner aspect of the orbital rim. It splits into superior and inferior branches that attach to the respective tarsal plates. Cutting, stretching, or disinsertion of either of the canthal tendons usually causes cosmetic or functional problems such as telecanthus and horizontal eyelid laxity. Horizontal eyelid instability is almost always the result of lateral canthal lengthening. Therefore, surgical correction should be directed at shortening the lateral canthus, rather than resecting the normal eyelid in the palpebral fissure. The lateral canthal tendon usually inserts 2 mm higher than does the medial canthal tendon, giving the normal horizontal palpebral fissure an upward slope medial to lateral. When the lateral canthal tendon inserts lower than the medial canthal tendon, an antimongoloid slant occurs.

Eyelid margin

The mucocutaneous junction of the eyelid margin is often erroneously referred to as the *gray line.* The actual gray line is clearly visible in most patients. It consists of an isolated section of pretarsal orbicularis muscle (Riolan's) just anterior to the tarsus. The mucocutaneous junction is located posterior to the meibomian gland orifices on the eyelid margin (see Fig 9-6). The horizontal palpebral fissure is approximately 30 mm long. The main portion of the margin, called the *ciliary margin,* has a rather well-defined anterior and posterior edge. Medial to the punctum, the eyelid is thinner because of the lack of ciliary follicles.

> Wulc AE, Dryden RM, Khatchaturian T. Where is the gray line? *Arch Ophthalmol.* 1987; 105:1092–1098.

Eyelashes

There are approximately 100 eyelashes in the upper eyelid and 50 in the lower eyelid. The lashes usually originate from the anterior aspect of the eyelid margin just anterior to the tarsal plate and form two or three irregular rows. A few cilia may be found on the caruncle.

Meibomian glands

The meibomian glands originate in the tarsus and number approximately 25 in the upper eyelid and 20 in the lower eyelid. Both the eyelashes and the meibomian glands differentiate during the second month of gestation from a common pilosebaceous unit. This dual potentiality explains why, following trauma or chronic irritation, a lash follicle may develop from a meibomian gland *(acquired distichiasis)*. Similarly, an extra row of lashes arising from the meibomian orifices may be present from birth *(congenital distichiasis)*.

Vascular supply

The extensive vascularity of the eyelids promotes healing and helps defend against infection. The arterial supply of the eyelids comes from two main sources: (1) the internal carotid artery by way of the ophthalmic artery and its branches (supraorbital and lacrimal) and (2) the external carotid artery by way of the arteries of the face (angular and temporal). Collateral circulation between these two systems is extensive, anastomosing throughout the upper and lower eyelid and forming the marginal and peripheral arcades in the eyelids.

Eyelid venous drainage may be divided into pretarsal and posttarsal. The *pretarsal* tissues drain into the angular vein medially and into the superficial temporal vein laterally. *Posttarsal* drainage is into the orbital veins and the deeper branches of the anterior facial vein and pterygoid plexus. Lymphatic vessels serving the medial portion of the eyelids drain into the submandibular lymph nodes. Lymph channels serving the lateral portions of the eyelids drain first into the superficial preauricular nodes and then into the deeper cervical nodes.

Nerve supply

Sensory nerve supply to the eyelids is provided by branches of the first and second divisions of cranial nerve V. Branches of the supraorbital nerve (V_1) innervate the forehead and lateral periocular region. Branches of the maxillary nerve (V_2) innervate the lower eyelid and cheek. The motor nerve supply to the eyelids is provided by cranial nerve III, cranial nerve VII, and the sympathetic nerves.

CHAPTER 10

Principles of Facial and Eyelid Surgery

Patient Preparation

Proper patient selection, adequate preoperative evaluation, and meticulous surgical techniques enhance surgical outcome and help ensure predictable results. A basic understanding of wound healing and postoperative infection is mandatory.

Facial and eyelid surgery should be approached with care. Adequate preoperative preparation includes properly informing the patient about the proposed benefit of the procedure and its potential complications. Although a surgeon might wish to put the patient at ease by using such words as *routine* or *simple,* downplaying possible problems is inappropriate and misleading. Such reassurances imply that surgery is free of complications when, in actuality, significant complications—including facial nerve paralysis and loss of vision—are potential risks.

The patient should be encouraged to read, understand, and sign an operative consent in the relaxed atmosphere of the office. It is preferable to obtain this consent prior to the day of surgery, when patient anxiety or preoperative medication may make informed consent impossible. The patient must have an opportunity to discuss with the surgeon any concerns about the permit or the procedure.

Care must be taken to minimize surgical trauma to the tissue. The surgeon must be thoroughly familiar with the specialized instruments necessary for facial surgery. Careful selection and meticulous care of instruments allows for gentle manipulation of facial soft tissue with minimal trauma.

Postoperatively, both the patient and home caregivers should be given detailed oral and written instructions. Grafts and flaps require attention to wound hygiene to reduce the risk of tissue necrosis or infection. Careful follow-up and appropriately timed suture removal are essential.

Few patients undergo surgery without some degree of apprehension, which can be minimized with the following measures:

- Preoperative counseling regarding the anticipated sequence of events, including the surgical procedure and postoperative care
- Careful attention to any general medical problems of the patient
- An ongoing calm, reassuring attitude on the part of the surgeon, nursing staff, and administrative personnel

Anesthesia

Local anesthesia with patient cooperation allows the surgeon to assess lid margin height during eyelid surgery, improving accuracy in ptosis repair and eyelid retraction procedures. Anesthesia may be obtained by local infiltration, regional block, or a combination of the two techniques. Local infiltration, however, is usually adequate.

The newer, long-acting anesthetics are useful in procedures that require more than an hour of operating time. The administration of epinephrine with the anesthetic agent prolongs the anesthetic duration and decreases the rate of systemic absorption, but potential cardiac side effects must be considered. Hemostasis is also enhanced by epinephrine, provided that the surgeon is willing to wait for approximately 10 minutes between injection and incision for maximum vasoconstriction. Adding hyaluronidase to the anesthetic solution improves the soft tissue dispersion of the anesthetic agent. Buffering of the local anesthetic with bicarbonate may decrease the pain of local infiltration.

Patient safety and comfort are priorities; therefore, the smallest amount of the lowest concentration of anesthetic agent that will provide the desired effect should be used. Routine monitoring of the electrocardiogram, pulse oximeter, and the vital signs throughout the procedure by experienced personnel and establishment of intravenous access for quick handling of any emergency increase the margin of safety. Monitored intravenous sedation is a helpful adjunct for more prolonged or invasive procedures. The use of selective hypnotics and analgesics can decrease the patient's anxiety level and enhance the effectiveness of local anesthesia.

General anesthesia is usually necessary for performing longer, more complex facial surgeries or procedures on children. Any family history of an unexplained anesthetic death should alert the surgeon to the possibility of malignant hyperthermia (MH), necessitating a preoperative anesthesiology consultation. Although MH is more common in association with musculoskeletal ocular conditions, such as ptosis or strabismus, the clinical use of skeletal muscle biopsy results as a predictor of MH is controversial. See BCSC Section 1, *Update on General Medicine,* or Section 6, *Pediatric Ophthalmology and Strabismus,* for fuller discussions of MH, including treatment protocols.

Careful attention to the patient's general medical problems is mandatory, whether or not such conditions are related to the planned surgery. Every patient should also be asked about any history of bleeding diatheses or use of anticoagulants (eg, warfarin sodium [Coumadin]), antiplatelet agents including aspirin, nonsteroidal anti-inflammatory drugs (NSAIDs), or a variety of over-the-counter preparations (eg, ginkgo biloba, vitamin E). Patients using anticoagulants such as warfarin are usually asked to discontinue the medication 5 days before elective surgery if approved by the patient's primary care physician. Aspirin, because of its irreversible platelet inhibitory function, should be stopped 2 weeks before elective surgery. NSAIDs, which are reversible platelet inhibitors, should be stopped 24–72 hours before surgery. Platelet inhibitors may lead to severe operative or postoperative bleeding with resultant cosmetic and functional adverse sequelae. Bleeding time is clinically helpful, although it is an inexact test. Prothrombin time and partial thromboplastin time may be useful tests if coagulation status is a concern. A more complicated history of poor clotting should be followed up with a preoperative hematologic and oncologic consultation.

For more extensive discussion of surgical considerations, see Chapter 15, Perioperative Management in Ocular Surgery, in BCSC Section 1, *Update on General Medicine*.

Ang-Lee MK, Moss J, Yuan C. Herbal medicines and perioperative care. *JAMA*. 2001;286: 208–216.

Eccarius SG, Gordon ME, Parelman JJ. Bicarbonate-buffered lidocaine-epinephrine-hyaluronidase for eyelid anesthesia. *Ophthalmology*. 1990;97:1499–1501.

Heiman-Patterson TD. Malignant hyperthermia. *Semin Neurol*. 1991;11:220–227.

CHAPTER 11

Classification and Management of Eyelid Disorders

Like the orbit, the eyelids can be affected by a variety of congenital, infectious, inflammatory, neoplastic, and traumatic conditions. These disorders and their management are discussed in this chapter. In addition, the eyelids are subject to various positional abnormalities and involutional changes; these disorders are discussed in Chapter 12.

Congenital Anomalies

Congenital anomalies of the eyelid may be isolated or associated with other eyelid, facial, or systemic anomalies. Careful evaluation of patients in cases of hereditary syndromes is helpful prior to proceeding with treatment. Most congenital anomalies of the eyelids occur during the second month of gestation because of a failure of fusion or an arrest of development. The majority of the defects described below are rare. (See also BCSC Section 6, *Pediatric Ophthalmology and Strabismus*.)

Blepharophimosis Syndrome

This congenital eyelid syndrome is an autosomal dominantly inherited blepharophimosis, usually presenting with telecanthus (widened intercanthal distance), epicanthus inversus (fold of skin extending from the lower to upper eyelid), and severe ptosis. Additional findings may include lateral lower eyelid ectropion secondary to anterior lamellar deficiency, a poorly developed nasal bridge, hypoplasia of the superior orbital rims, lop ears, and hypertelorism (Fig 11-1).

Reconstruction is often carried out in multiple stages. Initially, the telecanthus and epicanthus inversus are corrected by multiple Z-plasties or Y-V-plasties, sometimes combined with transnasal wiring of the elongated medial canthal tendons. In 3 or 4 months, a bilateral frontalis sling procedure is performed to correct the ptosis. Sufficient levator function may be present to allow ptosis correction using levator aponeurosis resection. Additional procedures may be needed to correct associated problems such as ectropion or hypoplasia of the orbital rims.

> Anderson RL, Nowinski TS. The five-flap technique for blepharophimosis. *Arch Ophthalmol*. 1989;107:448–452.

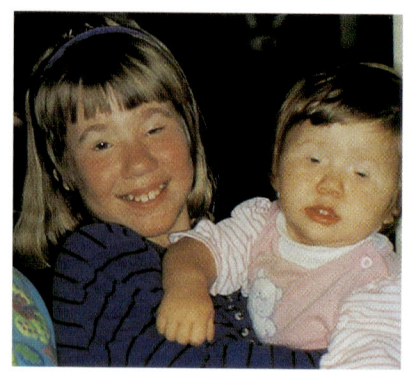

Figure 11-1 Blepharophimosis syndrome. *(Photograph courtesy of Jeffrey A. Nerad, MD.)*

Congenital Ptosis of the Upper Eyelid

Congenital ptosis of the upper eyelid is discussed in Chapter 12 as part of a general review of all types of blepharoptosis.

Congenital Ectropion

In rare cases, congenital ectropion occurs as an isolated finding. It is more often associated with blepharophimosis syndrome or with ichthyosis. Congenital ectropion is caused by a vertical insufficiency of the anterior lamella of the eyelid and, if severe, may give rise to chronic epiphora and exposure keratitis. Mild congenital ectropion usually requires no treatment. If it is severe and symptomatic, it is treated like a cicatricial ectropion, with horizontal tightening of the lateral canthal tendon and vertical lengthening of the anterior lamella using a full-thickness skin graft.

A complete eversion of the upper eyelids occasionally occurs in newborns (Fig 11-2). Topical lubrication and short-term patching of both eyes is often curative. Full-thickness sutures or a temporary tarsorrhaphy may be necessary. Possible causes include inclusion conjunctivitis, anterior lamellar inflammation or shortage, or Down syndrome.

Euryblepharon

Euryblepharon is a unilateral or bilateral horizontal widening of the palpebral fissure often associated with blepharophimosis syndrome. Euryblepharon usually involves the lateral portion of the lower eyelids and is associated with both vertical shortening and horizontal lengthening of the involved eyelids (Fig 11-3). The palpebral fissure often has an antimongoloid slant because of inferiorly displaced lateral canthal tendon. Impaired blinking, poor closure, and lagophthalmos may result in exposure keratitis. If symptoms necessitate treatment, reconstruction may include full-thickness resection of excess eyelid length with or without canthal tendon repositioning and vertical eyelid lengthening using a full-thickness skin graft.

Ankyloblepharon

Ankyloblepharon is partial or complete fusion of the eyelids by webs of skin (see Fig 11-3). These webs can usually be opened with scissors after the web is clamped for a few

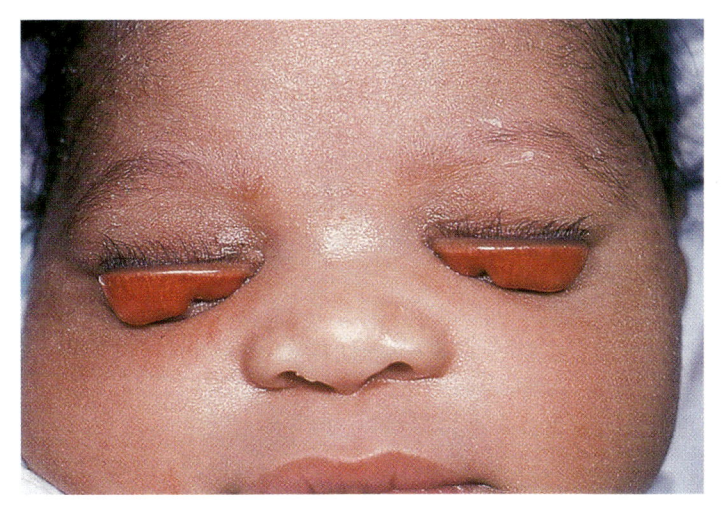

CHAPTER 11: Classification and Management of Eyelid Disorders • 155

Figure 11-2 Congenital eyelid eversion. *(Photograph courtesy of Thaddeus S. Nowinski, MD.)*

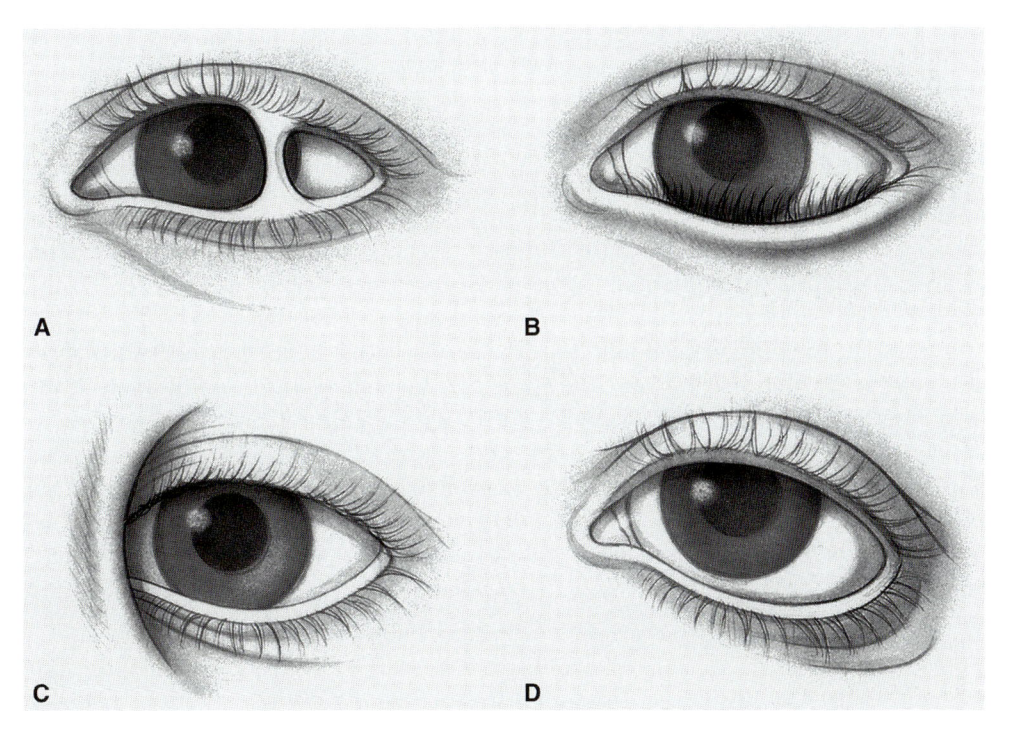

Figure 11-3 Congenital eyelid deformities. **A,** Ankyloblepharon. **B,** Epiblepharon. **C,** Epicanthus. **D,** Euryblepharon. *(Illustration by Christine Gralapp.)*

seconds with a hemostat. To prevent readhesion at the sites of operation, the skin and conjunctiva should be primarily apposed with sutures. More severe forms of ankyloblepharon that appear in conjunction with craniofacial deformities may require extensive reconstruction.

Epicanthus

Epicanthus is a medial canthal fold that may result from immature midfacial bones or a fold of skin and subcutaneous tissue (see Fig 11-3). The condition is usually bilateral. An affected child may appear esotropic because of decreased scleral exposure nasally *(pseudostrabismus)*. Traditionally, four types of epicanthus are described:

- *Epicanthus tarsalis* if the fold is most prominent in the upper eyelid
- *Epicanthus inversus* if the fold is most prominent in the lower eyelid
- *Epicanthus palpebralis* if the fold is equally distributed in the upper and lower eyelids
- *Epicanthus supraciliaris* if the fold arises from the eyebrow region running to the lacrimal sac

Epicanthus tarsalis is most frequently associated with the Asian eyelid, whereas epicanthus inversus is almost invariably associated with blepharophimosis syndrome.

Most forms of epicanthus resolve with normal growth of the facial bones. If no associated eyelid anomalies are present, treatment should be delayed until the face achieves maturity. Epicanthus inversus, however, rarely improves with facial growth. Most cases of isolated epicanthus requiring treatment respond well to linear revisions such as Z-plasty or Y-V-plasty. Epicanthus tarsalis in the Asian patient may be eliminated by a Y-V-plasty with or without construction of an upper eyelid crease.

Epiblepharon

In epiblepharon, the lower eyelid pretarsal muscle and skin ride above the lower eyelid margin to form a horizontal fold of tissue that causes the cilia to assume a vertical position (see Fig 11-3). The eyelid margin, therefore, is in normal position with respect to the globe. Epiblepharon is most common in Asian children.

Clinically, the cilia often do not touch the cornea except in downgaze. Epiblepharon usually requires no treatment because it tends to disappear with the maturation of the facial bones and the lashes rarely cause corneal staining. However, epiblepharon occasionally results in keratitis; in that case, the excess skin and muscle fold should be excised just inferior to the eyelid margin (in the case of the lower eyelid) and the skin edges approximated.

Congenital Entropion

In distinction from epiblepharon, eyelid margin inversion is present in congenital entropion. Developmental factors that lead to this rare condition include lower eyelid retractor dysgenesis, structural defects in the tarsal plate, and relative shortening of the posterior lamella. Congenital entropion often does not improve spontaneously and may require surgical correction.

Tarsal kink of the upper eyelid is an unusual form of congenital entropion. It may be repaired by incision of the kink combined with a marginal rotation (see Chapter 12, Fig 12-7).

Bartley GB, Nerad JA, Kersten RC, et al. Congenital entropion with intact lower eyelid retractor insertion. *Am J Ophthalmol.* 1991;112:437–441.

Congenital Distichiasis

Distichiasis is a rare, sometimes hereditary condition in which an extra row of eyelashes is present in place of the openings of the meibomian glands. Congenital distichiasis occurs when embryonic pilosebaceous units improperly differentiate into hair follicles. Treatment of this condition is indicated if the patient is symptomatic or if evidence of corneal irritation is present. Lubricants and soft contact lenses may be sufficient, but cryoepilation may be offered as an alternative. Eyelid splitting with cryoepilation or surgical removal of the abnormal follicles in the tarsal plate may preserve the normal eyelashes. Replacement of large areas of removed tarsal plate requires buccal mucosal grafting.

Boynton JR. Management of cicatricial entropion, trichiasis, and distichiasis. In: *Focal Points: Clinical Modules for Ophthalmologists.* San Francisco: American Academy of Ophthalmology; 1993: vol 11, no 12.

Vaughn GL, Dortzbach RK, Sires BS, et al. Eyelid splitting with excision or microhyfercation for distichiasis. *Arch Ophthalmol.* 1997;115:282–284.

Congenital Coloboma

A coloboma is an embryologic cleft that is usually an isolated anomaly when it occurs in the medial upper eyelid. When found in the lower eyelid, however, the coloboma is frequently associated with other congenital conditions such as facial clefts (eg, Goldenhar syndrome) and lacrimal deformities. A true coloboma includes a defect in the eyelid margin (Fig 11-4).

Full-thickness defects affecting up to one third of the eyelid can usually be repaired by creating a rectangular surgical wound between the eyelid crease line and the eyelid margin. The cut edges of the tarsus are then advanced along the eyelid crease line and repaired with direct closure. A lateral cantholysis may provide additional horizontal

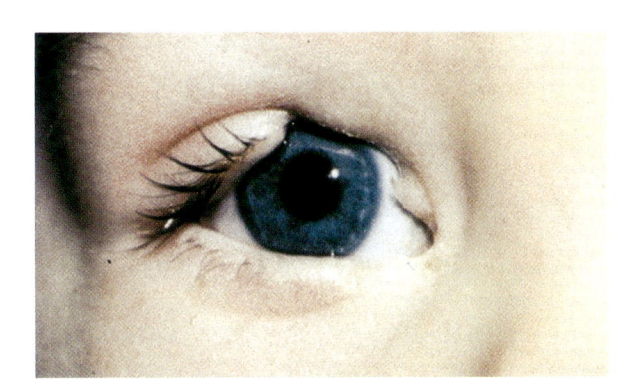

Figure 11-4 True coloboma of upper eyelid.

relaxation. Almost all large defects can be repaired using a variation of the lateral canthal semicircular flap (see Eyelid Defects Involving the Eyelid Margin later in this chapter).

To avoid deprivation amblyopia, eyelid-sharing procedures that occlude the visual axis should not be used in children unless no other reconstructive alternative will preserve the eye.

Congenital Eyelid Lesions

Although capillary hemangiomas sometimes occur as congenital eyelid lesions, most are not apparent at birth. Rather, they usually appear over the first weeks or months of life. Hemangiomas may also involve the orbit (see under Vascular Tumors in Chapter 5). They are associated with a high incidence of amblyopia; therefore, treatment is recommended for patients who present with occlusion of the visual axis, anisometropia, or strabismus, as well as for those with lesions causing significant disfigurement. In the typical natural course of capillary hemangioma, the lesion occurs shortly after birth, increases in size until the patient is 1 year old, and then decreases over the next 4–5 years.

Intralesional corticosteroid injection is the current treatment of choice in patients whose vision is threatened. Intralesional steroids presumably act by rendering the tumor's vascular bed more sensitive to the body's circulating catecholamines. This technique is relatively safe, simple, and repeatable. However, rare cases of eyelid necrosis, embolic retinal vascular occlusion, and systemic adrenal suppression may occur following even a single injection. Other treatment methods (such as external radiation, radioactive implants, and systemic corticosteroids) used for capillary hemangiomas in the past have all been associated with a significant incidence of complications. Alternatively, well-circumscribed lesions may be surgically excised.

> Kushner BJ. Intralesional corticosteroid injection for infantile adnexal hemangioma. *Am J Ophthalmol.* 1982;93:496–506.

Cryptophthalmos

Cryptophthalmos is a rare condition that presents with partial or complete absence of the eyebrow, palpebral fissure, eyelashes, and conjunctiva (Fig 11-5). The partially developed adnexa are fused to the anterior segment of the globe. Cryptophthalmos may be unilateral or bilateral. Histologically, the levator, orbicularis, tarsus, conjunctiva, and meibomian glands are attenuated or absent, making attempts at reconstruction difficult. Severe ocular defects are present in the underlying eye.

Acquired Eyelid Disorders

Chalazion

A type of focal inflammation of the eyelids, a chalazion can result from an obstruction of the meibomian glands (an internal posterior hordeolum). This disorder is commonly associated with rosacea and chronic posterior blepharitis. This common disorder may occasionally be confused with a malignant neoplasm.

CHAPTER 11: Classification and Management of Eyelid Disorders • 159

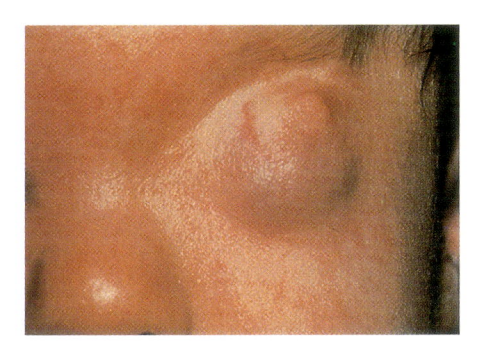

Figure 11-5 Cryptophthalmos.

The meibomian glands are oil-producing sebaceous glands located in the tarsal plates of both upper and lower eyelids. If the gland openings on the eyelid margin become plugged, the contents of the glands (sebum) are released into the tarsus and the surrounding eyelid soft tissue. This elicits an acute inflammatory response accompanied by pain and erythema of the skin. The exact role of bacterial agents (most commonly *Staphylococcus aureus*) in the production of chalazia is not clear. Histopathologically, these lesions are characterized by chronic lipogranulomatous inflammation.

Treatment

In the acute inflammatory phase, the treatment consists of warm compresses and appropriate eyelid hygiene, including scrubbing. Although topical antibiotic or anti-inflammatory ocular medications can be used, they may have minimal effect in resolving a chalazion. Systemic doxycycline may be appropriate when a significant secondary bacterial infection is suspected or when a case requires long-term suppression of meibomian gland inflammation associated with ocular rosacea.

Frequently, chalazia become chronic and cystlike, requiring surgical management to facilitate clearing of the inflammatory mass. Simple incision and curettage of the chalazion is often inadequate for permanent resolution. If the greatest inflammatory response is on the posterior eyelid margin, an incision through tarsus and conjunctiva is appropriate for drainage. Sharp dissection and excision of all necrotic material, including the posterior cyst wall, is indicated. This results in a posterior marsupialization of the chalazion (Fig 11-6). Extreme care is needed when removing inflammatory tissue at the eyelid margin or adjacent to the punctum. In the rare cases in which the greatest inflammatory response is anterior, incision through the skin and orbicularis muscle with appropriate removal of granulomatous tissue is possible. Because of the possibility of mistaking malignant lesions for chalazia, pathological examination is appropriate for any suspicious or atypical chalazion and for all recurrent chalazia. Local injection of corticosteroids in chalazia resistant to conservative management can cause depigmentation of the overlying skin and is not as effective as surgical treatment. Combining excision with steroid injection into the excisional bed results in a 95% resolution rate.

Epstein GA, Putterman AM. Combined excision and drainage with intralesional corticosteroid injection in the treatment of chronic chalazia. *Arch Ophthalmol.* 1988;106:514–516.

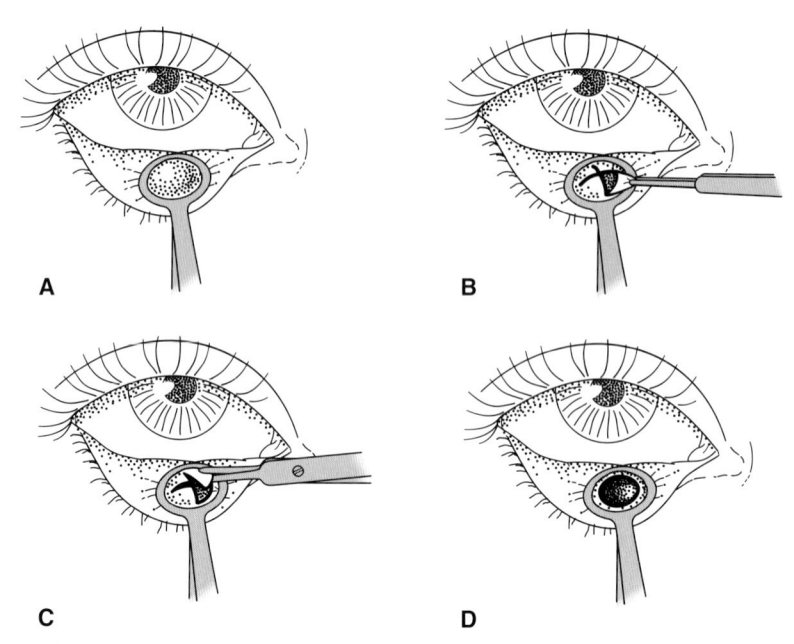

Figure 11-6 Excision of chalazion. **A,** After a clamp is placed around the chalazion, a blade is used to make a vertical incision into the tarsus. **B,** Cruciate incision of conjunctiva and cyst wall. **C,** Flaps are excised with a scissors. **D,** Defect is allowed to heal by secondary intention. *(Illustration by Jeanne C. Koelling.)*

Hordeolum (Stye)

An acute infection (usually staphylococcal) can involve the sebaceous secretions in the glands of Zeis *(external hordeolum,* or *stye)* or the meibomian glands *(internal hordeolum).* In the case of external hordeola, the infection often appears to center around an eyelash follicle, and the eyelash can be plucked to promote drainage. Spontaneous resolution often occurs. If needed, assiduous application of hot compresses and topical antibiotic ointment is usually curative. Rarely, hordeola may progress to true superficial cellulitis, or even abscesses, of the eyelid. In such cases, systemic antibiotic therapy and possible surgical incision and drainage may be required.

Eyelid Edema

Swelling of the eyelids may be caused by local conditions such as insect bites or allergy or by systemic conditions such as cardiovascular disease, renal disease, certain collagen vascular diseases, or Graves disease. Cerebrospinal fluid leakage into the orbit or eyelids following trauma may mimic eyelid edema. Lymphedema may be present after the lymph drainage system from the eyelid is interrupted; thus, surgeons should avoid eyelid incisions that transect the lymph channels in the lateral canthal area.

Floppy Eyelid Syndrome

The floppy eyelid syndrome is characterized by chronic papillary conjunctivitis; easily everted, flaccid upper eyelids; and nonspecific irritative symptoms (Fig 11-7). Associa-

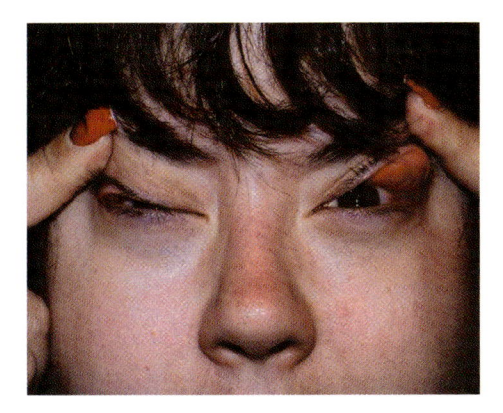

Figure 11-7 Floppy eyelid syndrome. Superolateral traction on the upper eyelid results in eversion of the tarsal plate. *(Photograph courtesy of Jerry Popham, MD.)*

tions have been reported with obesity, keratoconus, eyelid rubbing or mechanical pressure, hyperglycemia, and sleep apnea. A marked decrease of elastin fibers in the tarsus has been reported. Men are affected much more frequently than women. Patients often have a history of sleeping prone, which can cause mechanical upper eyelid eversion from contact with a pillow or bed sheets. Initial conservative treatment with either patching or an eyelid shield is helpful. Frequently, surgical treatment is indicated (central upper eyelid pentagonal block resection in order to facilitate horizontal tightening of the eyelid). In addition, sleep studies are recommended to rule out sleep apnea.

> McNab AA. Floppy eyelid syndrome and obstructive sleep apnea. *Ophthal Plast Reconstr Surg*. 1997;13:98–114.
> Netland PA, Sugrue SP, Albert DM, et al. Histopathologic features of the floppy eyelid syndrome. *Ophthalmology*. 1994;101:174–181.

Eyelid Imbrication Syndrome

Horizontal laxity of the upper eyelid may interfere with normal upper eyelid apposition against the globe during the blink cycle. In addition, the upper eyelid overrides the lower eyelid margin during eyelid closure, and this situation may result in chronic conjunctivitis of the palpebral conjunctiva of the upper eyelid. Further, keratinization of the posterior aspect of the upper eyelid margin and adjacent conjunctiva leads to corneal surface irritation and tear film abnormalities. Direct observation of the upper eyelid position during the blink cycle and with relaxed eyelid closure reveals a subtle upper eyelid override of the lower eyelid margin. Eyelid imbrication syndrome is pathophysiologically similar to floppy eyelid syndrome in that both have a lax upper eyelid. However, in eyelid imbrication syndrome, the upper eyelid does not easily evert and the tarsal plate is normal. Management consists of topical lubrication in mild cases. In more severe cases, horizontal tightening of the upper eyelid is indicated.

> Donnenfeld ED, Perry HD, Schrier A, et al. Lid imbrication syndrome: diagnosis with rose bengal staining. *Ophthalmology*. 1994;101:763–766.
> Karesh JW, Nirankari VS, Hameroff SB. Eyelid imbrication: an unrecognized cause of chronic ocular irritation. *Ophthalmology*. 1993;100:883–889.

Eyelid Neoplasms

Numerous benign and malignant cutaneous neoplasms may develop in the periocular skin, arising from the epidermis, dermis, or eyelid adnexal structures. However, most lesions, whether benign or malignant, develop from the epidermis, the rapidly growing superficial layer of the skin. Although many of these lesions may also occur elsewhere on the body, their appearance and behavior in the eyelids may be unique owing to the particular characteristics of eyelid skin and the specialized adnexal elements. The ophthalmologist's main goal in treating periocular lesions is to identify and appropriately diagnose malignancy. The malignant lesions most frequently affecting the eyelids are basal cell carcinoma, squamous cell carcinoma, sebaceous cell carcinoma, and melanoma. Only 15%–20% of periocular epithelial lesions actually are malignant. However, because clinical judgment has proved to be less than 100% accurate in distinguishing malignant from benign epithelial lesions, histopathologic examination of all excised cutaneous neoplasms is recommended.

> Kersten RC, Ewing-Chow D, Kulwin DR, et al. Accuracy of clinical diagnosis of cutaneous eyelid lesions. *Ophthalmology.* 1997;104:479–484.

Clinical Evaluation of Eyelid Tumors

The history and physical examination of eyelid lesions offer important clues regarding the likelihood of malignancy. Predisposing factors in the development of skin cancer include

- A history of prior skin cancer
- Excessive sun exposure, especially blistering sunburn during adolescence
- Previous radiation therapy
- History of smoking
- Celtic or Scandinavian ancestry, with fair skin, red hair, blue eyes

Signs suggesting eyelid malignancy are

- Slow, painless growth of a lesion
- Ulceration, with intermittent drainage, bleeding, and crusting
- Irregular pigmentary changes
- Destruction of normal eyelid margin architecture (especially meibomian orifices) and loss of cilia
- Heaped-up, pearly, translucent margins with possible central ulceration
- Fine telangiectasias
- Loss of fine cutaneous wrinkles

Palpable induration extending well beyond visibly apparent margins suggests tumor infiltration into the dermis and subcutaneous tissue.

Lesions near the puncta should be carefully examined to determine whether there is punctal or canalicular involvement. Probing and irrigation may be required to exclude lacrimal system involvement or to prepare for surgical resection.

Large lesions should be palpated for evidence of fixation to deeper tissues or bone. In addition, regional lymph nodes should be palpated for evidence of metastases in cases of suspected squamous cell carcinoma, sebaceous carcinoma, malignant melanoma, or Merkel cell carcinoma. Lymphatic tumor spread may produce rubbery swelling along the line of the jaw or in front of the ear. Restriction of ocular motility and proptosis suggest orbital extension of an eyelid malignancy, which can be evaluated via CT. Cranial nerve VII and cranial nerve V function should be carefully assessed to detect any deficiencies that may indicate perineural tumor spread, especially in cases of squamous cell carcinoma. Systemic evidence of liver, pulmonary, bone, or neurologic involvement should be sought in cases of sebaceous adenocarcinoma or melanoma of the eyelid.

It is important to obtain photographs prior to treatment. If photographs cannot be obtained, precise drawings and measurements of the lesion are necessary.

The following discussions of eyelid neoplasms are intended to provide a brief overview of the most prevalent lesions. For more extensive coverage and additional clinical and pathological photographs, see BCSC Section 4, *Ophthalmic Pathology and Intraocular Tumors*.

> Cook BE, Bartley GB. Epidemiologic characteristics and clinical course of patients with malignant eyelid tumors in an incidence cohort in Olmsted County, Minnesota. *Ophthalmology*. 1999;106:746–750.

Benign Eyelid Lesions

Epithelial hyperplasias

The terminology used by dermatopathologists to describe various benign epithelial proliferations is continuing to evolve and can be confusing. It is helpful to group the various benign epithelial proliferations under the clinical heading of *papillomas*. (This designation does not necessarily imply any association with the papillomavirus.) Clinical and histopathologic characterizations of the various benign epithelial proliferations overlap considerably. Included within this group are seborrheic keratoses, pseudoepitheliomatous hyperplasia, verrucae, acrochordons or skin tags, fibroepithelial polyps, squamous papillomas (Fig 11-8), seborrheic keratosis, basosquamous acanthoma, squamous acanthoma, and many others. These benign epithelial proliferations can all be managed with shave excision, removing them at the dermal–epidermal junction.

Seborrheic keratoses (Fig 11-9) are probably the most common of the various acquired benign eyelid papillomas. They tend to affect middle-aged and elderly patients. Their clinical appearance varies; they may be sessile or pedunculated and have varying degrees of pigmentation and hyperkeratosis. On facial skin, seborrheic keratoses typically appear as a smooth, greasy, stuck-on lesion; on the thinner eyelid skin, these lesions can be more lobulated, papillary, or pedunculated with visible excrescences on their surface. Even large lesions of this type remain totally superficial and can be managed by shaving the lesion at the dermal–epidermal junction with a scalpel. Deep excision is unnecessary, and the residual flat surface reepithelializes rapidly. Shaving a seborrheic keratosis from the thin eyelid skin may be more challenging. *Inverted follicular keratosis* is an older term that is now thought to represent an irritated seborrheic keratosis.

164 • Orbit, Eyelids, and Lacrimal System

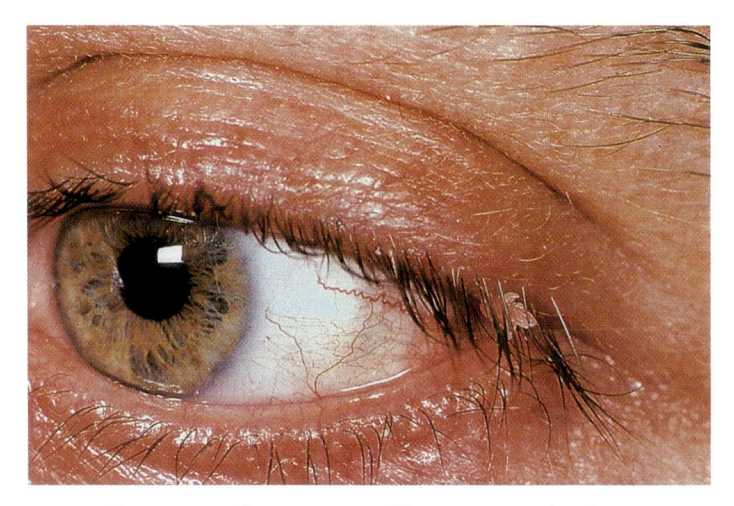

Figure 11-8 Squamous papilloma, or acrochordon.

Pseudoepitheliomatous hyperplasia is not a discrete lesion per se but rather refers to a pattern of reactive changes in the epidermis that may occur overlying areas of inflammation or neoplasia.

Verruca vulgaris (Fig 11-10), caused by epidermal infection with the human papillomavirus (type VI or XI), rarely occurs in thin eyelid skin. Cryotherapy may eradicate the lesion and minimizes the risk of viral spread.

A *cutaneous horn* is a clinically descriptive, nondiagnostic term referring to *exuberant hyperkeratosis.* This chronic lesion may be associated with a variety of benign or malignant histopathologic processes including seborrheic keratosis, verruca vulgaris, and squamous or basal cell carcinoma. Biopsy of the base of the cutaneous horn is required to establish definitive diagnosis.

Benign epithelial cysts

Cysts of the epidermis are the second most common type of benign periocular cutaneous lesions, accounting for approximately 18% of excised benign lesions. The large majority of these are *epidermal inclusion cysts* (Fig 11-11), which arise from the infundibulum of the hair follicle, either spontaneously or following traumatic implantation of epidermal tissue into the dermis. The lesions are slow-growing, elevated, round, and smooth. They often have a central pore, indicating the remaining pilar duct. Although these cysts are often called *sebaceous cysts* they are actually filled with keratin; rupture of the cyst wall may cause an inflammatory foreign body reaction. The cysts may also become secondarily infected. Recommended treatment for small cysts is marsupialization, excising around the periphery of the cyst but leaving the base of the cyst wall to serve as the new surface epithelium. Larger or deeper cysts may require a complete excision of the cyst, in which case the cyst wall should be removed intact in order to avoid recurrence.

Multiple tiny epidermal inclusion cysts are called *milia.* Milia may appear spontaneously, following trauma, or during the healing phase of a bullous disease process. They are particularly common in newborn infants. Generally, milia resolve spontaneously but

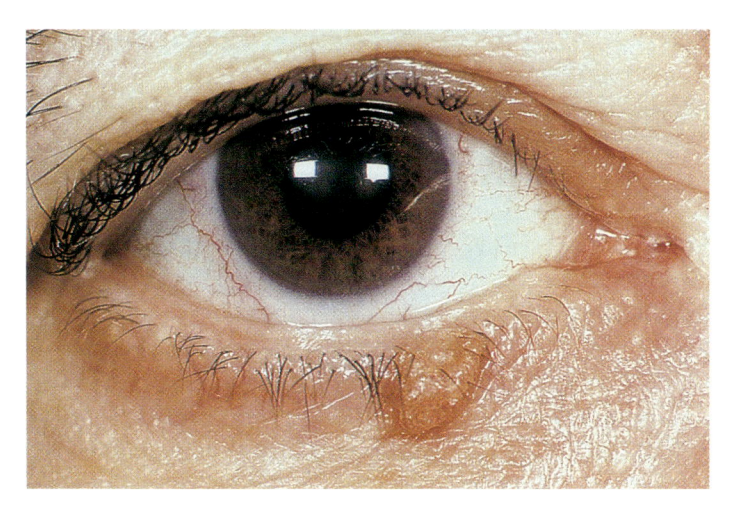

CHAPTER 11: Classification and Management of Eyelid Disorders • 165

Figure 11-9 Seborrheic keratosis.

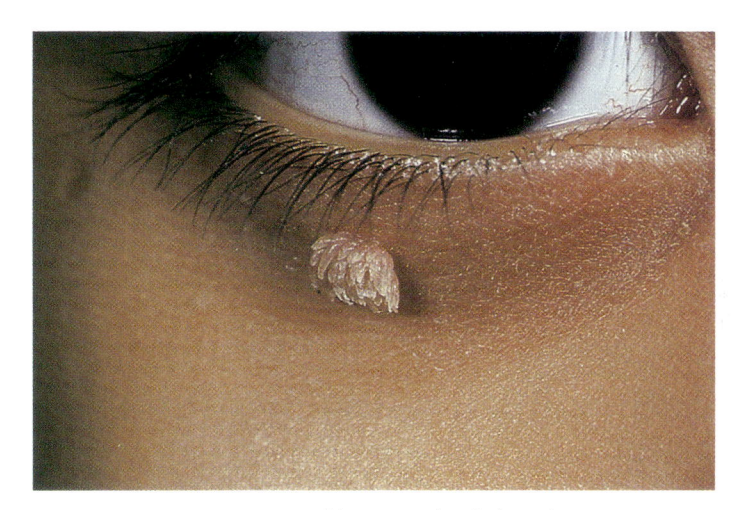

Figure 11-10 Verruca vulgaris (wart).

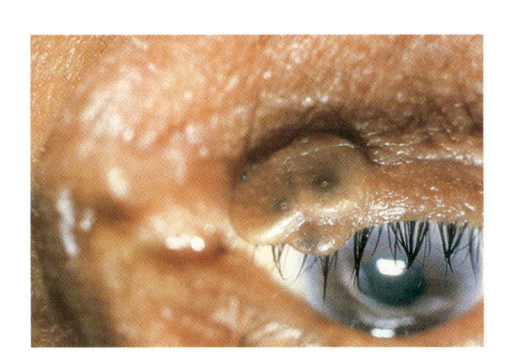

Figure 11-11 Epidermal inclusion cyst. *(Photograph courtesy of Robert C. Kersten, MD.)*

may be marsupialized with a sharp blade or needle. Multiple confluent milia may be treated with topical retinoic acid cream.

A less common epidermal cyst is the *pilar*, or *trichilemmal, cyst*. These cysts are clinically indistinguishable from epidermal inclusion cysts but tend to occur in areas containing large and numerous hair follicles. Approximately 90% of pilar cysts occur on the scalp; in the periocular region, they are generally found in the eyebrows. The cysts are filled with desquamated epithelium, and calcification occurs in approximately 25%.

Molluscum contagiosum is a viral infection of the epidermis that often involves the eyelid margin of children. Occasionally, multiple exuberant lesions appear in adult patients with acquired immunodeficiency syndrome (AIDS). The lesions are characteristically waxy and nodular, with a central umbilication. They may produce an associated follicular conjunctivitis. Treatment is observation, excision, controlled cryotherapy, or curettage with care taken to avoid damaging eyelash follicles or the eyelid margin or causing depigmentation of the skin.

Xanthelasmas are yellowish plaques that occur commonly in the medial canthal areas of the upper and lower eyelids. They represent collections of lipid-laden macrophages in the superficial dermis and subdermal tissues. Although xanthelasmas usually occur in patients with normal serum cholesterol levels, they are sometimes associated with hypercholesterolemia or congenital disorders of lipid metabolism. When excising these lesions, the surgeon must be careful to avoid removing too much of the anterior lamella of the eyelids, which can lead to cicatricial ectropion. Once excised, xanthelasma may recur. Other treatment options include serial excision, CO_2 laser ablation, or topical 100% trichloroacetic acid. Deep extension into the orbicularis muscle can occur, in which case the lesion may not be amenable to surface ablative therapies.

Benign Adnexal Lesions

The term *adnexa* refers to skin appendages that are located within the dermis but communicate through the epidermis to the surface. They include hair follicles, oil glands, and sweat glands. The eyelid contains both the specialized eyelashes and the normal vellus hairs found on skin throughout the body. Periocular adnexal oil glands include the *meibomian glands* within the tarsal plate, the *Zeis glands* associated with eyelash follicles, and normal *sebaceous glands* that are present as part of the pilosebaceous units in the skin hair. Sweat glands in the periocular region include the *eccrine sweat glands,* which have a general distribution throughout the body and are responsible for thermal regulation, and the *apocrine glands* (the *glands of Moll*) associated with the eyelash follicles.

Lesions of oil gland origin

Chalazia and hordeola These common eyelid lesions are discussed earlier in this chapter under Acquired Eyelid Disorders.

Sebaceous hyperplasia Sebaceous gland hyperplasia presents as multiple small yellow papules that may have central umbilication. They tend to occur on the forehead and cheeks and are common in patients older than 40 years. These lesions may sometimes be mistaken for basal cell carcinoma because of their tendency for central umbilication and fine telangiectasias. However, they have a yellow coloration and are soft on palpation. They may result from chronic dermatitis and can also be seen in patients with rosacea. Patients with multiple acquired sebaceous gland adenomas, adenomatoid sebaceous hyperplasia, or basal cell carcinomas with sebaceous differentiation have an increased incidence of visceral malignancy *(Muir-Torre syndrome)* and should be evaluated accordingly.

Sebaceous adenoma This rare tumor appears as a yellowish papule on the face, scalp, or trunk and may mimic a basal cell carcinoma or seborrheic keratosis. When sebaceous gland hyperplasia occurs in the involved meibomian glands in the tarsal plate, the eyelids may become thickened and ectropic. This condition may coexist with chronic blepharitis, and the possibility of sebaceous gland carcinoma must be considered.

Tumors of eccrine sweat gland origin

Syringomas Benign eccrine sweat gland tumors found commonly in young females, syringomas present as multiple, small, waxy, pale yellow nodules 1–2 mm in diameter on the lower eyelids (Fig 11-12). Syringomas occur at about the time of puberty and can also be found in the axilla and sternal region. Because the eccrine glands are located within the dermis, these lesions lie too deep to allow shave excision. Removal requires complete surgical excision, which is often best accomplished in a staged fashion.

Eccrine spiradenoma This uncommon benign tumor appears as a solitary nodule 1–2 cm in diameter that may be tender and painful. It tends to occur in early adulthood, and eyelid involvement is rare. Treatment is surgical excision.

Eccrine acrospiroma Also called *clear cell hidradenoma,* this rare tumor occurs as a solitary nodular lesion that is usually mobile beneath the skin. Treatment is surgical excision.

Eccrine hidrocystoma Eccrine hidrocystomas are common cystic lesions 1–3 mm in diameter that occur multiply and tend to cluster around the lower eyelids and on the face. They are considered to be ductal retention cysts, and they often enlarge in conditions such as heat and increased humidity, which stimulate perspiration. Treatment consists of surgical excision.

Pleomorphic adenoma This rare benign tumor occurs most commonly in the head and neck region and may involve the eyelids. Histologically, the tumor is identical to the pleomorphic adenoma of the salivary and lacrimal glands (discussed in Chapter 5). Treatment is complete surgical excision.

Tumors of apocrine sweat gland origin

Apocrine hidrocystoma A very common solitary smooth cyst arising from the glands of Moll along the eyelid margin, apocrine hidrocystoma is considered a true adenoma of the secretory cells of Moll rather than a retention cyst (Fig 11-13). These lesions typically are translucent or bluish and transilluminate. They may be multiple and often extend

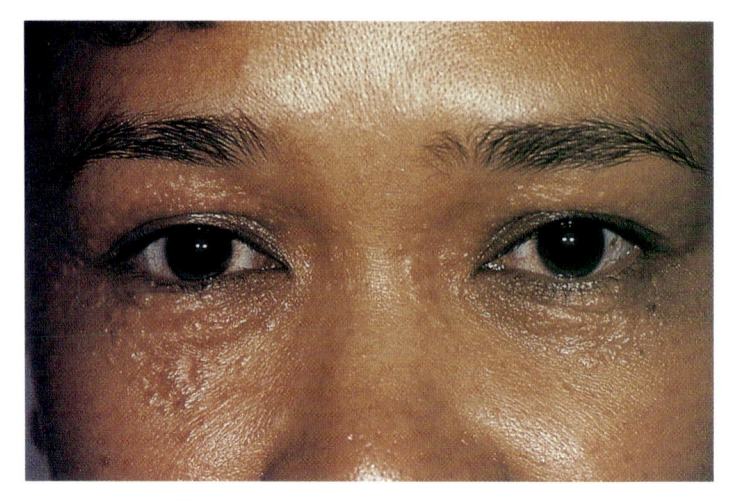

Figure 11-12 Syringomas. *(Photograph courtesy of Robert C. Kersten, MD.)*

deep beneath the surface, especially in the canthal regions. Treatment for superficial cysts is marsupialization. Deep cysts require complete excision of the cyst wall. These are also known as *cystadenomas* or *sudoriferous cysts*.

Cylindroma Cylindromas are rare tumors of sweat gland origin that may be solitary or multiple and may be dominantly inherited. Lesions are dome-shaped, smooth, flesh-colored nodules of varying size and tend to affect the scalp and face. They may occur so profusely in the scalp that the scalp is entirely covered with lesions, in which case they are called *turban tumors*. Treatment is surgical excision, but it may prove difficult if there are multiple lesions over a large surface area.

Tumors of hair follicle origin

Several rare benign lesions may arise from the eyelashes, eyebrows, or vellus hairs in the periocular region.

Trichoepitheliomas These lesions are small, flesh-colored papules with occasional telangiectasias that occur on the eyelids or forehead (Fig 11-14). Histopathologically, trichoepitheliomas appear as basaloid islands and keratin cysts with immature hair follicle structures. If keratin is abundant, they may clinically resemble an epidermal inclusion cyst. The individual histologic picture may be difficult to differentiate from that of basal cell carcinoma. Simple excision is curative.

Trichofolliculoma A trichofolliculoma is a single, sometimes umbilicated, lesion usually found in adults. Histopathologically, it represents a squamous cystic structure containing keratin and hair shaft components.

Trichilemmoma Another type of solitary lesion found in adults, trichilemmomas resemble verrucae. Histopathologically, they show glycogen-rich cells oriented around hair follicles.

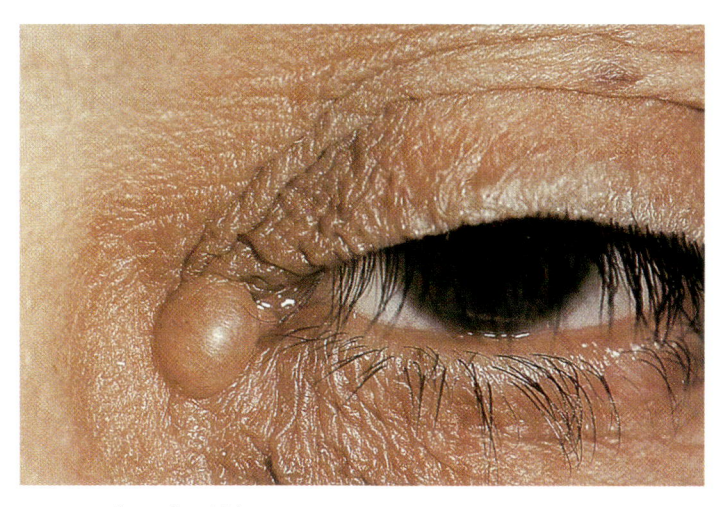

CHAPTER 11: Classification and Management of Eyelid Disorders • 169

Figure 11-13 Apocrine hidrocystoma. *(Photograph courtesy of Robert C. Kersten, MD.)*

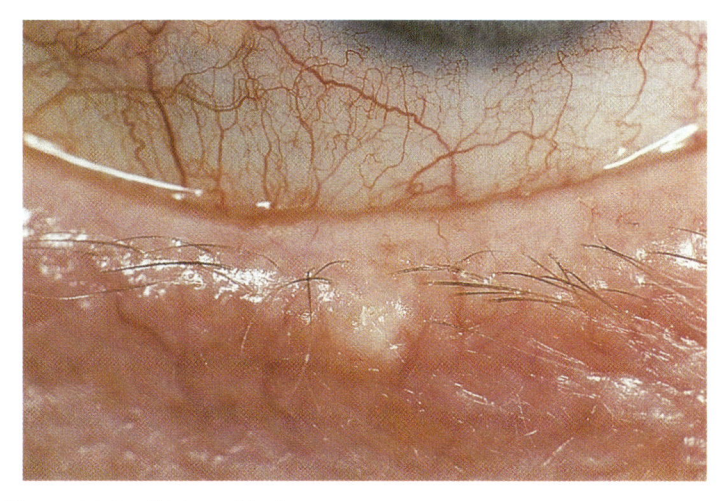

Figure 11-14 Trichoepithelioma. *(Photograph courtesy of Jeffrey A. Nerad, MD.)*

Pilomatrixomas These lesions affect young adults and usually occur in the eyebrow and central upper eyelid as a reddish purple subcutaneous mass attached to the overlying skin. They may become quite large. The tumor is composed of islands of epithelial cells surrounded by basophilic cells with shadow cells. Excision is curative.

Benign Melanocytic Lesions

Melanocytic lesions of the skin arise from three sources: nevus cells, dermal melanocytes, and epidermal melanocytes. *Virtually any benign or malignant lesion may be pigmented, and lesions of melanocytic origin do not necessarily have visible pigmentation.* For example, seborrheic keratoses are frequently pigmented, and basal cell carcinomas are occasionally pigmented, especially if they arise in persons with darker skin. In contrast, dermal nevi typically have no pigmentation in Caucasians. Melanocytes are normally found distributed at the dermal–epidermal junction throughout the skin. Melanocytes are similar to nevus cells, but nevus cells are arranged in clusters and have ultrastructural differences. Both nevus cells and melanocytes give rise to a number of benign lesions.

In addition to the individual lesions described below, diffuse eyelid skin hyperpigmentation called *melasma,* or *chloasma,* can occur in women who are pregnant or using oral contraceptives; in families with an autosomal dominant trait; and in patients with chronic atopic eczema, rosacea, and other inflammatory dermatoses.

Nevi

Nevi are the third most common benign lesions encountered in the periocular region after papillomas and epidermal inclusion cysts. They arise from *nevus cells,* which are incompletely differentiated melanocytes found in clumps in the epidermis and dermis and in the junction zone between these two layers. Nevi are not apparent clinically at birth but begin to appear during childhood and often develop increased pigmentation at the time of puberty.

All nevi tend to undergo evolution during life through three stages: *junctional* (located in the basal layer of the epidermis at the dermal–epidermal junction), *compound* (extending from the junctional zone up into the epidermis and down into the dermis), and *dermal* (caused by involution of the epidermal component and persistence of the dermal component). In children, nevi arise initially as junctional nevi, which are typically flat, pigmented macules. Beyond the second decade, most nevi become compound, at which stage they appear as elevated pigmented papules. Later in life, the epidermal pigmentation is lost and the compound nevus remains as an elevated but minimally pigmented or amelanotic lesion. By age 70 virtually all nevi have become dermal nevi and have lost pigmentation.

Nevi are frequently found on the eyelid margin, characteristically molded to the ocular surface (Fig 11-15). Benign nevi require no treatment, but malignant transfor-

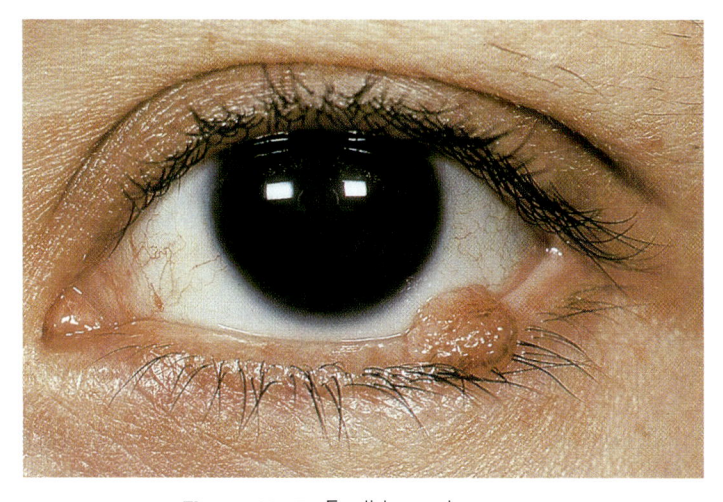

Figure 11-15 Eyelid margin nevus.

mation of a junctional or compound nevus can rarely occur. As long as there is no concern about malignant degeneration, nevi can be managed by shaving at the dermal–epidermal junction.

Freckle

An *ephelis,* or *freckle,* is a small, flat, brown spot on the skin. Ephelides appear from hyperpigmentation of the basal layer of the epidermis. The number of epidermal melanocytes is not increased, but they extrude more than the usual amount of pigment into the epidermal basal cell layer. Ephelides are common in fair-skinned persons, and their hue darkens with sunlight exposure. These small, circumscribed macules usually appear on the malar areas, but they occasionally present on the eyelids or conjunctiva. No treatment is necessary other than sun protection.

Lentigo simplex

Simple lentigines are flat, pigmented spots with a slightly larger area than ephelides. Occurring throughout life, lentigo simplex is not apparently related to sun exposure. This type of lentigo also differs from a freckle in that the number of epidermal melanocytes is increased, and melanin is found in adjacent basal keratinocytes. Individual lesions are evenly pigmented and measure a few millimeters in diameter. Eyelid lentigines may be associated with Peutz-Jeghers syndrome. No treatment is necessary for lentigo simplex. Melanin-bleaching preparations may achieve cosmetic improvement.

Solar lentigo

Multiple solar lentigines may occur in older persons, in which case they are called *senile lentigo* or, incorrectly, *liver spots*. Chronic sun exposure produces pigmented macules with an increased number of melanocytes. Solar lentigines are uniformly hyperpigmented and somewhat larger than simple lentigines. The dorsum of the hands and the forehead are the most frequently affected areas. No treatment is necessary, but sun protection is recommended. Melanin-bleaching preparations or cryotherapy may help fade their pigmentation.

Blue nevus

A blue nevus is a blue-gray, slightly elevated lesion that may be congenital or may develop during childhood. The blue nevus arises from a localized proliferation of dermal melanocytes. The dome-shaped, dark bluish-black lesions under the epidermis are usually 10 mm or less in diameter. Although the malignant potential is extremely low, these lesions are generally excised.

Dermal melanocytosis

Also known as *nevus of Ota,* this diffuse, congenital blue nevus of the periocular skin most often affects persons of African, Hispanic, or Asian descent, especially females. Dermal melanocytes proliferate in the region of the first and second dermatomes of cranial nerve V. The eyelid skin is diffusely brown or blue, and pigmentation may extend to the adjacent forehead. Approximately 5% of cases are bilateral. When patchy slate-gray pigmentation also appears on the episclera and uvea, as occurs in two thirds of affected patients, the condition is known as *oculodermal melanocytosis* (Fig 11-16).

172 • Orbit, Eyelids, and Lacrimal System

Although malignant transformation may occur, especially in white patients, no treatment is possible. Approximately 1 in 400 patients with oculodermal melanocytosis develop a uveal malignant melanoma.

Premalignant Epidermal Lesions

Actinic keratosis

Actinic keratosis is the most common precancerous skin lesion. It usually affects elderly persons with a fair complexion and a history of chronic sun exposure (Fig 11-17). These lesions are typically round, scaly, keratotic plaques that on palpation have the texture of sandpaper. They often develop on the face, head, neck, forearms, and dorsum of the hands. These lesions are in a state of continual flux, increasing in response to sunlight exposure and remitting with reduced sun exposure. It has been reported that up to 25% of individual actinic keratoses spontaneously resolve over a 12-month period, although new lesions tend to develop continually. The risk of malignant transformation from a given actinic keratosis is only 0.24% per year, but over extended follow-up, a patient with multiple actinic keratoses has a 12%–16% incidence of squamous cell carcinoma. Squa-

Figure 11-16 Oculodermal melanocytosis. *(Photograph courtesy of Jerry Popham, MD.)*

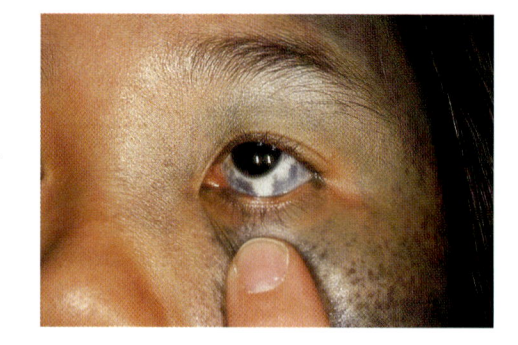

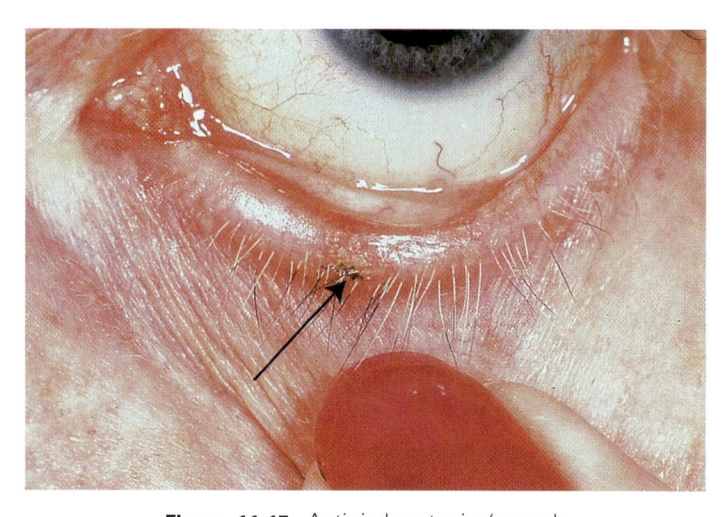

Figure 11-17 Actinic keratosis *(arrow).*

mous cell carcinomas arising from actinic keratoses are thought to be less aggressive than those developing de novo.

For lesions arising in the periocular region, incisional or excisional biopsy is recommended to establish definitive diagnosis. Excision or cryodestruction is recommended. Extensive lesions may require topical 5-fluorouracil (Fluoroplex) cream.

Bowen disease

The term *Bowen disease* refers to squamous cell carcinoma in situ of the skin. These lesions typically appear as elevated nonhealing erythematous lesions. They may present with scaling, crusting, or pigmented keratotic plaques. Pathologically, the lesions demonstrate full-thickness epidermal atypia without dermal invasion. In 5% of patients, Bowen disease may progress to vertically invasive squamous cell carcinoma; therefore, complete surgical excision is advised. Alternatively, cryotherapy of Bowen disease may be used, especially in larger areas of involvement.

Keratoacanthoma

Although keratoacanthoma was previously considered to be a benign self-limiting lesion, many authors now regard this entity as a low-grade squamous cell carcinoma. The lesion usually begins as a flesh-colored papule on the lower lid that develops rapidly into a dome-shaped nodule with a central keratin-filled crater and elevated rolled margins (Fig 11-18). Keratoacanthomas typically occur in middle-aged and elderly patients and show an increased incidence in immunosuppressed patients. Gradual involution over the course of 3–6 months has often been observed. The abundant keratin production in the center of the lesion may incite a surrounding inflammatory reaction, which may play a role in ultimate resolution. At present, incisional biopsy followed by complete surgical excision is recommended.

> Grossniklaus HE, Wojno TH, Yanoff M, et al. Invasive keratoacanthoma of the eyelid and ocular adnexa. *Ophthalmology*. 1996;103:937–941.

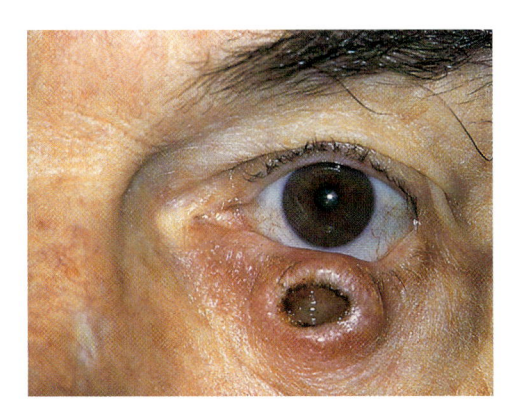

Figure 11-18 Keratoacanthoma.

Premalignant Melanocytic Lesions

Lentigo maligna

Also known as *Hutchinson melanotic freckle* or *precancerous melanosis,* lentigo maligna is a flat, irregularly shaped, unevenly pigmented, slowly enlarging lesion that typically occurs on the malar regions in older white persons. Unlike senile or solar lentigo, characteristics of lentigo maligna include significant pigmentary variation, irregular borders, and progressive enlargement. This represents a radial, intraepidermal, uncontrolled growth phase of melanocytes, which in 30%–50% of patients eventually progresses to nodules of vertically invasive melanoma.

The area of histopathologic abnormality often extends beyond the visible pigmented borders of the lesion; in the periocular region, cutaneous lentigo maligna of the eyelid may extend onto the conjunctival surface, where the lesion appears identical to primary acquired melanosis. Excision with adequate surgical margins is recommended, with permanent sections for final monitoring. Close observation for recurrence is warranted.

> Marines HM, Patrinely JR. Benign eyelid tumors. In: Liesegang TJ, ed. *Oculodermal Disease.* Ophthalmology Clinics of North America. Philadelphia: Saunders; 1992;5:243–260.

Malignant Eyelid Tumors

Basal cell carcinoma

Basal cell carcinoma, the most common eyelid malignancy, accounts for approximately 90%–95% of malignant eyelid tumors. Basal cell carcinomas are often located on the lower eyelid margin (50%–60%) and near the medial canthus (25%–30%). Less commonly, they may occur on the upper eyelid (15%) and lateral canthus (5%).

Patients at most risk for basal cell carcinoma are fair-skinned, blue-eyed, red-haired or blond, middle-aged and older people with English, Irish, Scottish, or Scandinavian ancestry. They may have a history of prolonged sun exposure during the first two decades of life. A history of cigarette smoking also increases the risk of basal cell carcinoma. Patients with prior basal cell carcinomas have a higher probability of developing additional skin cancers.

Basal cell carcinoma is being increasingly seen in younger patients, and discovery of malignant eyelid lesions in these patients or those with a positive family history should prompt inquiry into possible systemic associations such as basal cell nevus syndrome or xeroderma pigmentosum. *Basal cell nevus syndrome (Gorlin syndrome)* is an uncommon autosomal dominant multisystem disorder characterized by multiple nevoid basal cell carcinomas appearing early in life associated with skeletal anomalies, especially of the mandible, maxilla, and vertebrae. *Xeroderma pigmentosum* is a rare autosomal recessive disorder characterized by extreme sun sensitivity and a defective repair mechanism for UV light–induced DNA damage in skin cells.

> Nerad JA, Whitaker DC. Periocular basal cell carcinoma in adults 35 years of age and younger. *Am J Ophthalmol.* 1988;106:723–729.

Nodular basal cell carcinoma, the most common clinical appearance of basal cell carcinoma, is a firm, raised, pearly nodule that may be associated with telangiectasia and

CHAPTER 11: Classification and Management of Eyelid Disorders • 175

central ulceration (Fig 11-19). Histopathologically, tumors of this form demonstrate nests of basal cells that originate from the basal cell layer of the epithelium and may show peripheral palisading. As the nests of atypical cells break through to the surface of the epithelium, central necrosis and ulceration may occur.

A less common and more aggressive basal cell carcinoma is the *morpheaform*, or *fibrosing, type*. These lesions may be firm and slightly elevated. The margins of the tumor may be indeterminate on clinical examination (Fig 11-20). Histopathologically, these lesions do not show peripheral palisading but rather occur in thin cords that radiate peripherally. The surrounding stroma may show proliferation of connective tissue into a pattern of fibrosis.

Morpheaform tumors behave more aggressively than nodular basal cell carcinomas. Basal cell carcinoma may simulate chronic inflammation of the eyelid margin and is

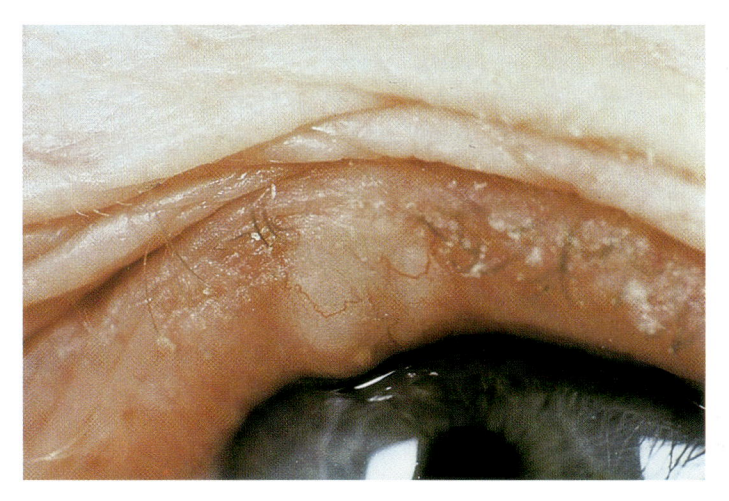

Figure 11-19 Basal cell carcinoma.

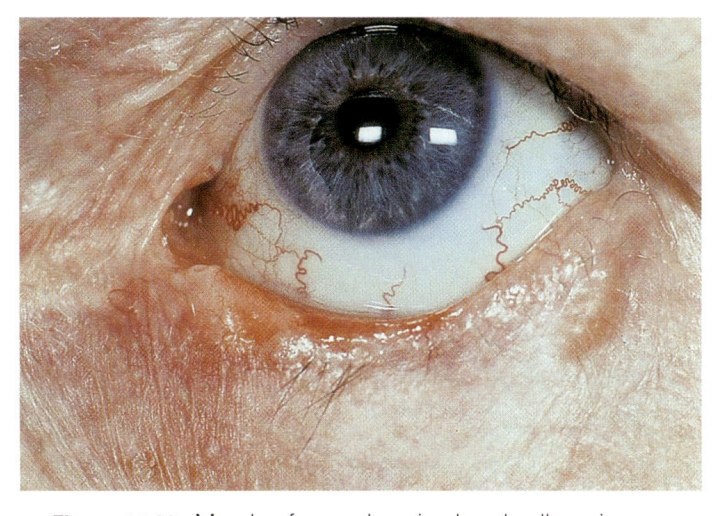

Figure 11-20 Morpheaform sclerosing basal cell carcinoma.

frequently associated with loss of eyelashes. Multicentric or superficial basal cell carcinoma may be mistaken for chronic blepharitis and can silently extend along the eyelid margin.

> Margo CE, Waltz K. Basal cell carcinoma of the eyelid and periocular skin. *Surv Ophthalmol.* 1993;38:169–192.
>
> Miller SJ. Biology of basal cell carcinoma (parts I and II). *J Am Acad Dermatol.* 1991;24: 1–13,161–175.

Management A biopsy is necessary to confirm any clinical suspicion of basal cell carcinoma (Fig 11-21). The most accurate diagnosis can be ensured if every incisional biopsy provides tissue that

- Is representative of the clinically evident lesion
- Is of adequate size for histologic processing
- Is not excessively traumatized or crushed
- Contains normal tissue at the margin to show the transitional area

An *incisional biopsy* can be used as a confirmatory office procedure for suspected malignant tumors. The site of the incisional biopsy should be photographed or sketched with measurements, because the site may heal so well that the original location of the tumor becomes difficult to find for subsequent additional tumor removal.

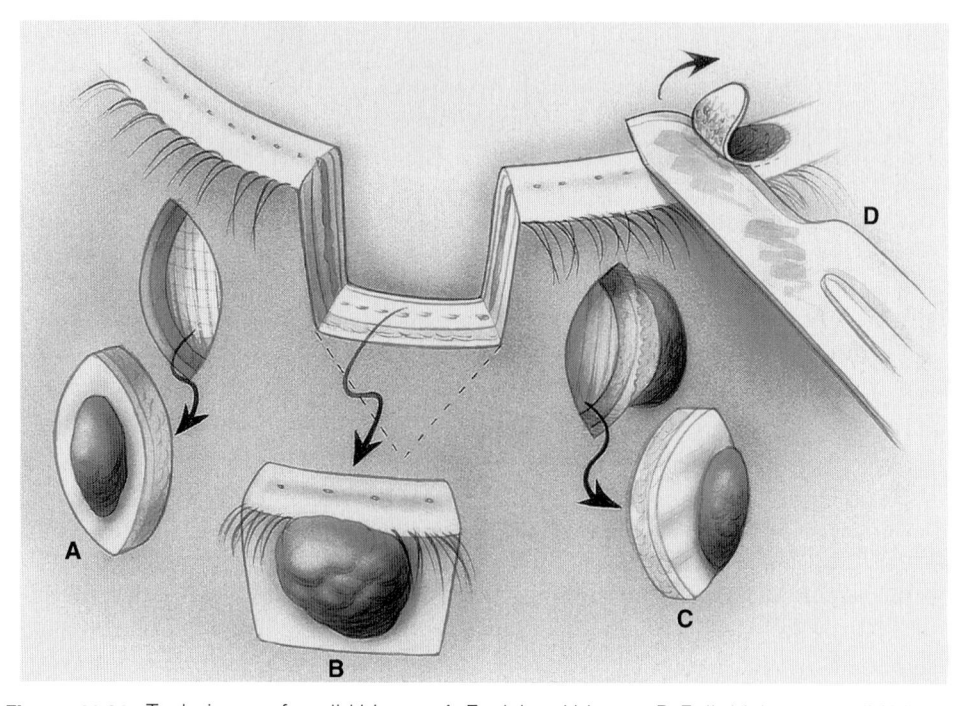

Figure 11-21 Techniques of eyelid biopsy. *A,* Excisional biopsy. *B,* Full-thickness eyelid biopsy. *C,* Incisional or punch biopsy including normal skin. *D,* Shave biopsy of eyelid margin lesion. *(Illustration by Christine Gralapp.)*

An *excisional biopsy* is reasonable when eyelid lesions are small and do not involve the eyelid margin or when eyelid margin lesions are centrally located, away from the lateral canthus or lacrimal punctum. However, histopathologic monitoring of tumor borders to ensure complete excision is mandatory. The borders of any excisional biopsy should be marked in case the excision is incomplete and further resection is thus necessary. Excisional biopsies should be oriented vertically so that closure does not put vertical traction on the eyelid. If the margins of the excised portion of the eyelid are positive for residual tumor cells, the involved area of the eyelid should be reexcised, with surgical monitoring of the margins by Mohs' micrographic technique (see below) or by frozen-section technique.

Occasionally, histopathologic examination of a clinically complete excision of a presumably benign lesion reveals an unsuspected basal cell carcinoma extending to the margins of resection. If reexamination of the patient at the slit lamp reveals no detectable residual lesion, the physician may elect to follow the patient closely for recurrence without additional initial excision of tissue. The importance of rigorous follow-up, especially for medial canthal excisional sites, must be stressed to the patient. Interestingly, less than half of incompletely excised basal cell carcinomas have been found to recur over inclusive long-term follow-up.

> Anscher M, Montana G. Management of periocular basal cell carcinoma. II, Radiotherapy. *Surv Ophthalmol.* 1993;38:203–210.
> Leshin B, Yeatts P. Management of periocular basal cell carcinoma. I, Mohs' micrographic surgery. *Surv Ophthalmol.* 1993;38:193–203.
> Warren RC, Nerad JA, Carter KD. Punch biopsy technique for the ophthalmologist. *Arch Ophthalmol.* 1990;108:778–779.

Surgery is the treatment of choice for all basal cell carcinomas of the eyelid. Surgical excision affords the advantages of complete tumor removal with histologic control of the margins. Excision has a lower recurrence rate than any other treatment modality. It also offers superior cosmetic results in most cases. Finally, surgery usually offers rapid resolution.

Caution: Basal cell carcinomas that arise in the medial canthal area and vertical midface *(H zone)* are more likely to be deeply infiltrative than those arising from the more central eyelid margins. Therefore, nonsurgical treatment such as radiation therapy or cryotherapy should be avoided with canthal tumors because these techniques offer no way to define the limits of the lesion.

When basal cell carcinomas involve the medial canthal area, the lacrimal drainage system may have to be removed in order to completely eradicate the tumor. If the lacrimal drainage system has been removed for tumor eradication, reconstruction of the lacrimal outflow system should not be undertaken until the patient has been tumor-free for at least 5 years. This waiting period reduces the possibility that unsuspected residual basal cell carcinoma will gain access to the nasal cavity through a surgically created conjunctivodacryocystorhinostomy tract.

Orbital invasion is particularly common in cases that have been inadequately treated, in clinically neglected tumors, or in morpheaform tumors. Orbital exenteration may be required in such cases. Retrospective studies show that the mortality rate from ocular adnexal basal cell carcinoma is 3%. The vast majority of patients who died from basal cell carcinoma had disease that started in the canthal areas, had undergone prior radiation therapy, or had clinically neglected tumors.

> Howard GR, Nerad JA, Carter KD, et al. Clinical characteristics associated with orbital invasion of cutaneous basal cell and squamous cell tumors of the eyelid. *Am J Ophthalmol.* 1992;113:123–133.

All tissue margins around an excised malignant tumor should be histologically examined to ensure complete removal. Frozen-section techniques permit such examination during the course of surgery. After the clinically apparent tumor has been removed, the surgeon should also excise strips that are 1–2 mm wide from the adjacent tissue for frozen-section examination. Alternatively, the surgeon may excise the clinically apparent tumor along with 1–2 mm of clinically uninvolved tissue, then send the entire specimen, oriented on a drawing, to the pathologist. The pathologist may then sample the margins with frozen-section technique. The surgeon must then communicate directly with the pathologist and ensure adequate examination of the tissue.

Reconstruction is undertaken only when all margins are found to be tumor-free. Some tumors have subcutaneous extensions that are not recognized clinically. Consequently, the surgeon must always be prepared to do a much larger reconstruction than originally anticipated from the surface appearance of the tumor.

Mohs' micrographic surgery is often used by dermatologists with special training to ensure complete removal of recurrent, deeply infiltrated, or morpheaform tumors and tumors in the medial canthal region. Tissue may be removed in lamellar layers that provide a three-dimensional mapping of the tumor excision. Mohs' micrographic tumor resection is most commonly used in the resection of morpheaform basal cell carcinoma and squamous cell carcinoma.

Micrographic excision preserves the maximal amount of healthy tissue while providing the best insurance of complete cancer removal. Preoperative planning between the micrographic surgeon and oculoplastic reconstructive surgeon allows for most efficient patient care. In some cases, micrographic excision may allow the preservation of a globe, whereas conventional surgical techniques might indicate the need for exenteration. However, a major limitation of Mohs' micrographic surgery is in identifying margins of the tumor when it has invaded orbital fat.

Following Mohs' micrographic surgery, the eyelid should be reconstructed by standard oculoplastic procedures. Urgent reconstruction is not critical, but surgery should be performed expeditiously. Early surgery affords maximum protection for the globe and allows reconstruction to take place while the remaining eyelid margins are still fresh. At times, it is not possible to proceed with immediate reconstruction. In such cases, the cornea should be protected by patching or temporarily suturing the remaining eyelids closed over the globe. Reconstruction then proceeds once the surgical team is assembled and the medical situation stabilized. Spontaneous granulation may be a treatment alternative when small defects are encountered. Best results have been reported for defects of the medial canthus, particularly when the defect extends equally above and below the medial canthal tendon.

Mohs FE. Micrographic surgery for microscopically controlled excision of eyelid tumors. *Arch Ophthalmol.* 1986;104:901–909.

Waltz K, Margo CE. Mohs' micrographic surgery. *Ophthalmol Clin North Am.* 1991;4: 153–163.

The recurrence rate following *cryotherapy* is higher than that following surgical therapy for well-circumscribed nodular lesions. When used to treat more diffuse sclerosing lesions, the recurrence rate with cryotherapy is unacceptably high. Consequently, this modality of treatment must be avoided for canthal lesions, recurrent lesions, lesions greater than 1 cm in diameter, and morpheaform lesions. Further, since cryotherapy may lead to depigmentation and tissue atrophy, it should not be used when final cosmesis is important. Accordingly, cryotherapy for eyelid basal cell carcinoma is generally reserved for patients who are otherwise unable to tolerate surgery, such as elderly patients confined to bed or those with serious medical conditions that prevent surgical intervention.

Radiation therapy should also be considered only a palliative treatment that should generally be avoided for periorbital lesions. In particular, it should not be used for canthal lesions in view of the risk of orbital recurrence. As with cryotherapy, histologic margins cannot be evaluated with radiation treatment. The recurrence rate following radiation treatment is higher than that following surgical treatment. Moreover, recurrence after radiation is more difficult to detect, occurs at a longer interval after initial treatment, and is more difficult to manage surgically because of the altered healing of previously irradiated tissues.

Complications of radiation therapy include cicatricial changes in the eyelids, lacrimal drainage scarring with obstruction, keratitis sicca, and radiation-induced malignancy. Radiation-induced injury to the globe may also occur if it is not shielded during treatment.

Squamous cell carcinoma

Squamous cell carcinoma of the eyelid is 40 times less common than basal cell carcinoma but is biologically more aggressive. Tumors can arise spontaneously or from areas of solar injury and actinic keratosis and may be potentiated by immunodeficiency (Fig 11-22). The treatment modalities available for squamous cell carcinoma are similar to those for

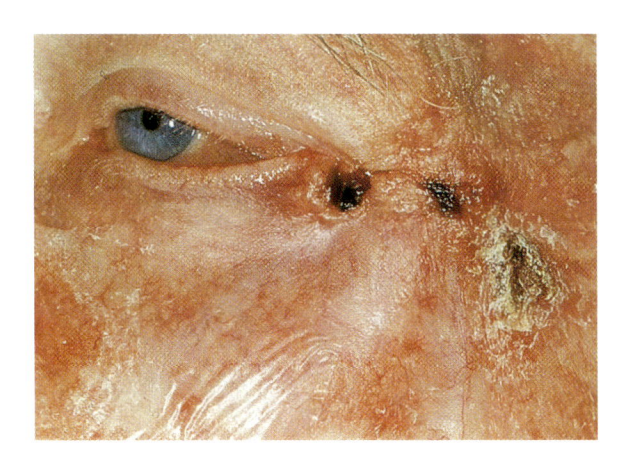

Figure 11-22 Infiltrative squamous carcinoma of the eyelid treated with medial wedge resection. *(Photograph courtesy of Jeffrey A. Nerad, MD.)*

basal cell carcinoma. The greater aggressiveness of squamous cell carcinoma and potential for metastatic spread make histologic control of margins following tumor resection even more important than for basal cell carcinoma. Mohs' micrographic resection or surgical excision with wide margins and frozen sections is preferred because of the potentially lethal nature of this tumor. Squamous cell carcinoma may metastasize through lymphatic transmission, blood-borne transmission, or direct extension, often along nerves. Recurrences of squamous cell carcinoma should be treated with wide surgical resection, possibly including orbital exenteration, and may require collaboration with a head and neck cancer surgeon.

> Reifler DM, Hornblass A. Squamous cell carcinoma of the eyelid. *Surv Ophthalmol.* 1986;30:349–365.

Sebaceous adenocarcinoma

Carcinoma of the sebaceous glands is a highly malignant and potentially lethal tumor that arises from meibomian glands of the tarsal plate; from glands of Zeis associated with the eyelashes; or from sebaceous glands of the caruncle, eyebrow, or facial skin. Unlike basal cell or squamous cell carcinoma, sebaceous gland carcinoma occurs more frequently in females and originates twice as often in the upper eyelid, reflecting the greater numbers of meibomian and Zeis glands there. Multicentric origin is common, and separate upper and lower eyelid tumors occur in 6%–8% of patients. The tumor often exhibits a yellow coloration as a result of lipid material within the neoplastic cells. Patients are commonly older than 50 years, but these tumors have been reported in younger patients.

These tumors often masquerade as benign eyelid diseases. Clinically, they may simulate chalazia, chronic blepharitis, basal cell or squamous cell carcinoma, ocular cicatricial pemphigoid, superior limbic keratoconjunctivitis, or pannus associated with adult inclusion conjunctivitis. Typically, effacement of the meibomian gland orifices with destruction of follicles of the cilia occurs, leading to loss of lashes (Figs 11-23, 11-24).

A feature of sebaceous carcinoma is the tendency for the tumor within the tarsal plate to progress to an intraepidermal growth phase, which may extend over the palpebral and bulbar conjunctiva. This pagetoid intraepidermal involvement mimics Paget disease of the breast. A fine papillary elevation of the tarsal conjunctiva may indicate pagetoid spread of tumor cells; intraepithelial growth may replace corneal epithelium as well. Sebaceous secretions from the intraepithelial cancer cells may cause marked conjunctival inflammation and injection.

Figure 11-23 Sebaceous gland carcinoma. *(Photograph courtesy of John B. Holds, MD.)*

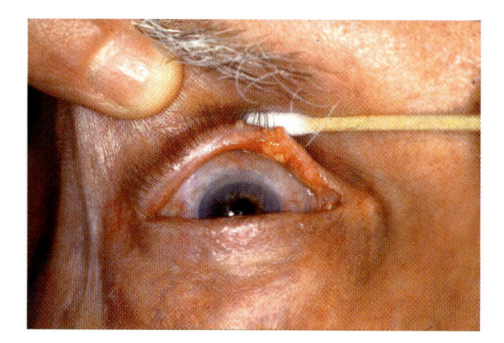

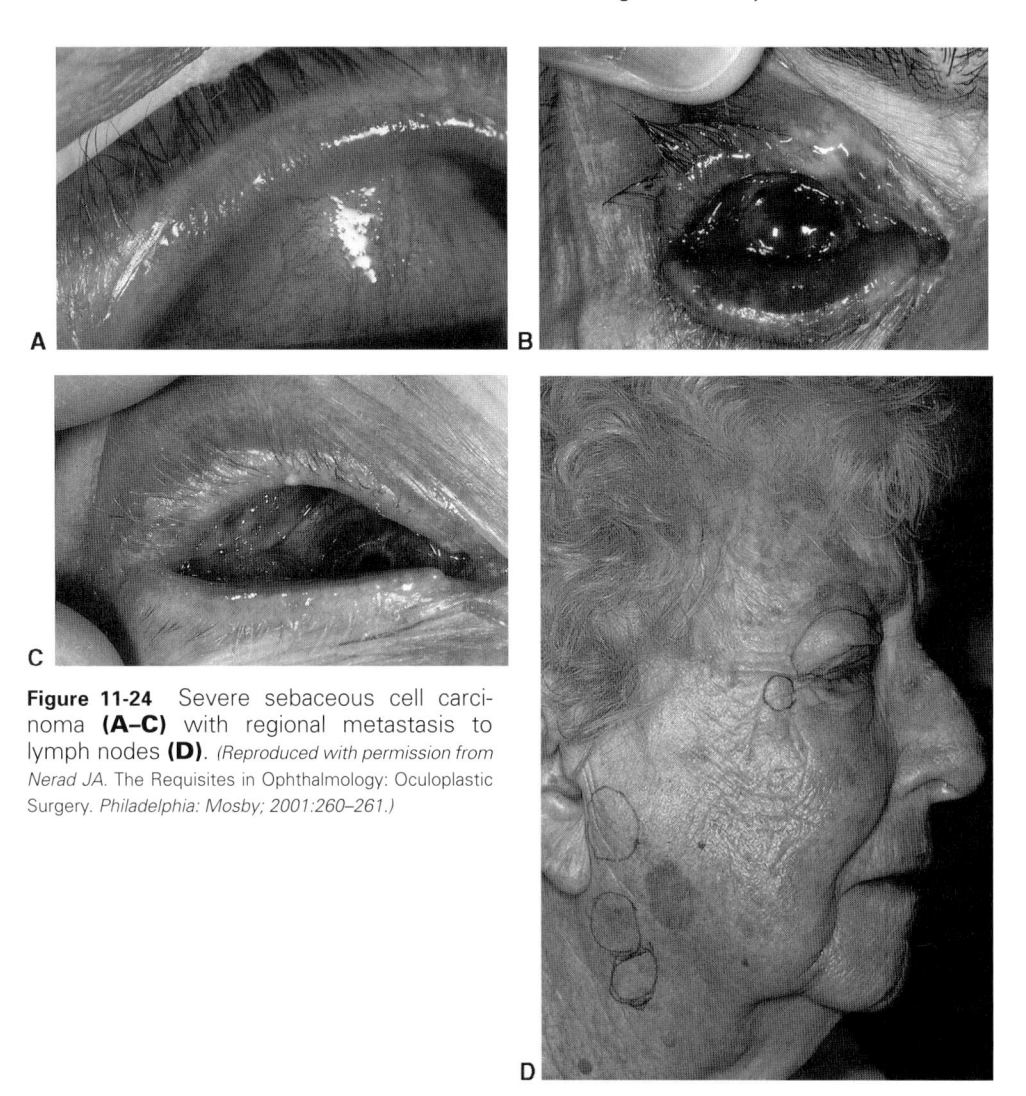

CHAPTER 11: Classification and Management of Eyelid Disorders • 181

Figure 11-24 Severe sebaceous cell carcinoma **(A–C)** with regional metastasis to lymph nodes **(D)**. *(Reproduced with permission from Nerad JA. The Requisites in Ophthalmology: Oculoplastic Surgery. Philadelphia: Mosby; 2001:260–261.)*

A nodule that initially simulates a chalazion but later causes loss of eyelashes and destruction of the meibomian gland orifices is characteristic of sebaceous gland carcinoma. Such a lesion warrants biopsy. Material from a chalazion that has been surgically excised more than once should be submitted for histopathologic examination. Because the rate of histopathological misdiagnosis is high among general pathologists, the clinician should maintain suspicion based on clinical findings and request special stains (lipid) or outside consultation. Any chronic unilateral blepharitis should also suggest the possibility of sebaceous gland carcinoma.

Because eyelid margin sebaceous carcinomas originate in the tarsal plate or the eyelash margin, superficial shave biopsies may reveal chronic inflammation but miss the underlying tumor. A full-thickness eyelid biopsy with permanent sections may be required to assist the correct diagnosis. Alternately, full-thickness punch biopsy of the tarsal plate may be diagnostic.

Wide surgical excision is mandatory for adequate treatment of sebaceous adenocarcinoma. Mohs' micrographic surgery has been used in some cases, but skip areas, pagetoid spread, and polycentricity characteristic of these tumors demand considerable caution. Map biopsies of the conjunctiva are helpful to eliminate the potential of pagetoid spread. If pagetoid spread is present, cryotherapy may be used. Orbital exenteration may be considered for recurrent or large tumors invading through the orbital septum (see Chapter 8). These tumors usually metastasize to regional lymph nodes but may also spread hematogenously or through direct extension. Radiation therapy is usually not appropriate, as sebaceous carcinomas are relatively radioresistant.

> Kass LG, Hornblass A. Sebaceous carcinoma of the ocular adnexa. *Surv Ophthalmol.* 1989;33:477–490.
>
> Khan JA, Doane JF, Grove AS Jr. Sebaceous and meibomian carcinomas of the eyelid: recognition, diagnosis, and management. *Ophthal Plast Reconstr Surg.* 1991;7:61–66.
>
> Lisman RD, Jakobiec FA, Small P. Sebaceous carcinoma of the eyelids. The role of adjunctive cryotherapy in the management of conjunctival pagetoid spread. *Ophthalmology.* 1989;96:1021–1026.

Malignant melanoma

Malignant melanoma accounts for about 5% of cutaneous cancers. The incidence of malignant melanoma has been steadily increasing over the last half century. Multiple factors, including sunlight exposure, genetic predisposition, and environmental mutagens, have been implicated in this increase. Cutaneous melanomas may develop de novo or from preexisting melanocytic nevi or lentigo maligna. Although malignant melanoma accounts for about 5% of all skin cancers, primary cutaneous malignant melanoma of the eyelid skin is rare (<1% of eyelid malignancies). Melanomas should be suspected in any patient with an acquired pigmented lesion beyond the first two decades of life. Melanomas typically have variable pigmentation with darker and lighter hues within the lesion. They usually have irregular borders and may also ulcerate and bleed.

There are four clinicopathologic forms of cutaneous melanoma:

- Lentigo maligna melanoma
- Nodular melanoma
- Superficial spreading melanoma
- Acrolentiginous melanoma

The eyelid is most often involved by either lentigo maligna melanoma or nodular melanoma.

Lentigo maligna melanoma represents the invasive vertical malignant growth phase that occurs in 10%–20% of patients with lentigo maligna. It accounts for 90% of head and neck melanomas. Clinically, the invasive areas are marked by nodule formation within the broader flat tan to brown irregular macule. The eyelid is usually involved by secondary extension from the malar region, and pigmentation may progress over the eyelid margin and onto the conjunctival surface. Surgical excision is recommended for a premalignant lentigo maligna and is mandatory in patients with lentigo maligna melanoma.

Nodular melanoma accounts for approximately 10% of cutaneous melanomas. These tumors may be amelanotic, but they are extremely rare on the eyelids. The vertical invasive growth phase is the initial presentation of these lesions, and they are therefore likely to have extended deeply by the time of the initial diagnosis.

Treatment for cutaneous melanoma includes wide surgical excision with histologic assurance (by means of permanent sections) of complete tumor removal. Regional lymph node dissection or sentinel lymph node biopsy should be performed in patients with melanomas that show microscopic evidence of vascular or lymphatic involvement. Complete preoperative metastatic workup is indicated for tumors with thickness greater than 1.5 mm. Thin lesions (<0.75 mm) confer a 5-year survival rate of 98%; thicker lesions (>4 mm) confer a less than 50% survival rate. Because tumor thickness has strong prognostic implications, these lesions should be biopsied with a disposable punch that allows a core to be taken through the full depth of the tumor. Biopsy of these lesions does not increase the risk of metastatic spread. Although cryotherapy may have a role in the treatment of acquired melanomas in the conjunctiva, it should not be considered for treatment of cutaneous melanoma.

> Grossniklaus HE, McLean IW. Cutaneous melanoma of the eyelid: clinicopathologic features. *Ophthalmology*. 1991;98:1867–1873.
>
> Tahery DP, Goldberg R, Moy RL. Malignant melanoma of the eyelid. A report of eight cases and a review of the literature. *J Am Acad Dermatol*. 1992;27:17–21.

Kaposi sarcoma

This previously rare tumor presents as a chronic reddish dermal mass and is a frequent manifestation of AIDS (Fig 11-25). The conjunctival lesions can be mistaken for foreign body granuloma or cavernous hemangioma. The lesion is composed of spindle cells of probable endothelial origin; it may be treated with cryotherapy, excision, radiation, or intralesional chemotherapeutic agents. Kaposi sarcoma may regress with adequate treatment of HIV infection.

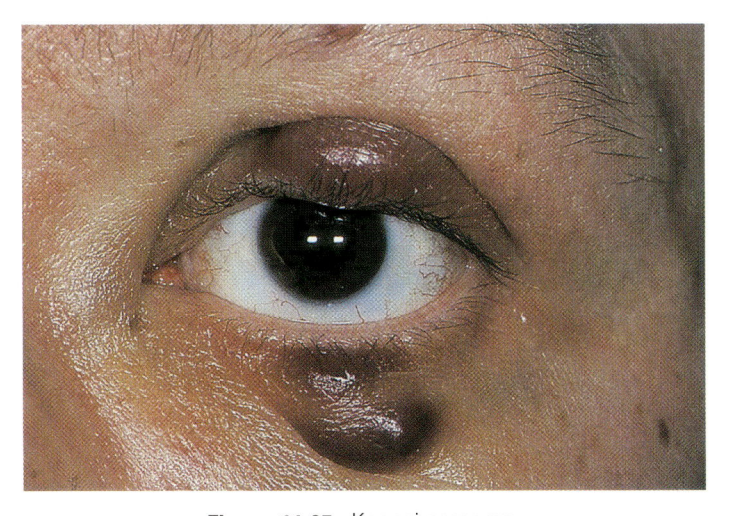

Figure 11-25 Kaposi sarcoma.

Shuler JD, Holland GN, Miles SA, et al. Kaposi sarcoma of the conjunctiva and eyelids associated with the acquired immunodeficiency syndrome. *Arch Ophthalmol.* 1989;107: 858–862.

Masquerading Neoplasms

Both basal cell carcinoma and sebaceous gland carcinoma may masquerade as chronic inflammatory disease of the eyelid (see earlier discussion under Acquired Eyelid Disorders).

Eyelid Trauma

Injury of the eyelid may be divided into blunt and penetrating trauma. Cardinal rules in the management of eyelid trauma include the following:
- Take a careful history.
- Record the best acuity for each eye.
- Thoroughly evaluate the globe and orbit.
- Obtain appropriate radiologic studies.
- Have a detailed knowledge of eyelid and orbital anatomy.
- Ensure the best possible primary repair.

Linberg JV. *Oculoplastic and Orbital Emergencies.* Norwalk, CT: Appleton & Lange; 1990.

Blunt Trauma

Ecchymosis and edema are the most common presenting signs of blunt trauma. Patients require a thorough biomicroscopic evaluation and a dilated fundus examination to rule out associated intraocular problems. CT, both axial and direct coronal, may be necessary to determine if an orbital fracture is present (see Chapter 6).

Penetrating Trauma

A detailed knowledge of eyelid anatomy helps the surgeon in repairing a penetrating eyelid injury and often reduces the need for secondary repairs. Generally, the treatment of eyelid lacerations depends on the depth and location of the injury.

Lacerations not involving the eyelid margin

Superficial eyelid lacerations involving just the skin and orbicularis muscle usually require only skin sutures. To avoid unnecessary scarring, however, basic principles of plastic repair must be followed. These include conservative debridement of the wound, use of small-caliber sutures, eversion of the wound edges, and early suture removal.

The presence of orbital fat in the wound means that the orbital septum has been violated. Superficial or deep foreign bodies should be searched for meticulously before these deeper eyelid lacerations are repaired. Copious irrigation lavages away contaminated material in the wound. Orbital fat prolapse in an upper eyelid wound is an indication for levator exploration. A lacerated levator muscle or aponeurosis must be carefully repaired to avoid postoperative ptosis. Upper eyelid lagophthalmos and tethering to the superior orbital rim are common if the orbital septum is inadvertently incorporated into the laceration repair. Orbital septum lacerations should not be sutured. Meticulous closure of overlying eyelid skin and orbicularis muscle is adequate in all cases and avoids possible vertical shortening of the sutured orbital septum.

Lacerations involving the eyelid margin

Eyelid margin lacerations require precise suture placement and critical suture tension to avoid notches in the margin. Many techniques have been described, but the most important principle is that tarsal approximation must be made in a meticulous, direct manner (Fig 11-26). Eyelid margin closure may be accomplished by two or three sutures for alignment through the lash line, the meibomian gland plane, and (optionally) the gray line. Surgeons differ as to whether they place the tarsal or the eyelid margin sutures first. Precise anatomic alignment of the margin and secure tarsal closure are the goals, and many variations of techniques are acceptable. To avoid corneal epithelial disruption, the tarsal sutures should not extend through the conjunctival surface, especially in the upper eyelid. The eyelid margin closure should result in a moderate eversion of the well-approximated wound edges.

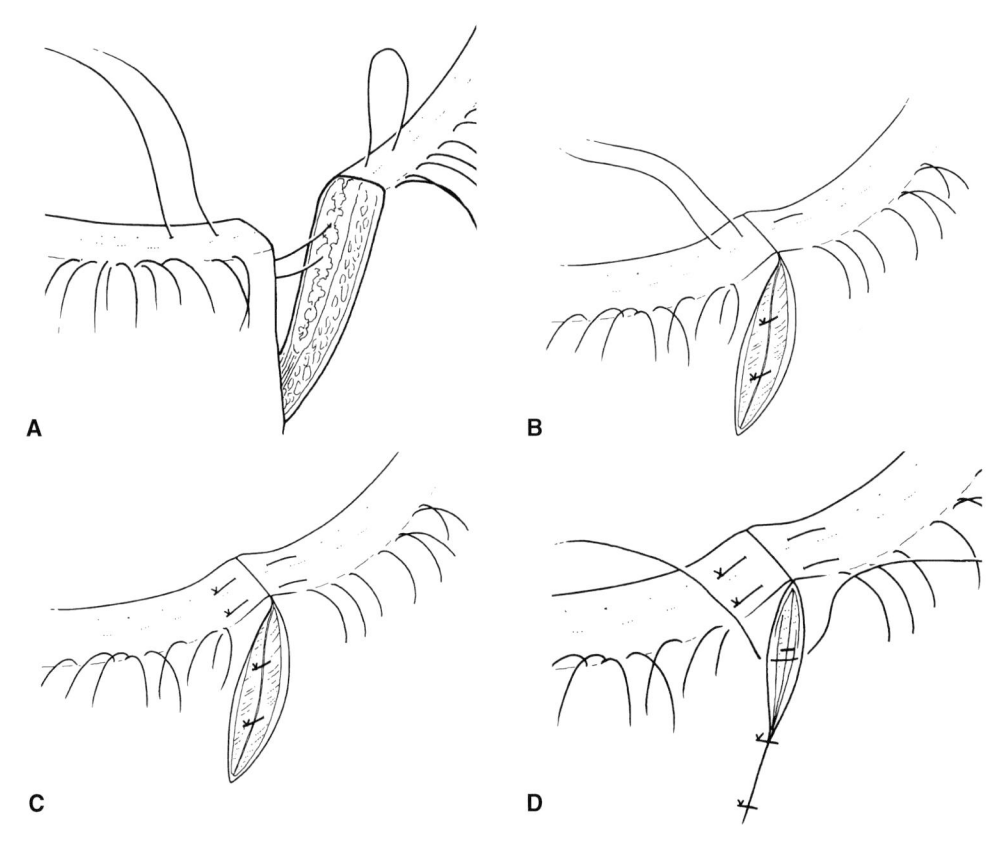

Figure 11-26 Lid margin repair. **A,** Align the lid margin using a vertical mattress suture passed through the meibomian gland orifices. **B,** Suture the tarsal plate using two or three interrupted sutures passed in a lamellar fashion. **C,** Suture the lid margin using an additional vertical mattress suture anterior to the gray line. **D,** Close the skin. *(Reproduced with permission from Nerad JA. The Requisites in Ophthalmology: Oculoplastic Surgery. Philadelphia: Mosby; 2001:319.)*

Trauma involving the canthal soft tissue

Trauma to the medial or lateral canthal areas is usually the result of horizontal traction on the eyelid, causing an eyelid avulsion at its weakest point, the medial or lateral canthal tendon. Careful review of the patient's history often confirms that an object or finger engaged the eyelid soft tissue in the central aspect of the eyelid, with subsequent horizontal traction of the eyelid. Hence, lacerations in the medial canthal area demand evaluation of the lacrimal drainage apparatus, which is always involved in an avulsion injury. Canalicular involvement is usually confirmed by inspection and gentle probing. Integrity of the inferior and superior limbs of medial or lateral canthal tendons can be assessed by grasping each lid with a toothed forceps and tugging away from the injury while palpating the insertion of the tendon. Even trivial medial canthal injuries can result in canalicular lacerations.

Medial canthal tendon avulsion should be suspected when there is a rounding of the medial canthal tendon and acquired telecanthus. Attention to the posterior portion of the tendon's attachment to the posterior lacrimal crest is critical.

Treatment of medial canthal tendon avulsions depends on the nature of the avulsion. If the upper or lower limb is avulsed but the posterior attachment of the tendon is intact, the avulsed limb may be sutured to its stump or to the periosteum overlying the anterior lacrimal crest. If the entire tendon, including the posterior portion, is avulsed but there is no naso-orbital fracture, the avulsed tendon should be wired through small drill holes in the ipsilateral posterior lacrimal crest. If the entire tendon is avulsed with a naso-orbital fracture, transnasal wiring or plating is necessary after reduction of the fracture.

   Devoto MH, Kersten RC, Teske SA, et al. Simplified technique for eyelid margin repair. *Arch Ophthalmol.* 1997;115:566–567.
   Howard GR, Nerad JA, Kersten RC. Medial canthoplasty with microplate fixation. *Arch Ophthalmol.* 1992;110:1793–1797.
   Shore JW, Rubin PA, Bilyk JR. Repair of telecanthus by anterior fixation of cantilevered miniplates. *Ophthalmology.* 1992;99:1133–1138.

A three-dimensional perspective is crucial in the evaluation and repair of canthal lacerations to ensure optimal functional and cosmetic repair—that is, the surgeon must always keep in mind the horizontal, vertical, and anteroposterior position of the canthal angle and medial canthal tendon. The different configurations of the medial and lateral canthal angles must also be considered. Whereas the lateral canthal angle is sharp, the medial canthal angle is slightly rounded. Failure to appreciate this difference gives rise to postoperative cosmetic and functional problems.

Secondary Repair

Secondary repair of eyelid trauma usually requires treatment of cicatricial changes that result from either the initial trauma or the subsequent surgical repair. Revision of scars may require simple fusiform excision with primary closure or a more complex rearrangement of tissue. The location of a particular scar in relation to the relaxed skin tension lines (which correspond to the facial wrinkles in most cases) determines the best technique or combination of techniques. An elliptical excision of the scar is most useful for revision of scars that follow the relaxed skin tension lines. Single Z-plasty or multiple Z-plasty reconstructive techniques can be used to revise scars that do not conform to relaxed skin tension lines.

Free skin grafts alone or in combination with various flaps are used when tissue has been lost. Although any non–hair-bearing skin can be used, full-thickness postauricular or preauricular skin is the most commonly used donor site for lower and upper eyelid reconstruction. Ipsilateral or contralateral upper eyelid, supra- or subclavicular areas, and even brachial or inner thigh areas are all potential donor sites for eyelid reconstruction.

Tarsoconjunctival grafts are good substitutes for posterior lamella eyelid defects when both the tarsal plate and the conjunctiva are deficient. Buccal mucosa may be used when only the conjunctiva is insufficient. Hard palate composite grafts have also become increasingly popular for posterior lamella defects. However, they should be avoided as a tarsal replacement in the upper eyelid because of the presence of keratinized epithelium that can irritate the cornea.

Before treatment is considered for traumatic ptosis, the patient should be observed for at least 6 months or until no further spontaneous return of function occurs. An exception to this general rule may be in a young child, in whom the possibility of deprivation amblyopia may necessitate early surgery to clear the visual axis.

Dog and Human Bites

Tearing and crushing injuries occur secondary to dog or human bites. Partial- and full-thickness eyelid lacerations, canthal avulsions, and canalicular lacerations are common. Serious facial and intracranial injury is possible, especially in infants, as bites generate hundreds of pounds of force per square inch. Irrigation and early wound repair are mandatory, and tetanus and rabies protocols should be observed. Systemic antibiotics are often recommended.

> Bartley GB. Periorbital animal bites. In: *Focal Points: Clinical Modules for Ophthalmologists.* San Francisco: American Academy of Ophthalmology; 1992: vol 10, no 3.

Burns

Burns of the eyelid are rare. Eyelid burns generally occur in patients who have sustained significant burns over large surface areas of the body. Often these patients are semiconscious or heavily sedated and require protection of the ocular surface to prevent corneal exposure, ulceration, and infection. Lubricating antibiotic drops and ointments, moisture chambers, and frequent evaluation of both the globes and the eyelids are part of the early treatment of these patients. Once cicatricial changes begin in the eyelids, a relentless and rapid deterioration of the patient's ocular status often ensues secondary to cicatricial eyelid retraction, lagophthalmos, and corneal exposure. If tarsorrhaphies are used, they should always be more extensive than seems to be immediately necessary. Unfortunately, with progression of the cicatricial traction, even the most aggressive eyelid adhesions may dehisce. In the past, skin grafting was usually delayed until the cicatricial changes stabilized, but the early use of full-thickness skin grafts and various types of flaps can effectively reduce ocular morbidity in selected patients.

Kulwin DR, Kersten RC. Management of eyelid burns. In: *Focal Points: Clinical Modules for Ophthalmologists.* San Francisco: American Academy of Ophthalmology; 1990: vol 8, no 2.

Meyer DR, Kersten RC, Kulwin DR, et al. Management of canalicular injury associated with eyelid burns. *Arch Ophthalmol.* 1995;113:900–903.

Eyelid and Canthal Reconstruction

The following discussion of eyelid reconstruction applies to defects resulting from tumor resection as well as congenital and traumatic defects. Several methods may be appropriate for reconstructing a particular eyelid defect. The surgeon's choice of procedure depends on the age of the patient, the character of the eyelids, the size and position of the defect, and personal experience and preference. Priorities in eyelid reconstruction are

- Development of a stable eyelid margin
- Provision of adequate vertical eyelid height
- Adequate eyelid closure
- Smooth, epithelialized internal surface
- Maximum cosmesis and symmetry

The following general principles guide the practice of eyelid reconstruction:

- Reconstruct either the anterior or the posterior eyelid lamella with a graft, but not both; one of the layers must provide the blood supply (pedicle flap). A graft placed on a graft has a high likelihood of failure.
- Maximize horizontal tension and minimize vertical tension.
- Maintain sufficient and anatomic canthal fixation.
- Match like tissue to like tissue.
- Narrow the defect as much as possible before sizing a graft.
- Choose the simplest technique.
- Don't create a defect you can't close.
- Get help from a subspecialist if you need it.

Eyelid Defects Not Involving the Eyelid Margin

Defects not involving the eyelid margins can be repaired by direct closure if this procedure does not distort the eyelid margin. If undermining does not allow direct closure, advancement or transposition of flaps of skin may be used. Tension of closure should be directed horizontally to avoid secondary deformity; vertical tension may cause eyelid retraction or ectropion. Avoidance of vertical tension requires placement of vertically oriented incision lines.

If the defect is too large to be closed primarily, several advancement or transposition techniques of local skin flaps may be used. The flaps most commonly used are rectangular advancement, rotation, and transposition. Flaps usually provide the best tissue match and aesthetic result but require planning to minimize secondary deformities. Although skin grafting procedures are generally easier to perform, the final texture, contour, and cosmesis are typically better with flaps.

Anterior lamella upper eyelid defects are best repaired with full-thickness skin grafts from the contralateral upper eyelid. Preauricular or retroauricular skin grafts may be used, but their greater thickness may limit upper eyelid mobility. Lower eyelid defects are best filled with preauricular or retroauricular skin grafts. If skin is not available from the upper eyelids or auricular areas, full-thickness grafts may be obtained from the supraclavicular fossa or the inner upper arm. It is important to avoid placement of hair-bearing skin grafts near the eyes.

Split-thickness grafts should be avoided in eyelid reconstruction. They are recommended only in treatment of severe burns of the face when adequate full-thickness skin is not available.

> Patrinely JR, Marines HM, Anderson RL. Skin flaps in periorbital reconstruction. *Surv Ophthalmol*. 1987;31:249–261.
>
> Teske SA, Kersten RC, Devoto MH, et al. The modified rhomboid transposition flap in periocular reconstruction. *Ophthal Plast Reconstr Surg*. 1998;14:360–366.

Eyelid Defects Involving the Eyelid Margin

Small upper eyelid defects

Small defects involving the upper eyelid margin can be repaired by direct closure if this technique does not place too much tension on the wound (Fig 11-27). Direct closure is usually employed when 33% or less of the eyelid margin is involved; if a larger area is involved, advancement of adjacent tissue or grafting of distant tissue may be required. The superior limb of the lateral canthal tendon can be cut to allow 3–5 mm of medial mobilization of the remaining lateral eyelid margin. Care is required to avoid the lacrimal ductules in the lateral third of the upper eyelid. Removal or destruction of these ductules may lead to dry eye problems. Postoperatively, the eyelid appears tight and ptotic because of bowstringing but relaxes over several weeks.

Moderate upper eyelid defects

Moderate defects of the upper eyelid margin (33%–50%) can be repaired by advancement of the lateral segment of the eyelid. The lateral canthal tendon is incised, and a semicircular skin flap is made below the lateral portion of the eyebrow and canthus to allow for further mobilization of the eyelid. Tarsal-sharing procedures in the upper eyelid have also been described.

Large upper eyelid defects

Upper eyelid defects involving more than 50% of the upper eyelid margin require advancement of adjacent tissues. A full-thickness lower eyelid flap may be advanced into the defect of the upper eyelid by passing it behind the remaining lower eyelid margin *(Cutler-Beard procedure)*. This procedure, however, results in a thick and relatively immobile upper eyelid. Alternatively, a free tarsoconjunctival graft taken from the contralateral upper eyelid can be positioned and covered with a skin-muscle flap if adequate redundant upper eyelid skin is present.

Small lower eyelid defects

Small defects of the lower eyelid (<33%) can be repaired by primary closure (Fig 11-28). In addition, the inferior crus of the lateral canthal tendon can be severed to allow an additional 3–5 mm of medial mobilization of the remaining lateral eyelid margin.

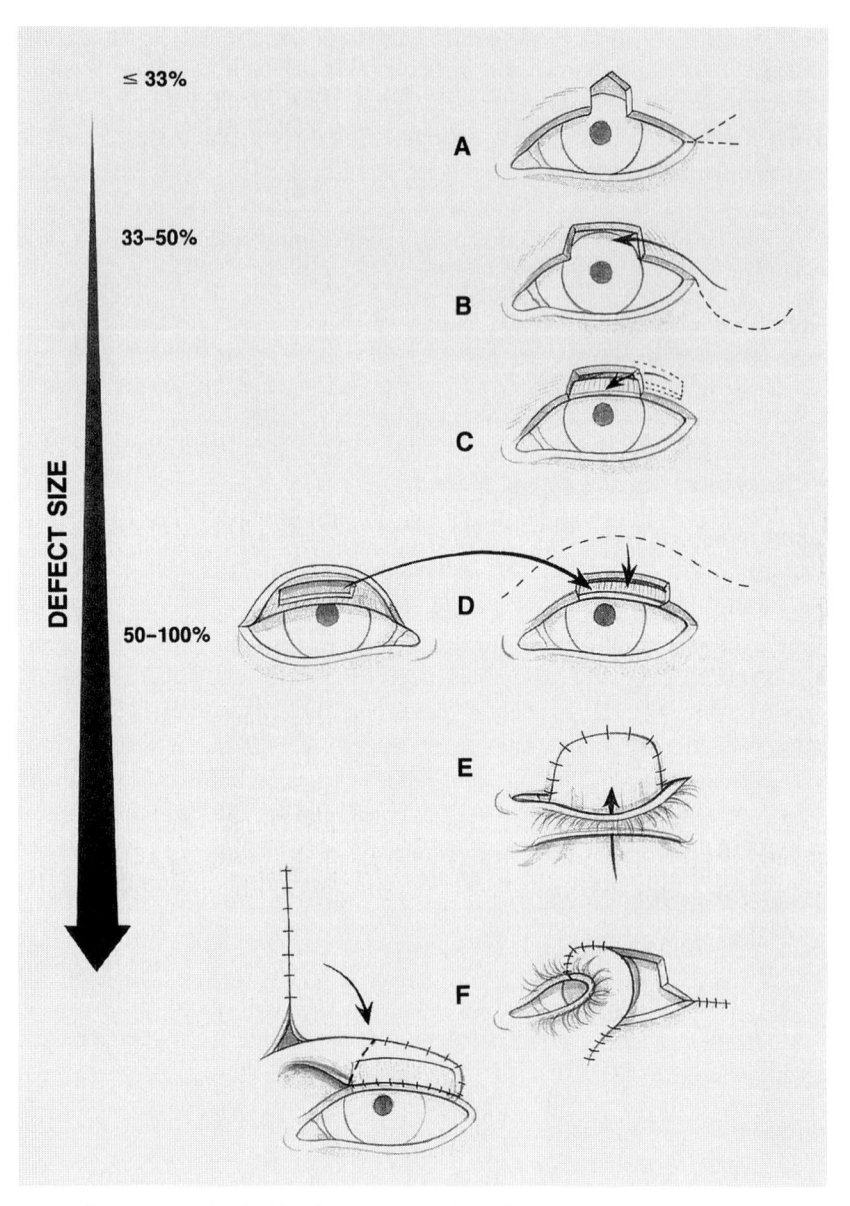

Figure 11-27 Reconstructive ladder for upper eyelid defect. *A,* Primary closure with or without lateral canthotomy or superior cantholysis. *B,* Semicircular flap. *C,* Adjacent tarsoconjunctival flap and full-thickness skin graft. *D,* Free tarsoconjunctival graft and skin flap. *E,* Full-thickness lower eyelid advancement flap (Cutler-Beard). *F,* Lower eyelid switch flap or median forehead flap. *(Illustration by Christine Gralapp.)*

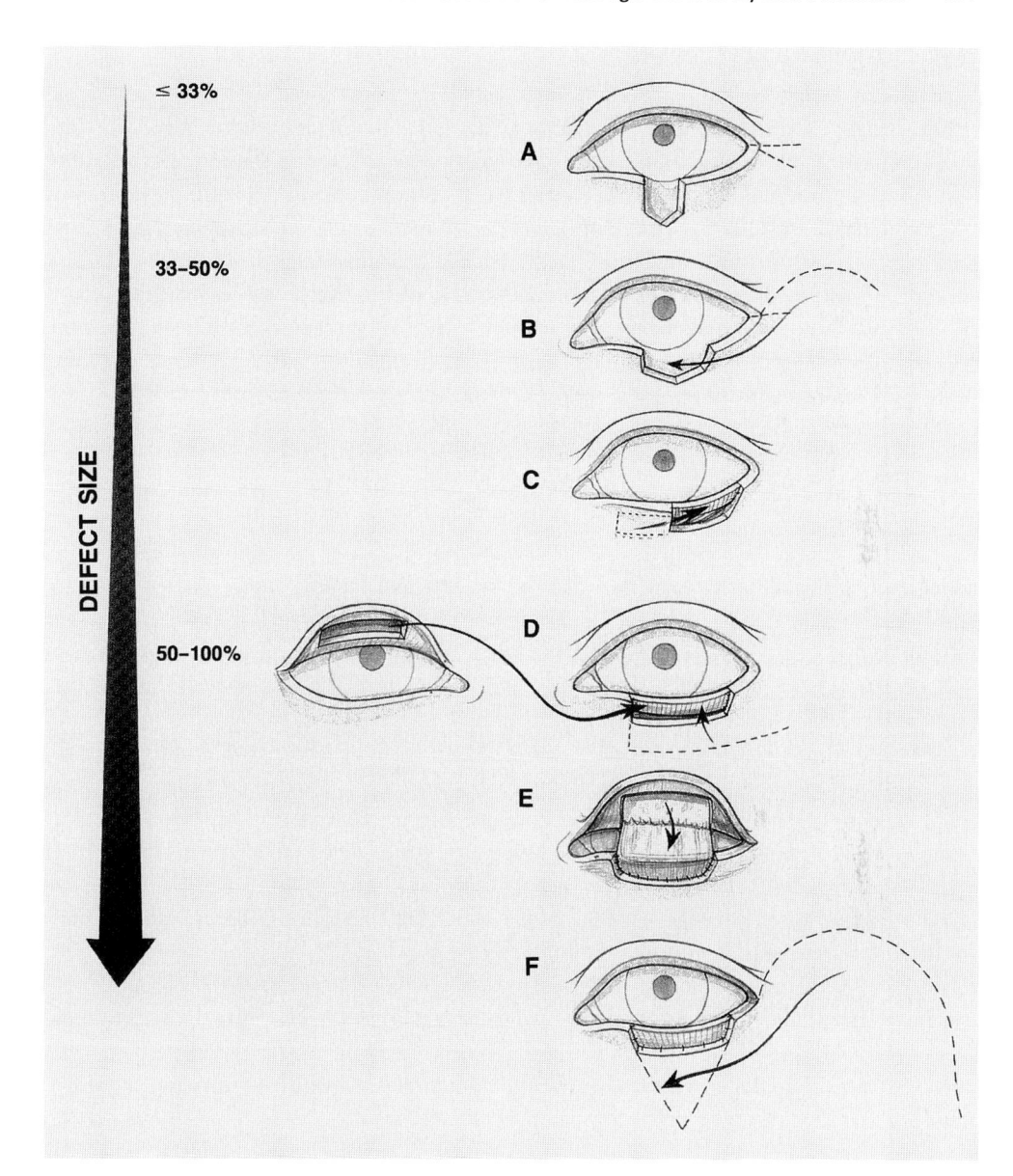

CHAPTER 11: Classification and Management of Eyelid Disorders • 191

Figure 11-28 Reconstructive ladder for lower eyelid defect. *A*, Primary closure with or without lateral canthotomy or superior cantholysis. *B*, Semicircular flap. *C*, Adjacent tarsoconjunctival flap and full-thickness skin graft. *D*, Free tarsoconjunctival graft and skin flap. *E*, Tarsoconjunctival flap from upper eyelid and skin graft (Hughes procedure). *F*, Composite graft with cheek advancement flap (Mustardé flap). *(Illustration by Christine Gralapp.)*

Moderate lower eyelid defects

Semicircular advancement or rotation flaps, which have been described for upper eyelid repair, can be used to reconstruct moderate defects in the lower eyelid as well. The flap most commonly used in such cases is a modification of the Tenzel semicircular rotation flap. Tarsoconjunctival autografts harvested from the underside of the upper eyelid may be transplanted into the lower eyelid defect to reconstruct the posterior lamella of the eyelid. When tarsal grafts are being harvested, the marginal 4–5 mm height of tarsus should be preserved in order to prevent distortion of the donor eyelid margin. Tarsoconjunctival autografts may be covered with skin flaps of various types. Cheek elevation may also be required in order to avoid vertical traction on the lid and ectropion. Alternatively, a tarsoconjunctival flap developed from the upper eyelid and a full-thickness skin graft can also be used.

Large lower eyelid defects

Defects larger than 50% of the lower eyelid margin can be repaired by advancement of a tarsoconjunctival flap from the upper eyelid into the posterior lamellar defect of the lower eyelid. The anterior lamella of the reconstructed eyelid is then created with an advancement skin flap or, in most cases, a free skin graft taken from the preauricular or retroauricular area *(modified Hughes procedure)*. The modified Hughes procedure therefore results in placement of a bridge of conjunctiva from the upper eyelid across the pupil for several weeks. The vascularized pedicle of conjunctiva is then released in a staged, second procedure once the lower eyelid flap is revascularized. Therefore, eyelid-sharing techniques should be avoided in children under age 7, who may develop occlusion amblyopia as a result. Large rotating cheek flaps *(Mustardé procedure)* can work well for repair of large anterior lamellar defects, but they require some tarsal substitute such as a free tarsoconjunctival autograft, hard palate mucosa, or a Hughes flap for posterior lamella replacement. Both the Mustardé cheek rotation flap and the Tenzel semicircular rotation flap frequently result in a rounded lateral canthus. The surgeon can reduce this problem by creating a very high incision toward the lateral end of the eyebrow where the incision emanates from the lateral commissure. Free tarsoconjunctival autografts from the upper eyelid covered with a vascularized skin flap have been used to repair large defects as well. This type of procedure has the advantage of requiring only one surgical stage and avoids even temporary occlusion of the visual axis.

Lateral Canthal Defects

Laterally based transposition flaps of upper eyelid tarsus and conjunctiva can be used for large lower eyelid defects extending to the lateral canthus. These flaps can be covered with free skin grafts. Semicircular advancement flaps of skin can also be used to repair defects extending to the lateral canthal area. Sometimes, strips of periosteum and temporalis fascia left attached at the lateral orbital rim can be swung over and attached to the remaining lateral eyelid margins to reconstruct the entire lateral canthal posterior lamella. A Y-shaped pedicle flap of periosteum is optimal to reconstruct the entire lateral canthal posterior lamella.

Medial Canthal Defects

The medial canthal area lends itself to a variety of reconstructive methods. Spontaneous granulation of anterior lamellar defects has been used with varying success. Full-thickness skin grafting or flap reconstructions are more widely accepted repair techniques for medial canthal defects. When full-thickness medial eyelid defects are present, the medial canthal attachments of the remaining eyelid margin must be fixed to firm periosteum. This fixation may be accomplished with heavy permanent suture, wire, or titanium miniplates. Defects involving the lacrimal drainage apparatus are more complex and require simultaneous microsurgical reconstruction and possible silicone intubation or marsupialization. If extensive sacrifice of the canaliculi has occurred in the resection of a tumor, the patient may have to tolerate epiphora until recurrence of the tumor is no longer a risk. Until tumor recurrence is ruled out, it is critical to avoid lacrimal surgery that could create a pathway for tumor to spread into the nose or sinuses. After a recurrence-free period of up to 5 years (based on clinical judgment), a conjunctivodacryocystorhinostomy with a Jones tube can be performed to eliminate the epiphora.

>Howard GR, Nerad JA, Kersten RC. Medial canthoplasty with microplate fixation. *Arch Ophthalmol.* 1992;110:1793–1797.
>
>Lowry JC, Bartley GB, Garrity JA. The role of second-intention healing in periocular reconstruction. *Ophthal Plast Reconstr Surg.* 1997;13:174–188.

Full-thickness skin grafts offer an excellent method of reconstruction of the medial canthus compared with the cicatrix resulting from spontaneous granulation. The full-thickness grafts are thin enough to allow for early detection of tumor recurrence. However, every effort should be made at the time of tumor resection to minimize the risk of recurrent medial canthal tumors. Frozen sections and wide margins or Mohs' micrographic resection techniques minimize the risk of recurrent medial canthal tumors and the risk of orbital or lacrimal extension of these tumors. Large medial canthal defects of anterior lamellar structures may be reconstructed through the transposition of forehead or glabellar flaps. However, such flaps have the disadvantage of being thick, thereby making early detection of recurrences difficult. In addition, they often require second-stage thinning in order to achieve the best cosmetic result. Mohs' micrographic resection of tumors offers the highest cure rates for eradication of medial canthal epithelial malignancies.

>Spinelli HM, Jelks GW. Periocular reconstruction: a systematic approach. *Plast Reconstr Surg.* 1993;91:1017–1024.

CHAPTER 12

Periocular Malpositions and Involutional Changes

Evaluation of all eyelid anomalies requires an assessment of what structural alterations are present. Determining whether the abnormality is associated with anterior lamella (skin and orbicularis muscle) or posterior lamella (tarsus and conjunctiva) facilitates treatment planning.

Ectropion

Ectropion (Fig 12-1) is an outward turning of the eyelid margin and may be classified as:

- Congenital
- Involutional
- Paralytic
- Cicatricial
- Mechanical

The majority of cases seen in a general ophthalmology practice are involutional, with horizontal eyelid laxity being the primary cause. Congenital ectropion of the eyelid is rare. Treatment errors and recurrences will be minimized if each case is accurately diagnosed before treatment is undertaken.

> Goldberg RA, Neuhaus RW. Eyelid malpositions associated with skin and conjunctival disease. *Ophthalmol Clin North Am.* 1992;5:227–241.

Congenital Ectropion

Congenital ectropion is discussed in Chapter 11, under the heading Congenital Anomalies.

Involutional Ectropion

Involutional ectropion results from tissue relaxation, with horizontal eyelid laxity usually in the medial or lateral canthal tendons. If untreated, this condition usually leads to loss of eyelid apposition to the globe with eversion of the eyelid margin. Chronic conjunctival inflammation with hypertrophy and keratinization results.

196 • Orbit, Eyelids, and Lacrimal System

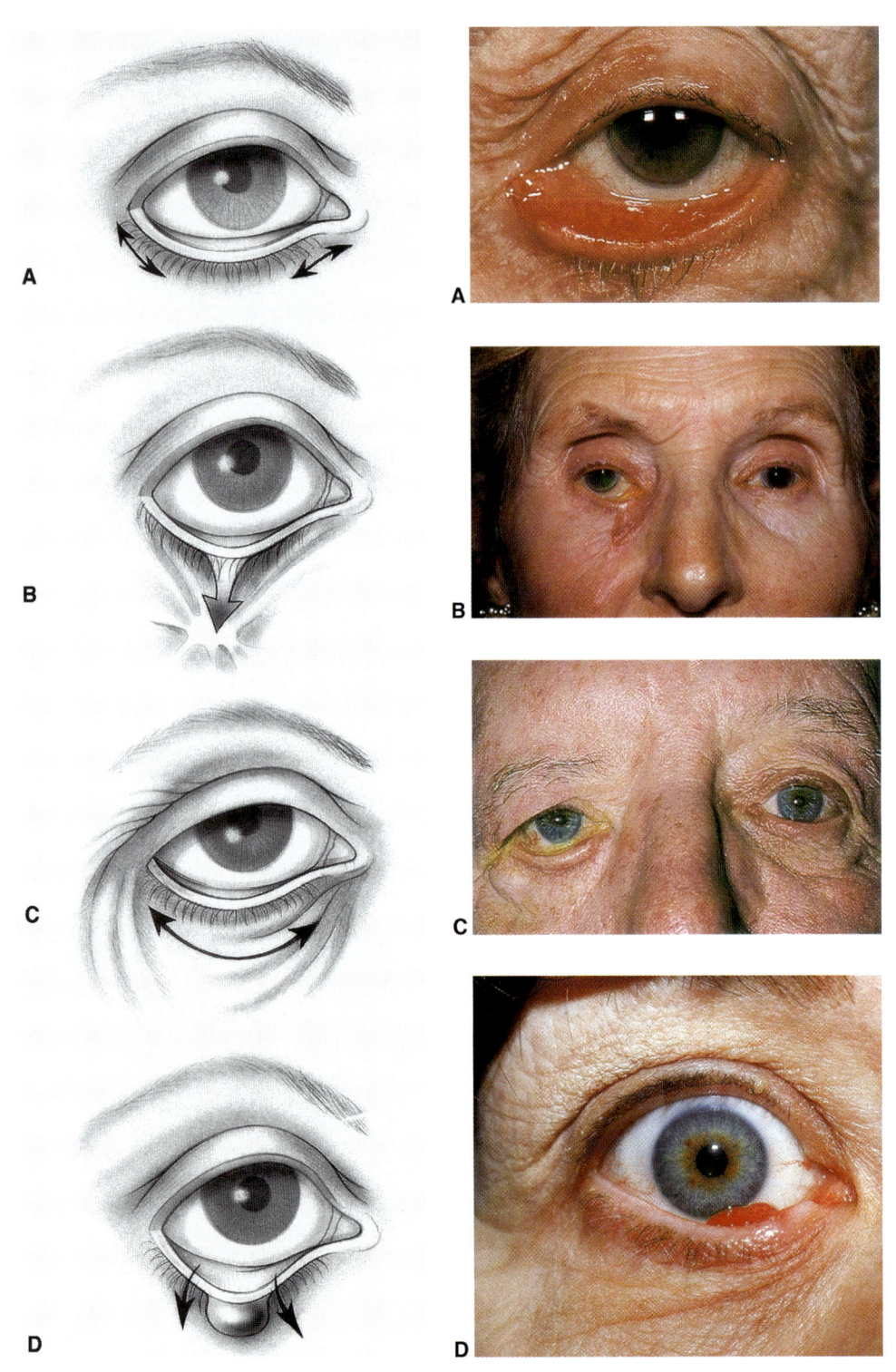

Figure 12-1 Types of ectropion. **A,** Involutional. **B,** Cicatricial. **C,** Paralytic. **D,** Mechanical. *(Illustration by Christine Gralapp; photographs A and B courtesy of James R. Patrinely, MD. Photograph D courtesy of Robert C. Kersten, MD.)*

CHAPTER 12: Periocular Malpositions and Involutional Changes • 197

Involutional ectropion usually occurs in the lower eyelid, probably because of the added effects of gravity on a horizontally lax lower eyelid. Horizontal laxity of the eyelid caused by disinsertion or stretching of the inferior limbs of the canthal tendons, especially laterally, is a common feature in involutional ectropion.

In cases of mild medial eyelid ectropion with punctal malposition, thermal cautery of the conjunctiva has historically been used and is still utilized in selected cases to cause inward rotation of the eyelid margin. However, recurrence of the ectropion is common. As an alternative surgical procedure, horizontal fusiform excision of conjunctiva and eyelid retractors 4 mm inferior to the puncta, with closure utilizing inverting sutures (*medial spindle procedure,* Fig 12-2A), usually corrects the punctal malposition. In cases with associated horizontal eyelid laxity, eyelid lateral canthal tightening may be used in conjunction with this operation.

If the involutional ectropion is more severe and involves more than the punctum, one of the following types of surgical procedures is generally used: (1) horizontal eyelid shortening, including horizontal resection of the lateral eyelid, plication of the canthal

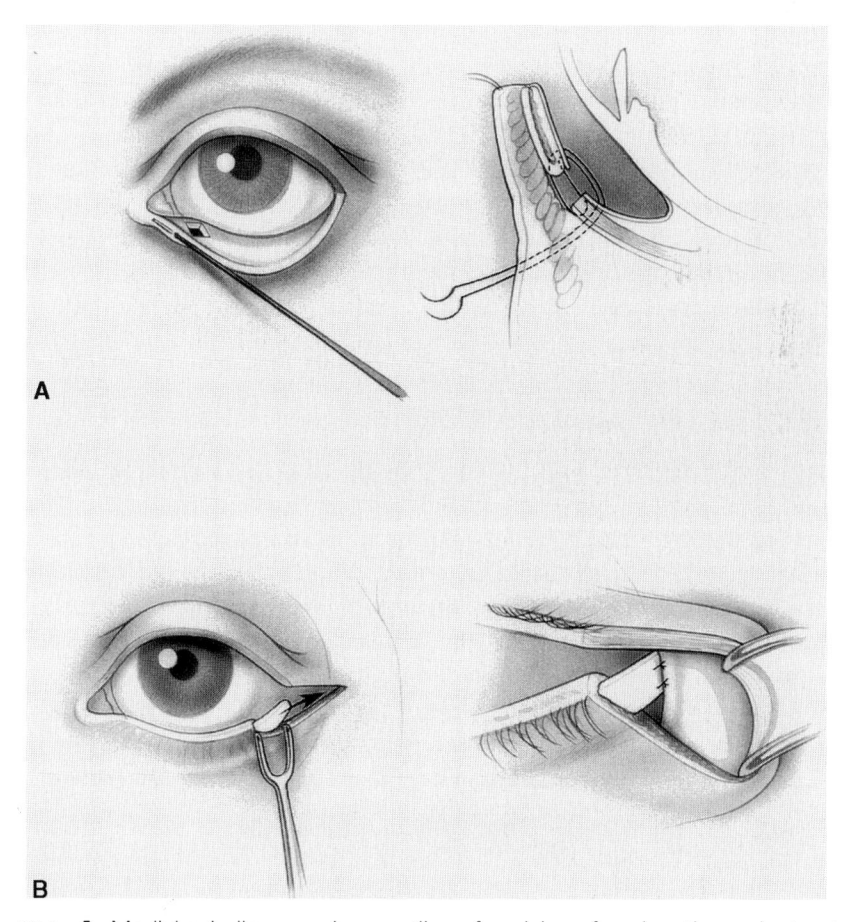

Figure 12-2 A, Medial spindle procedure: outline of excision of conjunctiva and retractors. **B,** Lateral tarsal strip procedure: anchoring of tarsal strip to periosteum inside lateral orbital rim. *(Illustration by Christine Gralapp.)*

tendons, and lateral canthoplasty (*tarsal strip procedure,* Fig 12-2B); or (2) reinsertion of the lower eyelid retractors.

Before selecting the procedure or combinations of procedures to use, the surgeon must take into account not only the etiologic factors but also the presence or absence of punctal malposition and secondary contraction of the anterior lamella. Combining more than one type of procedure to correct involutional ectropion is not unusual.

Horizontal eyelid shortening

Horizontal tightening can be achieved via a full-thickness excision of the eyelid just medial to the lateral canthal angle *(Bick procedure).* Resection of the eyelid in this location may cause rounding and medial displacement of the lateral canthal angle. Repair of the eyelid defect following full-thickness resection is similar to the process described in Chapter 11 for a full-thickness eyelid margin laceration (see Fig 11-28).

Laxity of the lower limb of the medial canthal tendon can be diagnosed by observing excessive lateral movement of the lower punctum with lateral eyelid traction. Lateral canthal tendon laxity or disinsertion can be similarly detected. Repair of medial canthal laxity is difficult at best. After placing a probe in the canaliculus for identification, the surgeon makes an infraciliary incision from the medial canthal angle temporally 4–5 mm beyond the puncta. The anterior origin of the medial canthal tendon and its inferior limb are then plicated with a 5-0 nonabsorbable mattress suture. This technique is often complicated by a kinking of the canaliculus or distraction of the punctum away from the globe with secondary epiphora.

Horizontal eyelid laxity may be treated by direct shortening of the lateral canthal tendon or the lateral edge of the tarsal plate utilizing a lateral tarsal strip operation. The horizontally shortened lateral canthal tendon is reattached to the lateral orbital rim periosteum. This does not compromise the horizontal dimension of the palpebral fissure and maintains a sharp, correctly positioned lateral canthal angle.

Repair of lower eyelid retractors

Retractor laxity, disinsertion, or dehiscence may be associated with ectropion, especially when the eyelid is completely everted, a condition known as *tarsal ectropion.* Attenuation or disinsertion of the inferior retractors may occur as an isolated defect or may accompany horizontal laxity in involutional ectropion. When both defects are present, repair of the retractors can be combined with a horizontal tightening of the eyelid. Reattachment of the retractors can be initiated directly through a conjunctival approach to advance the lower eyelid retractors to the inferior border of tarsus.

Long-standing involutional ectropion with contraction of the anterior lamella (skin) usually requires horizontal tightening of the eyelid combined with midface lifting or full-thickness skin grafting. (See discussion under the heading Cicatricial Ectropion, below.)

Anderson RL, Gordy DD. The tarsal strip procedure. *Arch Ophthalmol.* 1979;97:2192–2196.

Dailey RA, Jones LT. Rejuvenation of the aging face. In: *Focal Points: Clinical Modules for Ophthalmologists.* San Francisco: American Academy of Ophthalmology; 2003: vol 21, no 11.

Nowinski TS, Anderson RL. The medial spindle procedure for involutional medial ectropion. *Arch Ophthalmol.* 1985;103:1750–1753.

Tse DT, Kronish JW, Buus D. Surgical correction of lower-eyelid tarsal ectropion by reinsertion of the retractors. *Arch Ophthalmol.* 1991;109:427–431.

Paralytic Ectropion

Paralytic ectropion usually follows temporary or permanent seventh nerve paralysis or palsy. Concomitant upper eyelid lagophthalmos is usually present secondary to paralytic upper eyelid orbicularis dysfunction. Poor blinking and eyelid closure lead to chronic ocular surface irritation resulting from inferior corneal exposure together with poor tear film replenishment and distribution. Chronically stimulated reflex secretors (main or accessory lacrimal glands) along with atonic eyelids account for the frequent complaint of tearing in these patients. Eyelid excursion during the blink cycle is further limited in the setting of vertical eyelid shortening or Graves ophthalmopathy with eyelid retraction or proptosis.

Neurologic evaluation may be indicated to determine the cause of the seventh nerve paralysis. In cases resulting from stroke or intracranial surgery, clinical evaluation of corneal sensation is indicated because neurotrophic keratitis combined with paralytic lagophthalmos leads to extreme corneal exposure and early corneal decompensation.

Lubricating drops, viscous tear supplementation, ointments, taping of the temporal half of the lower eyelid, or moisture chambers may be used alone or in combination. Such measures may be the only treatment necessary, especially for temporary paralysis. In long-term or permanent paralysis, tarsorrhaphy, medial or lateral canthoplasties, and horizontal tightening procedures are useful in selected patients.

Tarsorrhaphies can be performed either medially or laterally. An adequate temporary tarsorrhaphy (1–3 weeks) can be achieved with nonabsorbable suture placement between the upper and lower eyelid margins without disruption of the eyelid epithelium. A permanent tarsorrhaphy requires careful removal of the epithelium along the upper and lower eyelid margins; the surgeon should exercise caution to avoid the lash follicles. Next, absorbable sutures are placed to unite the raw surfaces of the upper and lower eyelids (Fig 12-3). In general, patients dislike the tarsorrhaphy from a functional or cosmetic perspective; this procedure should be avoided if possible. Placement of a gold weight in the upper eyelid and repair of horizontal laxity or ectropion generally allows the patient to avoid permanent tarsorrhaphy.

Occasionally, a fascia lata or silicone suspension sling of the lower eyelid may be indicated. Lower eyelid vertical elevation may be useful in reducing exposure of the lower one third of the cornea. This elevation may be accomplished through inferior retractor muscle recession combined with full-thickness hard palate mucosal graft or ear cartilage graft.

Interest in gold weight loading of the upper eyelid for paralytic lagophthalmos has grown in recent years. The appropriate gold weight size is selected by preoperatively taping various sizes of weights to the upper eyelid skin to determine which one best achieves adequate relaxed eyelid closure while limiting eyelid ptosis in primary gaze. A standard upper eyelid incision is made through skin and orbicularis muscle. The gold weight is then sutured to the anterior surface of the tarsal plate. The gold weight implant (average weight, 0.8–1.6 g) reduces but does not usually eliminate lagophthalmos and

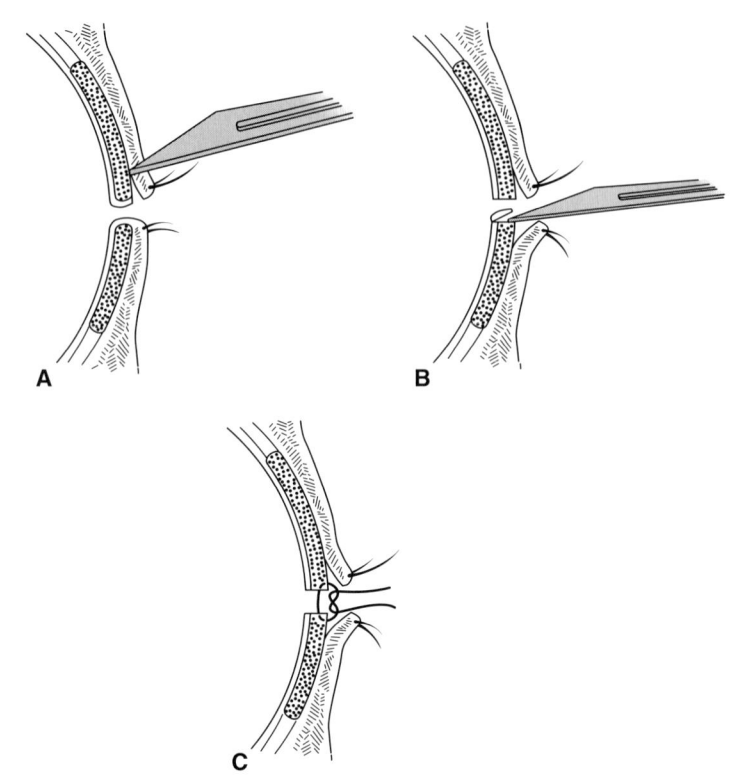

Figure 12-3 Tarsorrhaphy. **A,** Eyelid is split 2–3 mm deep. **B,** Epithelium is carefully removed along the upper and lower eyelid margins, avoiding the lash follicles. **C,** The raw surfaces are then united with absorbable sutures. *(Illustration by Christine Gralapp.)*

corneal exposure. A 2.2 g gold weight can be placed behind the orbital septum, superior to the tarsus, to avoid the inevitable mass effect of the pretarsal area if cosmesis is a concern. Implanted eyelid springs to provide dynamic eyelid closure are infrequently used because of limited long-term success.

> Gilliland G, Wobig JL, Dailey RA. A modified surgical technique in the treatment of facial nerve palsies. *Ophthal Plast Reconstr Surg.* 1998;14:94–98.
>
> Townsend DJ. Eyelid reanimation for the treatment of paralytic lagophthalmos: Historical perspectives and current applications of the gold weight implant. *Ophthal Plast Reconstr Surg.* 1992;8:196–201.

Cicatricial Ectropion

Cicatricial ectropion of the upper or lower eyelid may occur secondary to thermal or chemical burns, mechanical trauma, surgical trauma, or chronic actinic skin damage. Cicatricial ectropion can also be caused by chronic inflammation of the eyelid from dermatologic conditions such as rosacea, atopic dermatitis, eczematoid dermatitis, or herpes zoster infections. Treatment of the underlying cause along with conservative medical protection of the cornea is essential as primary management. Cicatricial ectropion of the lower eyelid is usually treated in a three-step procedure:

1. Vertical cicatricial traction is surgically incised and relaxed.
2. The eyelid is horizontally tightened with a lateral tarsal strip operation.
3. The anterior lamella is vertically lengthened via a midface lift or full-thickness skin graft.

Treatment of cicatricial ectropion or retraction of the upper eyelid usually requires only augmentation of the vertically shortened anterior lamella with a full-thickness skin graft.

Although skin from the opposite upper eyelid is the best color and texture match for skin grafting, this source is usually inadequate except in patients with significant dermatochalasis. Postauricular skin is the next most desirable donor site for eyelid reconstruction.

Mechanical Ectropion

Mechanical ectropion is usually caused by the effect of gravity on bulky tumors of the eyelid. Fluid accumulation, herniated orbital fat, or poorly fitted spectacles may also provide a mechanical component for lower eyelid ectropion.

Entropion

Entropion is an inversion of the eyelid margin. Lower eyelid entropion (usually involutional) is much more common than upper eyelid entropion (usually cicatricial). Entropion may be unilateral or bilateral and is often classified into the following categories:

- Congenital
- Acute spastic
- Involutional
- Cicatricial

More than 100 procedures have been described to correct entropion, and as in ectropion, causes must be identified before the most appropriate type of procedure can be selected.

Congenital Entropion

Congenital entropion is discussed in Chapter 11, under the heading Congenital Anomalies.

Acute Spastic Entropion

This condition follows ocular irritation or inflammation. It is most common after intraocular surgery in a patient who had unrecognized or mild involutional eyelid changes preoperatively. Sustained eyelid orbicularis muscle contraction causes inward rotation of the eyelid margin. A cycle of increasing entropion caused by corneal irritation secondary to the preexisting entropion perpetuates the problem. The acute entropion usually resolves when the irritation/entropion cycle is broken by treatment of both the underlying cause and the entropion.

Taping of the inturned eyelid to evert the margin, cautery, or various suture techniques afford temporary relief for most patients (Fig 12-4). However, because underlying

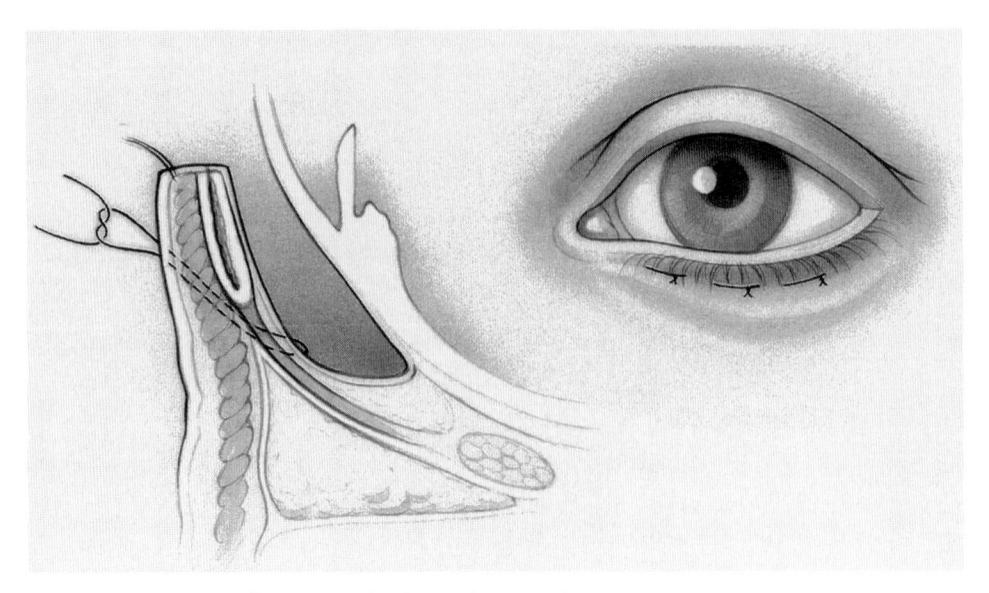

Figure 12-4 Suture repair of spastic entropion. *(Illustration by Christine Gralapp.)*

involutional changes are usually present in the eyelid, additional definitive surgical repair may be needed to permanently correct the entropion. In selected cases, botulinum toxin type A (Botox) can be used to paralyze the overriding preseptal orbicularis muscle.

Involutional Entropion

Involutional entropion is usually associated with the lower eyelids. The factors, alone or in combination, thought to play a role in the development of involutional entropion are horizontal laxity of the eyelid, attenuation or disinsertion of eyelid retractors, and overriding of the preseptal orbicularis. Horizontal laxity can be detected by a poor tone of the eyelid *(snapback test)* and ability to pull the eyelid more than 6 mm from the globe. Such laxity is a result of involutional stretching of the medial and lateral canthal tendons.

Normally, the lower eyelid retractors maintain the lower eyelid margin in proper orientation. However, attenuation of the eyelid retractors (capsulopalpebral fascia and inferior tarsal muscle) in the lower eyelids allows the inferior border of the tarsus to ride forward and superiorly with the eyelid margin rotating inward (Fig 12-5). Several clinical clues may be present to indicate disinsertion of the retractors:

- A white subconjunctival line several millimeters below the inferior tarsal border caused by the leading edge of the detached retractors
- An inferior fornix that is deeper than usual
- Ptosis of the lower eyelid (lower eyelid is higher than normal)
- Little or no inferior movement of the lower eyelid on downgaze

Superior migration of the preseptal orbicularis is detected by observation of the preseptal orbicularis as the patient squeezes his or her eyes closed after the entropic eyelid has been placed in its normal position (overriding orbicularis). Involutional changes in

CHAPTER 12: Periocular Malpositions and Involutional Changes • 203

the orbital soft tissues may also contribute to involutional entropion by reducing the lower eyelid posterior support.

Procedures to repair involutional entropion of the lower eyelid generally fall into one of three groups: temporizing measures, horizontal tightening procedures, and repair of the retractors (Fig 12-6). Often, a combination of procedures must be used to minimize recurrence. Trichiasis or malpositioned lashes may need specific treatment either in con-

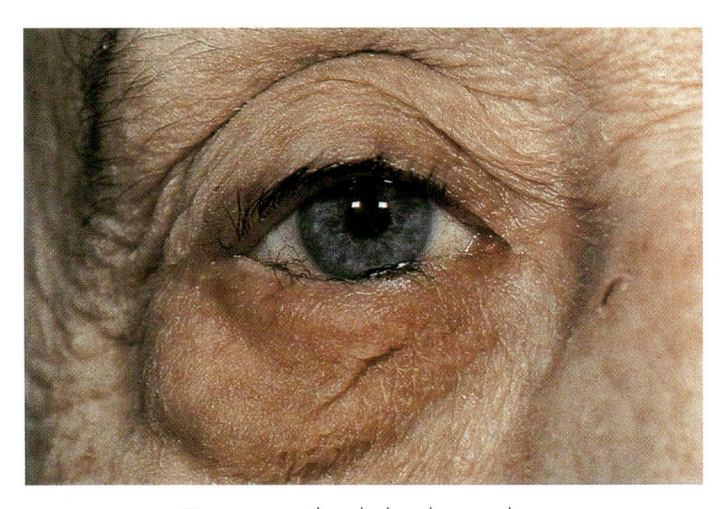

Figure 12-5 Involutional entropion.

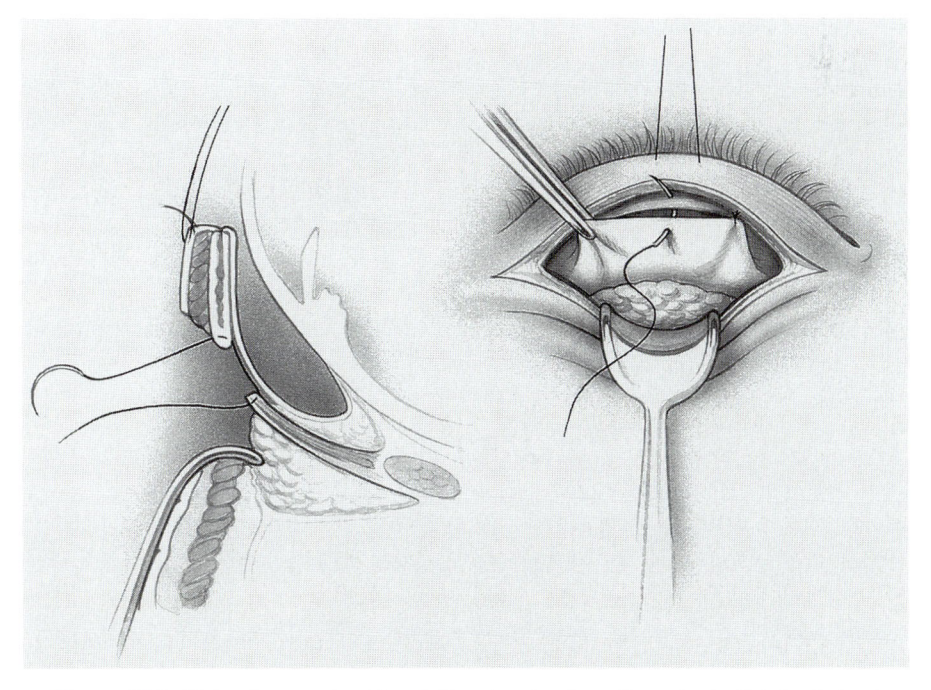

Figure 12-6 Retractor repair of involutional entropion. *(Illustration by Christine Gralapp.)*

junction with the entropion repair or subsequently if lashes remain misdirected after proper positioning of the eyelid margin.

Temporizing measures

Suture techniques (Quickert sutures—see Fig 12-4) are occasionally useful as temporizing measures in involutional entropion, but these procedures by themselves are associated with high recurrence rates. Thermal cautery is rarely successful as a means of tightening the anterior lamella.

Horizontal eyelid tightening

Horizontal tightening of the eyelid at the lateral canthus stabilizes the eyelid and often corrects the entropion. The lateral tarsal strip operation is useful (see Fig 12-2B).

Repair of retractors

The Quickert suture repair is a fast but often temporary means of reinserting the retractors. A marginal rotation by means of a full-thickness horizontal eyelid incision is used to advance the lower eyelid retractors (*Wies repair,* Fig 12-7). Although this procedure was originally described for the treatment of cicatricial entropion, it may also be appropriate for some cases of involutional entropion when used alone or in combination with horizontal tightening procedures. Marginal rotation can also be effective in upper entropion.

Direct exploration and repair of lower eyelid retractor defects through a skin incision or transconjunctival approach are designed to stabilize the inferior border of the tarsus. The retractor reinsertion operation is usually combined with a lateral canthal tightening of the eyelid. When retractor reinsertion is performed using an incision through the skin

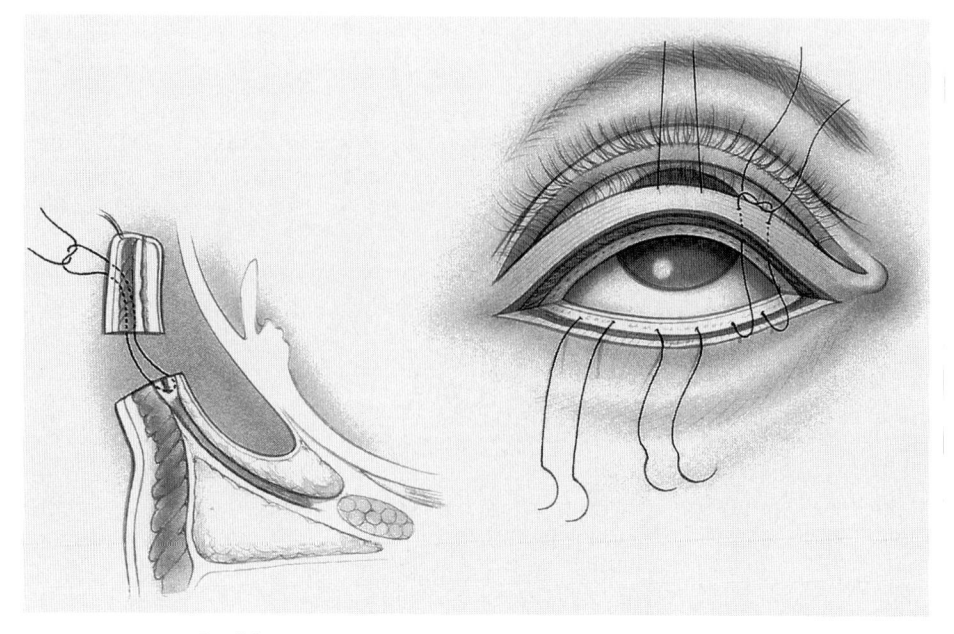

Figure 12-7 Eyelid margin rotation (Wies procedure). *(Illustration by Christine Gralapp.)*

and orbicularis muscles at or near the inferior tarsal border, the incisional scar helps prevent postoperative orbicularis override. A small amount of preseptal orbicularis muscle can also be removed in selected patients who have a large amount of override. Reinsertion of the retractor performed through the skin in conjunction with a lateral tarsal strip operation corrects all three etiologic factors in involutional entropion and is the combined approach of choice for many surgeons.

> Dresner SC, Karesh JW. Transconjunctival entropion repair. *Arch Ophthalmol.* 1993;111:1144–1148.
>
> Kersten RC, Hammer BJ, Kulwin DR. The role of enophthalmos in involutional entropion. *Ophthal Plast Reconstr Surg.* 1997;13:195–198.
>
> Nowinski TS. Orbicularis oculi muscle extirpation in a combined procedure for involutional entropion. *Ophthalmology.* 1991;98:1250–1256.

Cicatricial Entropion

Cicatricial entropion (Fig 12-8) is caused by vertical tarsoconjunctival contracture and internal rotation of the eyelid margin with resulting irritation of the globe from inturned cilia or the keratinized eyelid margin. A variety of conditions may lead to cicatricial entropion, including *autoimmune* (cicatricial pemphigoid), *inflammatory* (Stevens-Johnson syndrome), *infectious* (trachoma, herpes zoster), *surgical* (enucleation, posterior-approach ptosis correction), and *traumatic* (thermal or chemical burns, scarring). The chronic use of topical glaucoma medications, especially miotics, may cause chronic conjunctivitis with vertical conjunctival shortening and secondary cicatricial entropion.

The patient's history along with a simple diagnostic test (digital eversion) usually distinguishes cicatricial entropion from involutional entropion. Digital eyelid traction to attempt to return the eyelid to a normal anatomic position corrects the abnormal margin position in involutional entropion but not in cicatricial entropion. Inspection of the posterior aspect of the eyelid reveals subtle to severe scarring of the tarsal conjunctiva in cases of cicatricial entropion.

Effectiveness of treatment in cicatricial entropion depends primarily on cause and severity. When the cause is autoimmune or inflammatory disease, the prognosis is guarded because of frequent disease progression; when the cause is prior surgery or

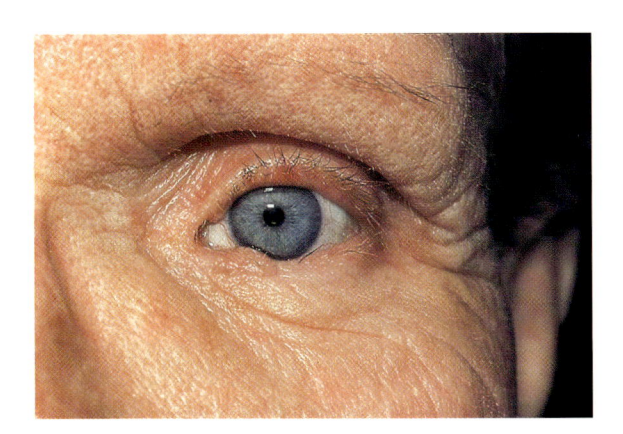

Figure 12-8 Cicatricial entropion. *(Photograph courtesy of Russell Neuhaus, MD.)*

trauma, prognosis is generally good because the process tends to be localized and reversible. Infectious causes fall somewhere in between.

Successful management of cicatricial entropion depends on thoughtful preoperative evaluation to determine the cause, severity, and prominent features in each patient. The goal of treatment is to eliminate the chronic ocular irritation by removing the lashes and keratinized tissue from contact with the cornea. Cicatricial entropion usually requires surgery, but lubricating drops and ointments, barriers to symblepharon formation, and cryotherapy are sometimes useful adjuncts. Indeed, surgery is contraindicated during the acute phase of autoimmune diseases, and topical and systemic medications are more appropriate until the disease stabilizes.

When there is only slight inversion of the margin (with or without trichiasis) and little distortion of other eyelid structures, resection of anterior lamellar tissue with or without mucous membrane grafting may be curative. The anterior lamellar repositioning slides the offending tissues away from the eye.

The tarsal fracture operation (Fig 12-9) is useful in cases of mild to moderate cicatricial entropion (marginal entropion) in the upper or lower eyelid. In this situation, lashes abrade the cornea, and careful examination shows that the ciliary eyelid margin has lost its square edges and is rotated posteriorly. A posterior horizontal tarsal incision is made 2 mm inferior to the eyelid margin. This full-thickness tarsal incision allows the eyelid margin to be fractured away from the globe in an everted position. The eyelid position is stabilized with everting sutures.

For marginal rotation to be effective, the tarsus should be intact and of reasonably good quality. Because it is advisable not to violate the conjunctiva in patients with active autoimmune disease, medical management of the inflammatory condition with systemic and topical anti-inflammatory medications is desirable. When surgery is indicated, maximal inflammatory suppression is achieved with pulsed systemic anti-inflammatory medications (corticosteroids and immunosuppressive agents).

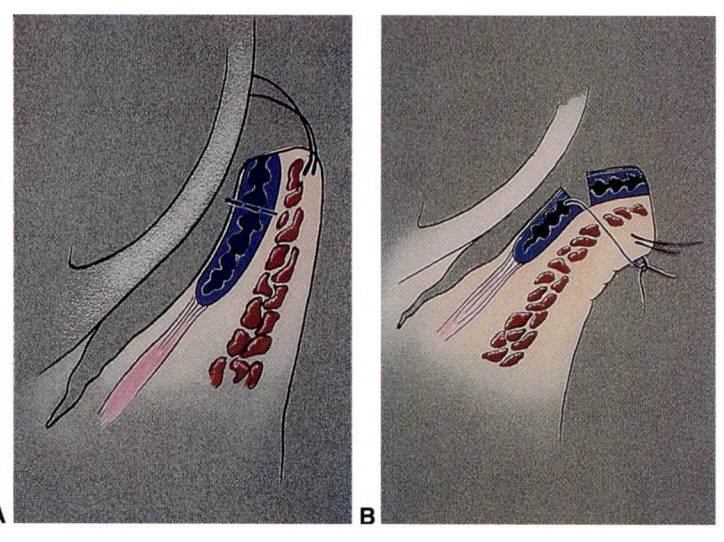

Figure 12-9 A, Tarsotomy. **B,** Margin rotation for cicatricial entropion.

Because it is usually scarred and distorted in patients with severe cicatricial entropion, the involved tarsus generally needs to be replaced. In the upper eyelid, tarsoconjunctival grafts are useful tarsal substitutes; in the lower eyelid, autogenous ear cartilage, preserved scleral grafts, and hard palate mucosa have been used.

> D'Ostroph AO, Dailey RA. Cicatricial entropion associated with chronic dipivefrin application. *Ophthal Plast Reconstr Surg.* 2001;17:328–331.
>
> Heiligenhaus A, Shore JW, Rubin PAD, et al. Long-term results of mucous membrane grafting in ocular cicatricial pemphigoid: implications for patient selection and surgical considerations. *Ophthalmology.* 1993;100:1283–1288.
>
> Kersten RC, Kleiner FP, Kulwin DR. Tarsotomy for the treatment of cicatricial entropion with trichiasis. *Arch Ophthalmol.* 1992;110:714–717.
>
> Shore JW, Foster S, Westfall CT, et al. Results of buccal mucosal grafting for patients with medically controlled ocular pemphigoid. *Ophthalmology.* 1992;99:383–395.

Symblepharon

A symblepharon is an adhesion between conjunctival surfaces that may be caused by inflammation, trauma, or previous surgery. Conjunctival Z-plasties are sometimes effective for localized contracted linear adhesions when vertical lengthening of the involved tissue is the primary objective. More extensive symblepharon formation requires a full-thickness conjunctival graft or flap or a partial-thickness buccal mucous membrane graft. The preferred technique for managing symblepharon formation associated with cicatricial entropion is determined by the area of conjunctiva involved in the entropion.

Trichiasis

Trichiasis is an acquired misdirection of the eyelashes. The method used for treating trichiasis is usually dictated by the pattern (segmental or diffuse) of the misdirected lashes and the quality of the posterior lamella of the involved eyelid. Inturned lashes are usually associated with posterior lamellar scarring (marginal cicatricial entropion). If the eyelid margin is misdirected, treatment should be directed at correcting the entropion.

Mechanical Epilation

The usual method for initially treating a few misdirected lashes is removal with forceps under the slit lamp. Following mechanical removal of the eyelash, recurrence is anticipated in 3–4 weeks because of eyelash regrowth. Short cilia regrowth is often mechanically more irritating to the cornea than mature longer lashes.

Electrolysis

Standard electrolysis is probably no longer indicated for the treatment of trichiasis. The recurrence rate is high, adjacent normal lashes may be damaged, and scarring of the adjacent eyelid margin tissue too often worsens the problem. Radiofrequency epilation with an insulated probe is an excellent alternative to electrolysis because the success rate is high and the collateral damage is minimal, which limits scarring.

Cryotherapy

Segmental trichiasis can be treated with a nitrous oxide probe using a double freeze/thaw technique. Cryotherapy is an office procedure that requires only local infiltrative anesthesia. The involved area is frozen for 25 seconds, allowed to thaw, and then refrozen for 20 seconds. The lashes are mechanically removed with forceps after treatment. Edema lasting several days, loss of skin pigmentation, notching of the eyelid margin, and possible interference with goblet cell function are disadvantages of cryotherapy. This method may be combined with various surgical techniques and repeated if offending lashes persist or recur.

Argon Laser

Argon laser treatment of trichiasis is less effective than cryotherapy but useful when only a few scattered eyelashes require ablation or when the stimulation of larger areas of inflammation is undesirable.

Surgery

Full-thickness pentagonal resection with primary closure may be considered when trichiasis is confined to a segment of the eyelid. A cantholysis with or without a semicircular advancement flap (see Eyelid Defects Involving the Eyelid Margin in Chapter 11) may be useful with more extensive full-thickness resections. When entropion is present, the treatment is dictated by the severity of the entropion.

> Bartley GB, Bullock JD, Olsen TG, et al. An experimental study to compare methods of eyelash ablation. *Ophthalmology*. 1987;94:1286–1289.
> Bartley GB, Lowry JC. Argon laser treatment of trichiasis. *Am J Ophthalmol*. 1992;113:71–74.
> Elder MJ, Bernauer W. Cryotherapy for trichiasis in ocular cicatricial pemphigoid. *Br J Ophthalmol*. 1994;78:769–771.
> Hurwitz J, Johnson D, Howarth D, et al. Experimental treatment of eyelashes with high-frequency radio wave electrosurgery. *Can J Ophthalmol*. 1993;28:62–64.

Blepharoptosis

The term *ptosis* refers to drooping or inferodisplacement of any anatomic structure. This shortened form is often used in place of the more accurate term, *blepharoptosis*, to describe drooping or inferodisplacement of the upper eyelid.

Two helpful classification systems are used to describe upper eyelid ptosis. It may be categorized by onset: congenital or acquired. Alternatively, it may be classified by the cause: myogenic, aponeurotic, neurogenic, mechanical, or traumatic. The most common type of *congenital* ptosis results from a poorly developed levator muscle (myogenic cause); the most common type of *acquired* ptosis is caused by stretching or even disinsertion of the levator aponeurosis (aponeurotic cause).

Blepharoptosis is an important cause of visual loss. Although the superior visual field is primarily involved, central vision can also be affected. Many patients with ptosis complain of difficulty with reading because the ptosis is worsened in downgaze. Such exacerbation of ptosis in downgaze is caused by relaxation of the frontalis muscle, whose chronic contracture might have been masking full expression of the ptosis in primary gaze. Blepharoptosis has also been shown to decrease the overall amount of light reaching the macula and therefore can reduce visual acuity as well, especially at night.

> Bergin DJ. *Management and Surgery of Congenital and Acquired Ptosis.* Continuing Ophthalmic Video Education. San Francisco: American Academy of Ophthalmology; 1990.
>
> Meyer DR, Rheeman CH. Downgaze eyelid position in patients with blepharoptosis. *Ophthalmology.* 1995;102:1517–1523.

Evaluation

The patient's ocular, medical, and surgical history helps identify appropriate candidates for surgical repair of ptosis. The surgeon should be aware of any history of dry eye syndrome and should temper any blepharoptosis repair in the presence of significant dry eye problems. Patients should be questioned about their coagulation status (see Chapter 10). Other pertinent historical queries should include the presence of thyroid eye disease, previous eye or eyelid surgery, and prior periorbital trauma.

The patient's history usually distinguishes congenital from acquired ptosis. Patients with congenital or acquired blepharoptosis may be aware of a family history of the condition. Marked variability in the degree of ptosis during the day and complaints of diplopia should suggest ocular myasthenia gravis (MG). Complaints of dysphonia, dyspnea, dysphagia, or proximal muscle weakness suggest systemic MG.

Physical Examination

Physical examination of the ptosis patient begins with four clinical measurements:

- Vertical interpalpebral fissure height
- Margin–reflex distance
- Upper eyelid crease position
- Levator function (upper eyelid excursion)

The physician can record these data by means of a drawing of the cornea, pupil size, and the position of the upper and lower eyelids in relation to these structures (Fig 12-10).

Vertical interpalpebral fissure height

The vertical interpalpebral fissure is measured at the widest point between the lower eyelid and the upper eyelid. This measurement is taken with the patient fixating on a distant object in primary gaze.

Margin–reflex distance (MRD)

The MRD, which is the distance from the upper eyelid margin to the corneal light reflex in primary position, is probably the single most effective measurement in describing the amount of ptosis. The light reflex may be obstructed by the eyelid in severe cases of ptosis and therefore have a zero or negative value. If the patient complains of visual obstruction while reading, the MRD should also be checked in the reading position. Lower eyelid retraction (or scleral show) should be noted separately as the *margin–reflex distance 2*

210 • Orbit, Eyelids, and Lacrimal System

Palpebral Fissure Height	9.5	7.5
Margin–Reflex Distance	+4	+2
Upper Eyelid Crease	8	11
Levator Function	15	14

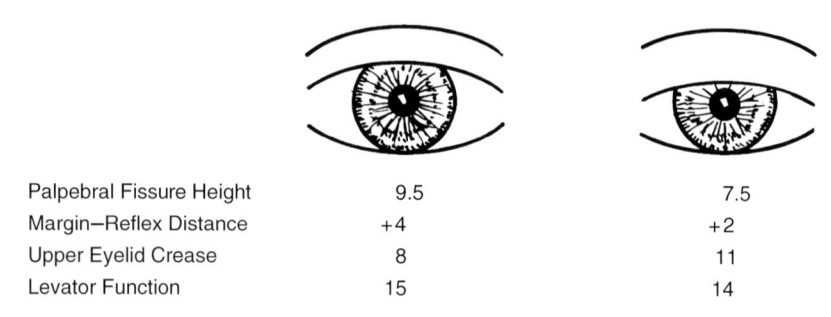

Figure 12-10 Example of ptosis data sheet.

(MRD2). The MRD2 is the distance from the corneal light reflex to the lower eyelid margin. The sum of the MRD1 and the MRD2 should equal the vertical interpalpebral fissure height.

Upper eyelid crease

The distance from the upper eyelid crease to the eyelid margin is measured. Because the insertion of fibers from the levator muscle into the skin contributes to formation of the upper eyelid crease, high, duplicated, and asymmetric creases may indicate abnormal insertions or disinsertions of the levator aponeurosis. The crease is usually elevated in patients with involutional ptosis. The upper eyelid crease is often shallow or absent in patients with congenital ptosis. The upper eyelid crease is typically lower or obscured in the Asian eyelid, with or without ptosis.

Levator function

The levator function is estimated by measuring the upper eyelid excursion from downgaze to upgaze with frontalis muscle function negated. Care should be taken to minimize contributions from accessory elevators of the eyelids such as the frontalis muscle by fixating the brow with digital pressure. Failure to negate the influence of the frontalis muscle results in incorrect evaluations of true levator function. Accurate analysis of the amount of levator function is crucial in determining the cause and treatment plan (Fig 12-11).

> Frueh BR, Musch DC. Evaluation of levator muscle integrity in ptosis with levator force measurement. *Ophthalmology.* 1996;103:244–250.

Other

Physical examination also includes checking head position, chin elevation, brow position, and brow action in attempted upgaze. These features help to show the patient how ptosis affects function. The quantity and quality of the tear film and the presence or absence of lagophthalmos (incomplete closure of the eyelids) must be evaluated and documented as part of the initial evaluation. Lagophthalmos and poor tear film quantity or quality may predispose a patient to complications of ptosis repair such as dryness and exposure keratitis. The examiner should also note the presence or absence of a normal Bell's phenomenon and assess whether corneal sensation is normal; these factors may also affect the treatment plan.

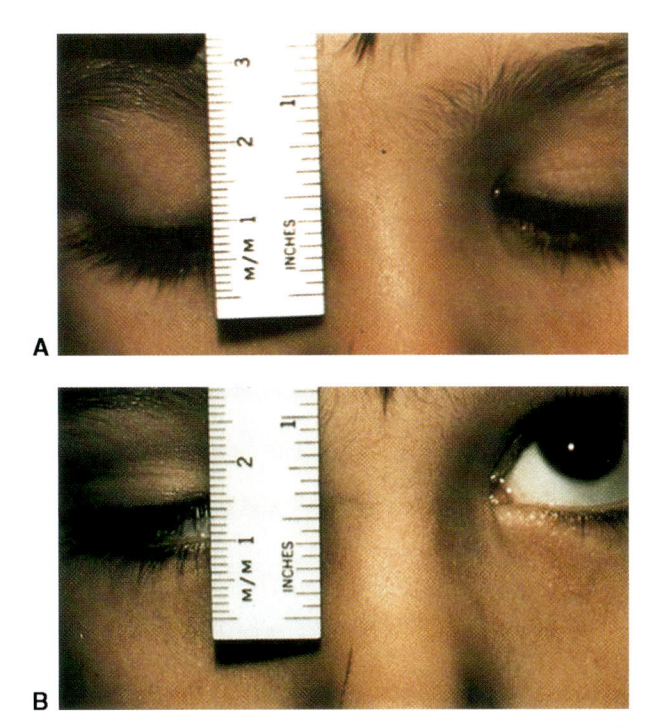

CHAPTER 12: Periocular Malpositions and Involutional Changes • 211

Figure 12-11 Measurement of levator excursion. **A,** Downgaze. **B,** Upgaze.

Variation in the amount of ptosis with extraocular muscle or jaw muscle movements *(synkinesis)* must also be assessed. Synkinesis may be seen in Marcus Gunn jaw-winking ptosis, aberrant regeneration of the oculomotor nerve or the facial nerve, and some types of Duane syndrome. The examiner should attempt to elicit synkinesis as part of the evaluation of patients with congenital blepharoptosis or those with possible aberrant regeneration.

The position of the ptotic eyelid in downgaze should be checked as an aid in differentiating between congenital and acquired causes. The congenitally ptotic eyelid is often higher in downgaze than the contralateral, normal eyelid as a result of eyelid lag. The congenitally ptotic eyelid may also manifest lagophthalmos. In contrast, the affected eyelid in acquired, involutional ptosis remains ptotic in all positions of gaze and may even worsen in downgaze with relaxation of the frontalis muscle.

In all cases of congenital or childhood ptosis, visual function and refractive error must be assessed in order to identify and treat the child with concomitant amblyopia resulting from anisometropia, high astigmatism, strabismus, or occlusion of the pupil. Amblyopia occurs in about 20% of patients with congenital ptosis but is attributable to the ptosis in only about 4% of cases. About 75% of cases of congenital ptosis are unilateral.

It is also important to assess extraocular muscle function because extraocular muscle dysfunction associated with blepharoptosis occurs in various congenital conditions (combined superior rectus/levator muscle maldevelopment, congenital oculomotor palsy) and acquired conditions (ocular or systemic MG, chronic progressive external ophthalmoplegia, oculopharyngeal dystrophy, and oculomotor palsy with or without aberrant regeneration).

In addition, pupillary examination is important in the evaluation of ptosis. Pupil abnormalities are present in some acquired and congenital conditions associated with ptosis (eg, Horner syndrome, cranial nerve III palsy). Miosis that is most apparent in dim illumination is one finding in Horner syndrome; mydriasis is seen in some cases of oculomotor nerve palsy.

External examination may reveal other abnormalities as well. For example, severe bilateral congenital ptosis may be associated with telecanthus, epicanthus inversus, flattening of the superior orbital rim, horizontal shortening of the eyelids, and hypoplasia of the nasal bridge. These findings characterize an autosomal dominant condition known as *blepharophimosis syndrome* (discussed in Chapter 11, under the heading Congenital Anomalies).

Ancillary tests

Visual field testing with the eyelids untaped (in the natural, ptotic state) and taped (artificially elevated as if the blepharoptosis has been repaired) helps determine the patient's level of functional impairment and potential for visual improvement. Comparison of the taped visual field with the untaped visual field gives an estimate of the superior visual field improvement that can be anticipated following surgery. Visual field testing and external full-face photography may be required as a part of the initial evaluation in order to distinguish *functional* from *cosmetic* blepharoptosis repair.

> Meyer DR, Stern JH, Jarvis JM, et al. Evaluating the visual field effects of blepharoptosis using automated static perimetry. *Ophthalmology*. 1993;100:651–659.

Pharmacologic testing may be helpful in confirming the clinical diagnosis of Horner syndrome. Because cocaine blocks the reuptake of norepinephrine at the neuromuscular junction, topical application of 4%–10% cocaine to a normal eye increases the availability of norepinephrine to the iris dilator muscle and results in pupillary dilation. In contrast, the pupil affected by Horner syndrome fails to dilate after application of cocaine because of the absence of norepinephrine in the synaptic cleft (Fig 12-12). A variety of other pharmacologic tests may help to localize the lesion causing the Horner syndrome (see

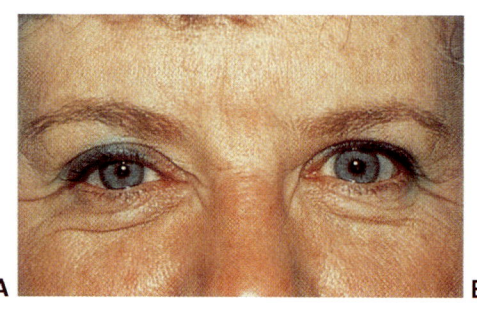

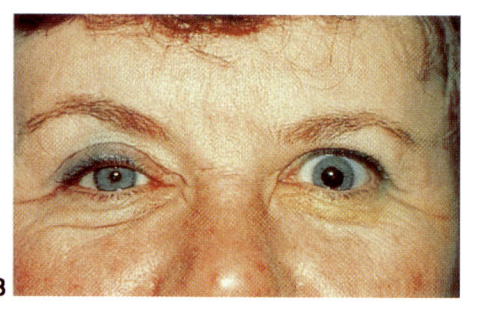

Figure 12-12 Horner syndrome. **A,** Before instillation of topical cocaine. **B,** Pupil of normal left eye dilates after instillation of cocaine, but right pupil does not respond. *(Photographs courtesy of Robert C. Kersten, MD.)*

BCSC Section 5, *Neuro-Ophthalmology*). Although the differentiation among first-, second-, and third-order neuron dysfunction in the cause of Horner syndrome is important to the patient's general medical assessment, this information does not affect the choice of treatment for the ptosis. Third-order neuron dysfunction resulting in Horner syndrome is typically benign. Neuron dysfunction of the first or second order, however, is more often associated with malignant neoplasms such as an apical lung (Pancoast) tumor, aneurysm, or dissection of the carotid artery.

Because blepharoptosis is the most common presenting sign of MG, the ophthalmologist may order or perform tests to rule out this diagnosis in appropriate patients. Fluctuating ptosis that seems to worsen with fatigue or prolonged upgaze, especially when accompanied by diplopia or other clinical manifestations of systemic MG, is an indication for further diagnostic testing. Testing with edrophonium chloride (Tensilon), an acetylcholinergic agent, has traditionally been used to diagnose MG. In the myasthenic patient whose acetylcholine receptors have been compromised through autoimmune destruction, the infusion of edrophonium chloride typically results in improvement in the ptosis or motility. Clinicians administering the Tensilon test should be aware of potential adverse effects such as lacrimation, salivation, flushing, abdominal cramping, bradycardia, or even respiratory arrest and should be prepared to administer atropine and other appropriate care in case of adverse reactions. (The Tensilon test is described more fully in BCSC Section 5, *Neuro-Ophthalmology*.)

The *ice pack test* is an alternative approach that may obviate routine Tensilon testing in the diagnosis of MG. The ice pack test is a simple procedure with few potential side effects that can be performed in the office. An ice pack is applied to the patient's eyelid(s) for about 2 minutes. If MG is present, the ptosis often improves because of the enhancement of neuromuscular transmission that occurs with inhibition of acetylcholinesterase under cold conditions.

Another alternative to Tensilon testing is the *acetylcholine receptor antibody test*, a serum assay designed to detect the autoimmune antibody responsible for the destruction of the muscle motor end-plate receptors in patients with MG. Binding antibodies are detectable in about 90% of patients with systemic MG and in about 70% of patients with ocular myasthenia. The ophthalmologist should be aware that some laboratories set their reference ranges artificially high, thus essentially assessing for systemic MG. The antibody levels in ocular myasthenia are presumably lower. Therefore, the detection of very small amounts of acetylcholine receptor antibodies may be suggestive or diagnostic of ocular MG.

Classification

As discussed above, ptosis may be classified according to the time of onset or the underlying abnormality. The vast majority of cases of congenital ptosis result from a localized myogenic dysgenesis. Most cases of acquired ptosis result from involutional stretching or disinsertion of the levator aponeurosis (aponeurotic abnormality). The cause of blepharoptosis is therefore commonly presumed to be myogenic in congenital ptosis and aponeurotic in acquired ptosis, and these cases are often referred to simply as congenital or acquired ptosis. However, a more specific and accurate classification system is based on a defined underlying abnormality and includes the additional categories of neurogenic, mechanical, and traumatic ptosis.

> Clark BJ, Kemp EG, Behan WM, et al. Abnormal extracellular material in the levator palpebrae superioris complex in congenital ptosis. *Arch Ophthalmol.* 1995;113:1414–1419.

Myogenic ptosis

Congenital myogenic ptosis results from dysgenesis of the levator muscle. Instead of normal muscle fibers, fibrous or adipose tissue is present in the muscle belly, diminishing the ability of the levator to contract and relax. Therefore, congenital ptosis caused by maldevelopment of the levator muscle is characterized by decreased levator function, eyelid lag, and sometimes lagophthalmos (Fig 12-13). The amount of levator function is an indication of the amount of normal muscle. Congenital myogenic ptosis with an associated poor Bell's phenomenon or vertical strabismus may indicate concomitant maldevelopment of the superior rectus muscle (*double elevator palsy,* or *monocular elevation deficiency*).

Acquired myogenic ptosis is uncommon and results from localized or diffuse muscular disease such as muscular dystrophy, chronic progressive external ophthalmoplegia, MG, or oculopharyngeal dystrophy. Because of the underlying muscle dysfunction, surgical correction may be difficult. The choice of surgical technique is most often based on the amount of levator function. Surgical procedures directed toward levator shortening are more effective in patients whose levator function is relatively good. If the levator function is relatively poor, frontalis suspension can be carried out by various surgical techniques designed to attach the eyelid to the frontalis muscle so that elevation of the brow results in elevation of the eyelid. Although shortening the levator muscle aponeurosis or frontalis

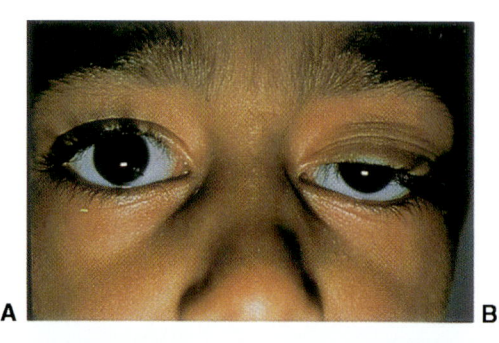

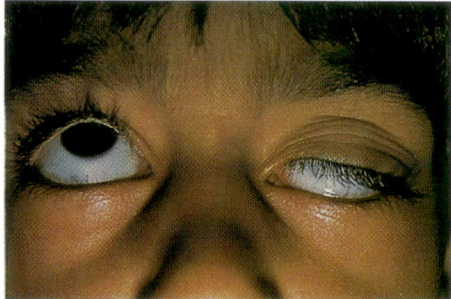

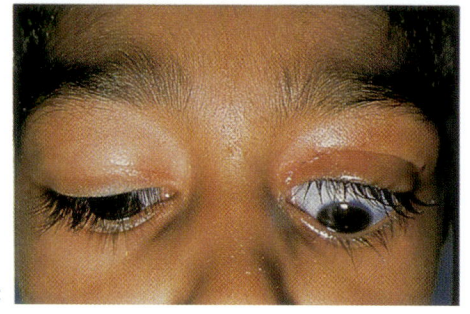

Figure 12-13 Bilateral asymmetric congenital ptosis. **A,** Note margin–reflex distance (MRD = 5.0 mm OD, 1.0 mm OS). Normal = 4.5 mm. **B,** Upgaze accentuates ptosis. **C,** Downgaze exhibits eyelid lag. *(Photographs courtesy of Robert C. Kersten, MD.)*

suspension may help to raise the eyelid to a functional level just above the pupil, too much elevation can lead to secondary keratitis due to lagophthalmos and exposure. Therefore, a compromise between cosmetic and functional results is sometimes required. Associated orbicularis oculi dysfunction in patients with myogenic blepharoptosis reduces the ability to close the eyelids and may further increase the risk of postoperative exposure keratitis. Silicone rod frontalis suspension may be more useful if removal or adjustment of the sling is anticipated.

> Holds JB, McLeish WM, Anderson RL. Whitnall's sling with superior tarsectomy for the correction of severe unilateral blepharoptosis. *Arch Ophthalmol.* 1993;111:1285–1291.

Aponeurotic ptosis

The levator aponeurosis transmits levator force to the eyelid. Thus, any disruption in its anatomy or function can lead to ptosis. *Congenital aponeurotic ptosis* is caused by failure of the aponeurosis to insert in its normal position on the anterior surface of the tarsus. This condition is characterized by good upper eyelid excursion and a high or indistinct upper eyelid crease. It is a rare cause of congenital ptosis and may be associated with birth trauma, especially in deliveries requiring forceps.

Acquired aponeurotic ptosis is the most common of all forms of ptosis. It is caused by stretching, dehiscence, or disinsertion of the levator aponeurosis from its normal position. Common causes are involutional attenuation or repetitive traction on the eyelid. Such repetitive traction may result from frequent eye rubbing or wearing of rigid contact lenses. Aponeurotic ptosis may also be caused or exacerbated by intraocular surgery or eyelid surgery through multiple mechanisms (Fig 12-14).

Eyelids with aponeurotic defects characteristically have a high or absent upper eyelid crease secondary to upward displacement or loss of the insertion of levator fibers into the skin. Thinning of the eyelid superior to the upper tarsal plate is often an associated finding and may allow visualization of the iris through the eyelid. Because the levator muscle itself is healthy, levator function in aponeurotic ptosis is usually normal (approximately 15 mm). Acquired aponeurotic ptosis may worsen in the reading position and therefore interfere with the patient's ability to read as well as limiting the superior visual field. Table 12-1 compares acquired aponeurotic ptosis with congenital myogenic ptosis.

> Kersten RC, de Conciliis C, Kulwin DR. Acquired ptosis in the young and middle-aged adult population. *Ophthalmology.* 1995;102:924–928.

Neurogenic ptosis

Congenital neurogenic ptosis is caused by innervational defects that occur during embryonic development. This condition is relatively rare and is most commonly associated with congenital cranial nerve III palsy, congenital Horner syndrome, or the Marcus Gunn jaw-winking syndrome.

Congenital oculomotor nerve (cranial nerve III) palsy is manifested as blepharoptosis together with inability to elevate, depress, or adduct the globe. The pupils may also be dilated. This nerve palsy may be partial or complete, but blepharoptosis is very rarely an isolated finding in cranial nerve III palsy. It is uncommon to find aberrant innervation

216 • Orbit, Eyelids, and Lacrimal System

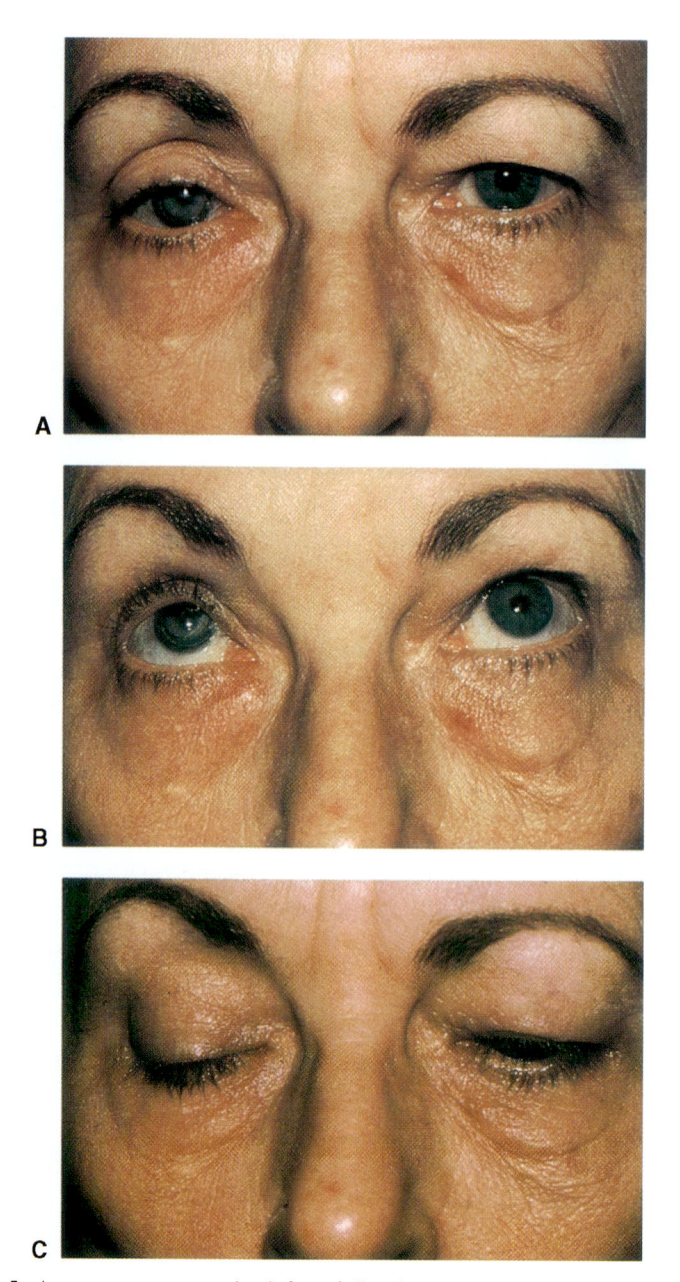

Figure 12-14 A, Levator aponeurosis defect following cataract surgery. Similar aponeurotic ptosis can occur following various other intraocular and eyelid surgical procedures as well. **B,** Excellent levator function on upgaze. **C,** Depression is greater than normal (eyelid drop) in downgaze.

Table 12-1 Blepharoptosis Comparison

	Congenital Myogenic Ptosis	Acquired Aponeurotic Ptosis
Palpebral fissure height	Mild to severe ptosis	Mild to severe ptosis
Upper eyelid crease	Weak or absent crease in normal position	Higher than normal crease
Levator function	Reduced	Near normal
On downgaze	Eyelid lag	Eyelid drop

in congenital cranial nerve III palsies. Management of strabismus and amblyopia is difficult in many cases of congenital third nerve palsy; moreover, management of the associated ptosis is also complicated. The ptosis repair usually requires a frontalis suspension procedure, which often leads to some degree of lagophthalmos. As a result of the lagophthalmos, poor motility of the globe, and poor postoperative eyelid excursion, postoperative management may be complicated by diplopia, exposure keratitis, and corneal ulceration.

> Malone TJ, Nerad JA. The surgical treatment of blepharoptosis in oculomotor nerve palsy. *Am J Ophthalmol.* 1988;105:57–64.

Congenital Horner syndrome is a manifestation of an interrupted sympathetic nervous chain and may cause mild ptosis associated with miosis, anhidrosis, and decreased pigmentation of the iris and areola on the involved side. The mild blepharoptosis of Horner syndrome is due to an innervational deficit to the sympathetic Müller's muscle, an eyelid elevator second in importance to the levator muscle. Decreased sympathetic tone to the lower eyelid tarsal muscle, the analogue of Müller's muscle in the upper eyelid, results in elevation of the lower eyelid, sometimes called *lower eyelid ptosis.* The combined upper and lower eyelid ptosis decreases the vertical interpalpebral fissure and may falsely suggest enophthalmos. The pupillary miosis is most apparent in dim illumination, when the contralateral pupil dilates more effectively (see the earlier subheading, Ancillary tests).

Congenital neurogenic ptosis may also be synkinetic. Marcus Gunn jaw-winking syndrome (Fig 12-15) is the most common form of congenital synkinetic neurogenic ptosis. In this synkinetic syndrome, the unilaterally ptotic eyelid elevates with jaw movements. The movement that most commonly causes elevation of the ptotic eyelid is lateral mandibular movement to the contralateral side. This phenomenon is usually first noticed by the mother when she is feeding or nursing the baby. This synkinesis is thought to be caused by aberrant connections between the motor division of cranial nerve V and the levator muscle. Infrequently, this syndrome is associated with abnormal connections between other cranial nerves and cranial nerve III. Some forms of Duane retraction syndrome also cause elevation of a ptotic eyelid with movement of the globe. This congenital syndrome is also thought to result from aberrant nerve connections.

Acquired neurogenic ptosis results from interruption of normally developed innervation and is most often secondary to an acquired cranial nerve III palsy, to an acquired Horner syndrome, or to MG.

Delineation of the cause of acquired oculomotor nerve palsy is important. Distinction must be made between *vasculopathic* and *compressive* causes. The majority of acquired

218 • Orbit, Eyelids, and Lacrimal System

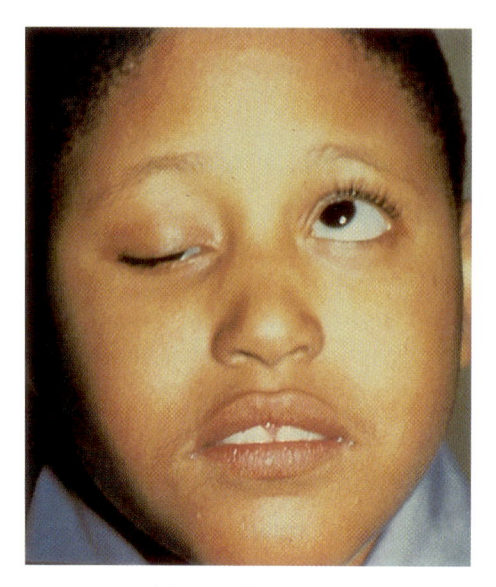

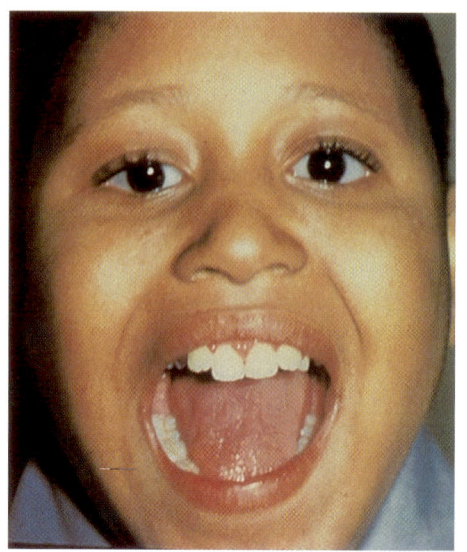

Figure 12-15 Marcus Gunn jaw-winking ptosis (synkinesis linking cranial nerve V to cranial nerve III). *(Photographs courtesy of Jeffrey A. Nerad, MD.)*

oculomotor palsies are vasculopathic and associated with diabetes, hypertension, or arteriosclerotic disease. Typically, vasculopathic acquired cranial nerve III palsies do not include pupillary abnormalities, and they resolve spontaneously with satisfactory levator function within 3 months. If a pupil-sparing third nerve palsy fails to resolve spontaneously within 3–6 months, further workup for a compressive lesion is indicated. However, if a patient presents with a cranial nerve III palsy involving the pupil, an immediate workup (including neuroimaging) should commence to rule out a compressive neoplastic or aneurysmal lesion. Surgical correction of ptosis related to cranial nerve III palsy usually requires frontalis suspension and should be reserved for patients in whom strabismus surgery allows single binocular vision in a useful field of gaze.

As discussed previously, the ice pack test, acetylcholine receptor antibody assay, or Tensilon test is indicated when the history or clinical examination suggests MG. MG is an autoimmune disorder in which autoantibodies attack the receptors of the neuromuscular junction. The disease is most often generalized and systemic. About 10% of patients with MG have thymomas; thus, scanning is indicated for all patients with MG to rule out these lesions. Early manifestation of MG is often ophthalmologic, with ptosis being the most common presenting sign. Diplopia is also common. When the effects of MG are isolated to the periocular musculature, the condition is called *ocular myasthenia gravis*. Other autoimmune disorders may occur in myasthenic patients. For example, Graves disease occurs in 5%–10% of patients with MG.

The ptosis of ocular myasthenia often responds poorly to systemic anticholinesterase medications or steroids. Neuro-ophthalmologic consultation is useful in the evaluation and treatment of difficult cases. Surgical treatment of blepharoptosis in the myasthenic patient should be delayed until medical improvement has been maximized. Because of the variability of levator function, frontalis suspension is usually preferred. (See BCSC Section 5, *Neuro-Ophthalmology*, for further discussion.)

> Sethi KD, Rivner MH, Swift TR. Ice pack test for myasthenia gravis. *Neurology*. 1987;37:1383–1385.
> Weinberg DA, Lesser RL, Vollmer TL. Ocular myasthenia: a protean disorder. *Surv Ophthalmol.* 1994;39:169–210.
> Wong JF, Theriault JF, Bouzouaya C, Codere F. Marcus Gunn jaw-winking phenomenon: a new supplemental test in the preoperative evaluation. *Ophthal Plast Reconstr Surg.* 2001;17:412–418.

Other, more unusual, causes of acquired neurogenic ptosis include myotonic dystrophy, chronic progressive external ophthalmoplegia, Guillain-Barré syndrome, oculopharyngeal dystrophy, and iatrogenic botulism. Botulinum toxin injection in the forehead or orbital region to ameliorate benign essential blepharospasm or to reduce facial rhytids may result in infiltration of the neurotoxin into the levator muscle complex. The resultant neurogenic ptosis is temporary, usually resolving after a few weeks.

Mechanical ptosis

Mechanical ptosis usually refers to the condition in which a neoplasm weighs or pulls down the upper eyelid, resulting in inferodisplacement. It may be caused by a *congenital abnormality*, such as plexiform neuroma or hemangioma, or by an *acquired neoplasm*, such as a large chalazion or basal cell or squamous cell carcinoma. Postsurgical or posttraumatic edema may result in temporary mechanical ptosis.

Traumatic ptosis

Blunt or sharp trauma to the levator aponeurosis or the levator muscle may also cause ptosis. The underlying histologic defects may be a combination of myogenic, aponeurotic, and cicatricial elements. Eyelid lacerations exposing preaponeurotic fat indicate that the orbital septum has been transected and suggest the possibility of damage to the levator aponeurosis. Exploration of the levator muscle or aponeurosis is indicated in these patients if levator function is diminished or ptosis is present. Orbital and neurosurgical procedures may also lead to traumatic ptosis. Because such ptosis may resolve or improve spontaneously, the ophthalmologist normally observes the patient for approximately 6 months before considering surgical intervention.

Pseudoptosis

Pseudoptosis—apparent eyelid drooping—should be differentiated from *true* ptosis. An eyelid may appear to be abnormally low in various conditions, including hypertropia, enophthalmos, microphthalmos, anophthalmos, phthisis bulbi, or a superior sulcus defect secondary to trauma or other causes. Contralateral upper eyelid retraction may also simulate ptosis. The term *pseudoptosis* is also sometimes used to describe *dermatochalasis*, the condition in which excess upper eyelid skin overhangs the eyelid margin, transects the pupil, and gives the appearance of a true ptosis of the eyelid margin (Fig 12-16).

Figure 12-16 A, Patient with apparent ptosis of left upper eyelid. **B,** Manual elevation of dermatochalasis reveals this to be pseudoptosis; the underlying palpebral fissure is actually within normal limits. **C,** Clearance of visual axis is achieved following blepharoplasty alone. *(Photographs courtesy of Robert C. Kersten, MD.)*

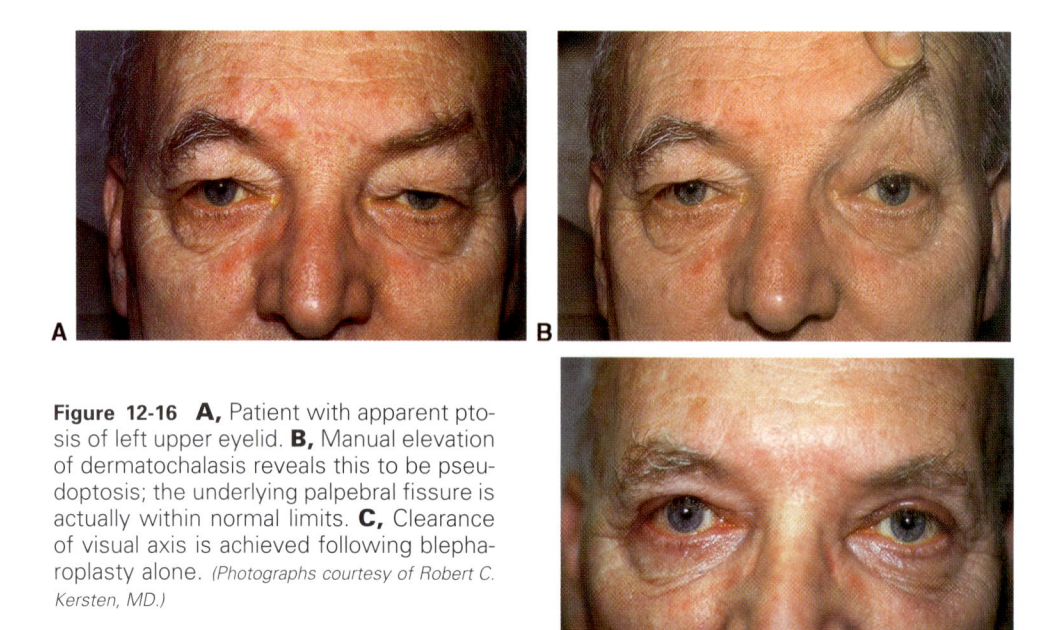

Treatment of Ptosis

Ptosis repair is a challenging oculoplastic surgical procedure that requires correct diagnosis, thoughtful planning, thorough understanding of eyelid anatomy, and good surgical technique. Although an inexperienced ptosis surgeon (and sometimes even the patient) may think that ptosis repair is straightforward and predictable, the experienced ptosis surgeon realizes and anticipates the potential complexities.

After the patient has been evaluated and the cause and nature of the ptosis have been determined, treatment plans may be formulated. Blepharoptosis that causes significant superior visual field loss or difficulties with reading is considered a functional problem, and correction of this defect often improves the ability of patients to perform the activities of daily living. In many instances, ptosis is considered to be a cosmetic issue, causing a tired or sleepy appearance in the absence of a true visual function deficit. Because ptosis repair is often an elective surgical procedure, it is particularly important for the surgeon to have a preoperative discussion with the patient to communicate the alternatives, potential risks, and benefits.

Nonsurgical treatment options are unusual but may include devices called *eyelid crutches* that are attached to eyeglass frames. Eyelid crutches are occasionally useful in patients with acquired neurogenic and myogenic ptosis in whom surgical correction could lead to severe exposure-related corneal defects. Taping the upper eyelid open during appropriate times is also a simple, but often impractical, treatment method. These methods have largely been supplanted by better homologous and synthetic materials for frontalis suspension.

Surgical procedures designed to correct ptosis fall into three broad categories and should be directed toward correction of the underlying pathological condition (Fig

CHAPTER 12: Periocular Malpositions and Involutional Changes • 221

12-17). The three categories of surgical procedures most commonly used in ptosis repair are

- External (transcutaneous) levator advancement
- Internal (transconjunctival) levator/tarsus/Müller's muscle resection approaches
- Frontalis muscle suspensions

The amount and type of ptosis and the degree of levator function are the most common determining factors in the choice of the surgical procedure for blepharoptosis repair. The surgeon's comfort level and experience with various procedures is also an important factor. In patients with good levator function, surgical correction is generally directed toward the levator aponeurosis: the levator muscle is the most potent and most useful elevator of the eyelid in most patients. However, if levator function is poor or absent, frontalis muscle suspension techniques become the preferred repair procedures.

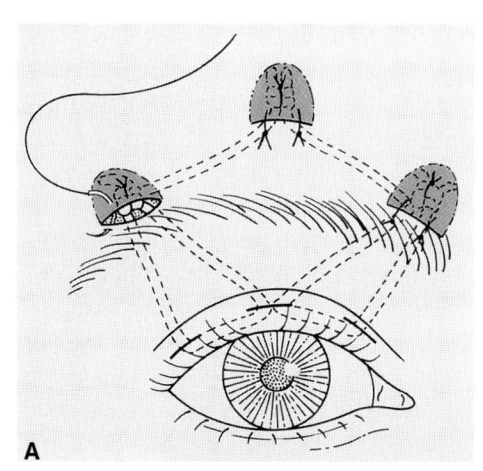

Figure 12-17 A, Frontalis suspension: Crawford method. *(Reprinted by permission from Stewart WB. Surgery of the Eyelid, Orbit, and Lacrimal System. Ophthalmology Monograph 8, vol 2. San Francisco: American Academy of Ophthalmology; 1994:120.)* **B,** Transconjunctival frontalis suspension. *(From Dailey RA, Wilson DJ, Wobig JL. Transconjunctival frontalis suspension [TCFS]. Ophthal Plast Reconstr Surg. 1991;7:289–297.)*

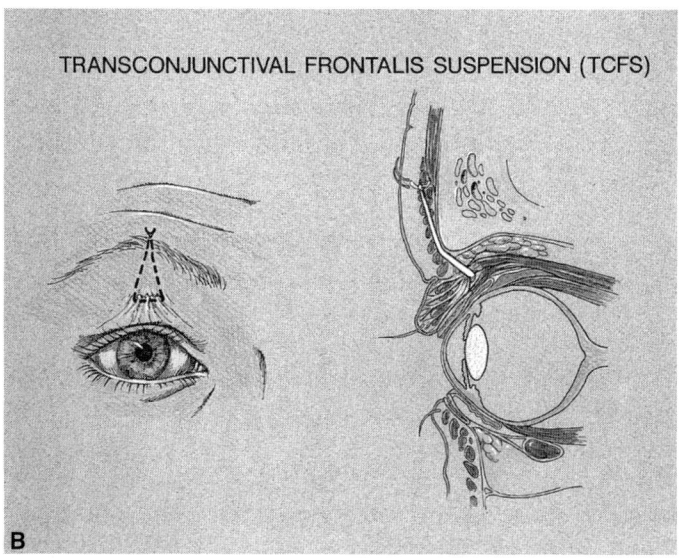

External (transcutaneous) levator advancement surgery is most commonly used when levator function is normal and the upper eyelid crease is high. In this setting, the levator muscle itself is normal, but the levator aponeurosis (its tendinous attachment to the tarsal plate) is stretched or pulled loose (disinserted). The levator aponeurosis is approached from the outside of the eyelid through the upper eyelid crease. This approach is the one used most commonly for acquired aponeurotic ptosis repair and is particularly useful because it allows the surgeon to remove excess eyelid skin (dermatochalasis) at the same time. Typically, the levator aponeurosis is attenuated or stretched and requires advancement. Occasionally, the redundant aponeurosis must be reduced to avoid a thickened or irregular eyelid. In some cases, the distal end of the aponeurosis may be found to be higher than its normal position on the lower anterior surface of the tarsus. Reinsertion of the aponeurosis usually produces an excellent result.

The *internal (transconjunctival)* approach to ptosis repair may be directed toward Müller's muscle, the tarsus, or the levator aponeurosis. Müller's muscle resections may be indicated when the sympathetic nerve supply to this smooth muscle has been interrupted, as in Horner syndrome. This type of muscle resection is also used by some surgeons on patients who have an adequate upper eyelid position following instillation of a drop of 2.5% phenylephrine hydrochloride. Müller's muscle resections are typically used for minimal ptosis (<2 mm) and are superior to the Fasanella-Servat procedure (tarsoconjunctival müllerectomy) in maintaining eyelid contour and preserving the superior tarsal border. (The Fasanella-Servat ptosis repair procedure, though also directed toward small amounts of ptosis, requires removal of the superior tarsal border.)

When levator function is essentially absent, the surgeon should consider utilizing the accessory elevators of the eyelid in ptosis repair. This type of surgery is most commonly required in congenital ptosis with poor levator function or in various forms of neurogenic ptosis with poor levator function.

Most patients with significant ptosis automatically elevate the forehead and brow on the affected side in an attempt to raise the eyelid and clear the visual axis; however, this maneuver is normally very inefficient because of the elasticity of the eyelid skin. In *frontalis suspension surgery* (the most common solution to this problem), the eyelid is suspended directly from the frontalis muscle so that movement of the brow is efficiently transmitted to the eyelid; thus, the patient is able to elevate the eyelid by using the frontalis muscle to lift the brow. This procedure can be performed transcutaneously or transconjunctivally (see Fig 12-17).

Autogenous tensor fascia lata, banked fascia lata, and synthetic materials have been used for this purpose. *Autogenous fascia lata* has shown the best long-term results but requires harvesting and additional surgery. Generally, patients need to be at least 3 years old or weigh 35 pounds or more. *Banked fascia lata* may be obtained from a variety of sources and obviates the need for additional operative sites and harvesting. However, this material may incite immune reactions or inflammation and have poorer long-term outcomes than autogenous tissue. *Synthetic materials* such as polytetrafluoroethane (GORE-TEX) and Silastic rods are being increasingly used and may improve eyelid elasticity and allow easier adjustment or removal if necessary.

There is some controversy about whether bilateral frontalis suspension should be performed in patients with unilateral ptosis. Unilateral frontalis suspension results in asymmetry in downgaze due to upper eyelid lag induced by the sling. Bilateral surgery may improve the patient's symmetry, especially in downgaze, but it subjects the normal eyelid to surgery and its attendant risks. The decision to modify a normal eyelid in an attempt to gain symmetry must be discussed by the surgeon and patient (or the parents if the patient is a child).

Complications

The most common complication of blepharoptosis surgery is undercorrection. This has led some ptosis surgeons to use adjustable suture techniques or to advocate early adjustment in the office during the first postoperative week when indicated. Judgment is required to differentiate true undercorrection from apparent undercorrection resulting from postoperative edema. Other potential complications include overcorrection, unsatisfactory or asymmetric eyelid contour, scarring, wound dehiscence, eyelid crease asymmetry, conjunctival prolapse, tarsal eversion, and lagophthalmos with resultant exposure keratitis. Lagophthalmos following ptosis repair is most common in patients with decreased levator function. This condition is usually temporary, but it requires treatment with lubricating drops or ointments until it resolves.

> Callahan MA, Beard C. *Beard's Ptosis*. 4th ed. Birmingham, AL: Aesculapius; 1990.
> Dailey RA, Wilson DJ, Wobig JL. Transconjunctival frontalis suspension (TCFS). *Ophthal Plast Reconstr Surg*. 1991;7:289–297.
> Dortzbach RK, Kronish JW. Early revision in the office for adults after unsatisfactory blepharoptosis correction. *Am J Ophthalmol*. 1993;115:68–75.

Eyelid Retraction

Eyelid retraction is present when the eyelids are displaced toward the respective superior or inferior orbital rim, exposing sclera between the limbus and the eyelid margin. Lower eyelid retraction may also be a normal anatomic variant in patients with shallow orbits or certain genetic orbital or eyelid characteristics. Retraction of the eyelids often leads to lagophthalmos and exposure keratitis. The effects of these conditions can range from ocular irritation and discomfort to vision-threatening corneal decompensation.

Eyelid retraction can have local, systemic, or central nervous system causes. The most common causes of eyelid retraction are Graves ophthalmopathy, recession of the vertical rectus muscles, overly aggressive skin excision in blepharoplasty, and overcompensation for a contralateral ptosis (in accordance with Hering's law).

Graves ophthalmopathy is the most common cause of both superior and inferior eyelid retraction (Fig 12-18), as well as the most common cause of unilateral or bilateral proptosis. Because proptosis commonly coexists with and may mimic eyelid retraction in patients with Graves ophthalmopathy, these conditions must be distinguished from each another through eyelid measurements and exophthalmometry. A common finding in Graves-related eyelid retraction is lateral flare. In this condition, the eyelid retraction is more severe laterally than medially, resulting in an abnormal upper eyelid contour that appears to flare along the lateral half of the eyelid margin. The histopathological changes in the eyelid in Graves ophthalmopathy are secondary to inflammatory infiltration and fibrous contraction of the eyelid retractors. The sympathetically innervated

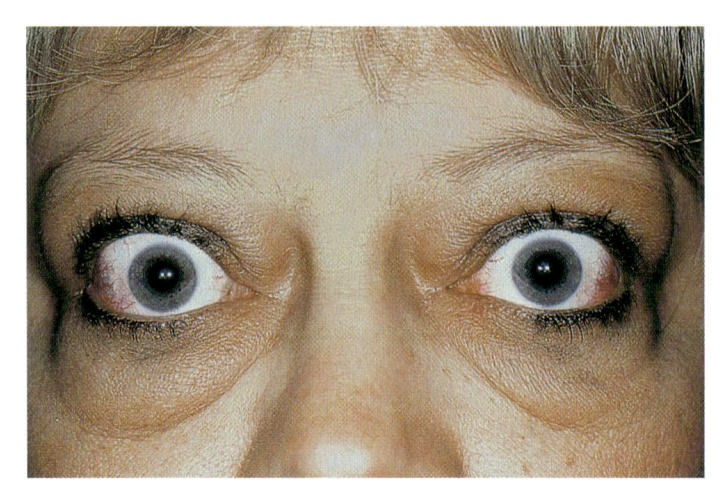

Figure 12-18 Thyroid eyelid retraction.

eyelid retractor muscles (Müller's muscle in the upper eyelid and the analogous eyelid retractor muscle in the lower eyelid) are preferentially affected by the inflammation and fibrosis of Graves ophthalmopathy (see Chapter 4 for a more extensive discussion of Graves ophthalmopathy).

Eyelid retraction may also be caused by recession of the vertical rectus muscles owing to anatomic connections between the superior rectus and the levator muscles in the upper eyelid and between the inferior rectus muscle and capsulopalpebral fascia in the lower eyelid. Eyelid retraction, therefore, is a common complication of vertical strabismus surgery.

Another common cause of eyelid retraction (especially of the lower eyelids) is excessive resection of skin during cosmetic lower blepharoplasty. This surgical complication is more common in patients with preexisting lower eyelid laxity and may even manifest as frank ectropion. Endoscopic midface lifting or full-thickness skin grafting may be required to correct this iatrogenic deformity. Conservative excision of skin in lower blepharoplasty along with concomitant correction of any lower eyelid laxity minimizes the risk of this problem.

Overcompensation for a contralateral ptosis (Hering's law) may also give the appearance of upper eyelid retraction. The surgeon must distinguish this condition from true eyelid retraction by observing the position of the supposedly retracted eyelid while the contralateral, presumably ptotic eyelid is either manually elevated or occluded.

> Meyer DR, Wobig JL. Detection of contralateral eyelid retraction associated with blepharoptosis. *Ophthalmology*. 1992;99:366–375.

Parinaud syndrome is an example of eyelid retraction caused by a central nervous system lesion. Congenital eyelid retraction may also occur as a rare, isolated entity.

Treatment of Eyelid Retraction

Management of eyelid retraction is based on the underlying etiologic factors. Artificial tears, lubricants, and ointments may be sufficient to protect the cornea and minimize symptoms in cases of mild eyelid retraction. Mild eyelid retraction following lower blepharoplasty or in Graves ophthalmopathy frequently resolves spontaneously with time. A variety of surgical techniques have been developed to correct eyelid retraction if the condition fails to resolve spontaneously or if the eyelid retraction causes an immediate threat to vision or the cornea. Various techniques involve release or recession of the eyelid retractors with or without spacers or grafts.

Eyelid retraction in Graves ophthalmopathy can be managed by means of several surgical procedures. Unless there is severe exposure keratopathy, surgical intervention is indicated only after serial measurements have established stability of the disease over at least 6 months. Upper eyelid retraction can be corrected by excising or recessing Müller's muscle (anterior or posterior approach), recessing the levator aponeurosis with or without hang-back sutures, performing a measured myotomy of the levator muscle, or inserting a spacer between the distal end of the levator aponeurosis and the tarsus. Spacers may include fascia lata, donor sclera, ear cartilage, or alloplastic materials.

If the patient has lateral flare (common in Graves ophthalmopathy), a small eyelid-splitting lateral tarsorrhaphy combined with recession of the upper and lower eyelid retractors can improve the upper eyelid contour. This technique should be used only if the release of the lateral horn of the levator aponeurosis has failed to correct the flare, because lateral tarsorrhaphy may limit the patient's lateral visual field.

Surgical correction of lower eyelid retraction is also directed by the etiologic factors or deficiency. *Anterior lamellar deficiency* (eg, excess skin resection from blepharoplasty) requires addition of vertical skin length by means of a direct or endoscopic midface lift or full-thickness skin graft. *Middle lamellar deficiency* (eg, posttraumatic septal scarring) requires scar release and possible placement of a rigid spacer graft. *Posterior lamellar deficiency* from congenital scarring or conjunctival shortage (eg, ocular cicatricial pemphigoid) may require a full-thickness mucous membrane graft.

Severe retraction of the lower eyelids, common in patients with Graves ophthalmopathy, requires grafting of spacer materials between the lower eyelid retractors and the inferior tarsal border. Autogenous auricular cartilage or hard palate mucosa are good spacer materials for this type of surgery. Preserved sclera and fascia lata have also been used, but autogenous materials are less likely to produce a significant inflammatory reaction. Some form of horizontal eyelid or lateral canthal tightening or elevation is also often required. Because horizontal tightening of the lower eyelid in a patient with proptosis may exacerbate the eyelid retraction, this technique requires caution.

>Bartley GB. The differential diagnosis and classification of eyelid retraction. *Ophthalmology.* 1996;103:168–176.
>Harvey JT, Corin S, Nixon D, et al. Modified levator aponeurosis recession for upper eyelid retraction in Graves' disease. *Ophthalmic Surg.* 1991;22:313–317.
>Kersten RC, Kulwin DR, Levartovsky S, et al. Management of lower-lid retraction with hard-palate mucosa grafting. *Arch Ophthalmol.* 1990;108:1339–1343.
>Putterman AM. Surgical treatment of thyroid-related upper eyelid retraction. Graded Müller's muscle excision and levator recession. *Ophthalmology.* 1981;88:507–512.

Facial Dystonia

Benign Essential Blepharospasm

Benign essential blepharospasm is a bilateral focal dystonia that affects about 300 of every 1 million people. The condition is characterized by increased blinking and involuntary spasms of the orbicularis oculi, procerus, and corrugator muscles. The spasms generally start as mild twitches and progress over time to forceful contractures. The involuntary episodes of forced blinking or contracture may severely limit the patient's ability to drive, read, or perform activities of daily living. With time, this condition can progress until the patient is functionally blind as a result of episodic inability to open the eyelids. Women are affected more frequently than men. The age of onset is usually over 40 years. Neuroimaging is rarely necessary in the workup because the diagnosis is usually made clinically. Severe dry eye syndrome may also result in contracture of the periorbital musculature and must be differentiated from benign essential blepharospasm.

Other muscles of the face may also be involved with blepharospasm. The cause of blepharospasm is unknown; however, it is probably of central origin, in the basal ganglia. Blepharospasm can be managed by medical or surgical approaches. Oral medications have very limited usefulness.

> Aramideh M, Ongerboer de Visser BW, Devriese PP, et al. Electromyographic features of levator palpebrae superioris and orbicularis oculi muscles in blepharospasm. *Brain.* 1994;117:27–38.
>
> Hallett M, Daroff RB. Blepharospasm: report of a workshop. *Neurology.* 1996;46:1213–1218.
>
> Jordan DR, Patrinely JR, Anderson RL, et al. Essential blepharospasm and related dystonias. *Surv Ophthalmol.* 1989;34:123–132.

Botulinum toxin injection

Repeated periodic injection of botulinum toxin type A (Botox) is the treatment of choice for benign essential blepharospasm. Botulinum toxin is a potent neurotoxin derived from *Clostridium botulinum.* Botulinum toxin type A blocks receptor sites in the neuromuscular junction, inhibiting the release of acetylcholine. Injection of this agent at therapeutic doses results in chemical denervation and localized muscle paralysis. Botulinum toxin injection is typically effective but temporary. Average onset of action is 2–3 days, and average peak effect occurs at about 2 weeks following injection. Duration of effect also varies but is typically 3–4 months, at which point recurrence of the spasms and reinjection can be anticipated. Orbicularis oculi subtotal myectomy and facial nerve ablation are considered secondary procedures for patients unresponsive to botulinum therapy. Surgical subtotal myectomy may result in improved patient responsiveness to botulinum toxin therapy. Complications associated with botulinum toxin injection include bruising, blepharoptosis, ectropion, epiphora, diplopia, lagophthalmos, dryness, and superficial punctate keratitis. These adverse reactions are usually transient and typically result from spread of the toxin to adjacent muscles.

> Dutton JJ, Buckley EG. Long-term results and complications of botulinum A toxin in the treatment of blepharospasm. *Ophthalmology.* 1988;95:1529–1534.

Price J, Farish S, Taylor H, et al. Blepharospasm and hemifacial spasm: randomized trial to determine the most appropriate location for botulinum toxin injections. *Ophthalmology.* 1997;104:865–868.

Surgical myectomy

This treatment is reserved for patients unresponsive to botulinum therapy who are incapacitated by the spasms. Meticulous removal of orbicularis fibers in the upper and lower eyelids, including the orbital as well as palpebral portions of the muscle, can be an effective and permanent treatment for blepharospasm. Complications of surgical myectomy include lagophthalmos, chronic lymphedema, or periorbital contour deformities. Limited myectomy is helpful in patients with less severe disease.

Surgical ablation of the facial nerve

Though effective in eliminating blepharospasm, this treatment has been largely discontinued. Recurrence rates may be as high as 30%, and hemifacial paralysis frequently results from facial nerve dissection. Subsequent complications include brow ptosis, inadequate eyelid closure, and weakness of the lower face. The results obtained with facial nerve dissection are, therefore, less satisfactory than with direct orbicularis oculi myectomy. Some surgeons have had greater success with microsurgical ablation of selected facial nerve branches.

Muscle relaxants and sedatives

These have proved to be of marginal or no benefit in the treatment of blepharospasm. Psychotherapy also has little or no value for the patient with blepharospasm.

Bates AK, Halliday BL, Bailey CS, et al. Surgical management of essential blepharospasm. *Br J Ophthalmol.* 1991;75:487–490.

Frueh BR, Musch DC, Bersani TA. Effects of eyelid protractor excision for the treatment of benign essential blepharospasm. *Am J Ophthalmol.* 1992;113:681–686.

Gillum WN, Anderson RL. Blepharospasm surgery. An anatomical approach. *Arch Ophthalmol.* 1981;99:1056–1062.

McCord CD Jr, Coles WH, Shore JW, et al. Treatment of essential blepharospasm. Comparison of facial nerve avulsion and eyebrow-eyelid muscle stripping procedure. *Arch Ophthalmol.* 1984;102:266–268.

Many patients with blepharospasm have an associated dry eye condition that may be aggravated by any treatment modality that decreases eyelid closure. Punctal plugs or occlusion, artificial tears, ointments, moisture chamber shields, and tinted spectacle lenses may help minimize discomfort from ocular surface problems.

Hemifacial Spasm

Blepharospasm should be differentiated from hemifacial spasm. Hemifacial spasm is characterized by intermittent synchronous gross contractures of the entire side of the face and is rarely bilateral. Unlike essential blepharospasm, the spasms are present during sleep. Hemifacial spasm is often associated with ipsilateral facial nerve weakness. In the vast majority of cases, the cause of hemifacial spasm is vascular compression of the facial nerve at the brain stem. Magnetic resonance imaging (MRI) often documents the ectatic vessel. MRI also helps rule out other lesions (eg, pontine glioma) that may be the cause in 1% of cases. Neurosurgical decompression of the facial nerve may be curative in hemifacial spasm. Periodic injection of botulinum toxin is another treatment option. Aberrant regeneration after facial nerve palsy also presents with unilateral aberrant synkinetic facial movements. The history (eg, previous Bell palsy, trauma) and clinical examination are distinctive.

> Sprik C, Wirtschafter JD. Hemifacial spasm due to intracranial tumor. An international survey of botulinum toxin investigators. *Ophthalmology*. 1988;95:1042–1045.

Involutional Periorbital Changes

Dermatochalasis

Dermatochalasis refers to redundancy of eyelid skin and is often associated with orbital fat protrusion or prolapse *(steatoblepharon)*. Although more common in older patients, dermatochalasis can also occur in middle-aged people, particularly if a familial predisposition exists. Dermatochalasis of the upper eyelids is often associated with an indistinct or lower-than-normal eyelid crease. It also may be associated with true ptosis of the upper eyelids (Fig 12-19).

Significant dermatochalasis of the upper lids leads to complaints of a heavy feeling around the eyes, brow ache, complaint of eyelashes in the visual axis, and, eventually, reduction in the superior visual field. This is often made worse by associated brow ptosis, especially if patients do not use their frontalis muscle to elevate the brows to relieve visual obscuration by the excess skin. Lower lid dermatochalasis is considered a cosmetic issue unless the excess skin and prolapsed fat is so severe that the patient cannot be fit with bifocals.

Blepharochalasis

Although blepharochalasis is not an involutional change, it is included in this discussion because it can simulate, and must be differentiated from, dermatochalasis. Rather, ble-

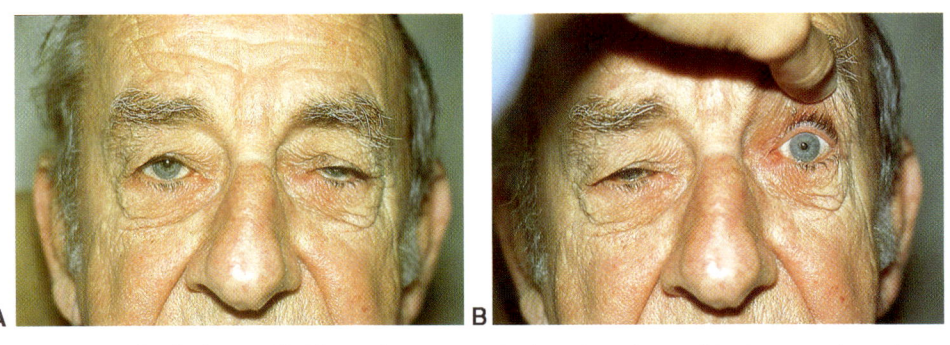

Figure 12-19 A, Patient with bilateral asymmetric drooping due to blepharoptosis and dermatochalasis. **B,** Elevation of more ptotic left upper eyelid reveals increased blepharoptosis on right, which had been masked by the effect of Hering's law of equal innervation to each levator muscle. *(Photographs courtesy of Robert C. Kersten, MD.)*

pharochalasis is a rare familial variant of angioneurotic edema occurring in younger persons that is characterized by idiopathic episodes of inflammatory edema of the eyelids. Because of the recurrent bouts of inflammation and edema, the eyelid skin of a patient with blepharochalasis becomes thin and wrinkled, simulating the appearance of dermatochalasis. In addition, true ptosis, herniation of the orbital lobe of the lacrimal gland, atrophy of the orbital fat pads, and prominent eyelid vascularity may be associated with blepharochalasis secondary to the repeated attacks of edema. This condition is most common in young females. Surgical repair of the eyelid skin changes and ptosis that result from blepharochalasis may be complicated by repeated episodes of inflammation and edema, causing recurrence of the ptosis and other eyelid changes.

    Collin JR. Blepharochalasis. A review of 30 cases. *Ophthal Plast Reconstr Surg.* 1991;7: 153–157.

Blepharoplasty

Upper Eyelid

Upper eyelid blepharoplasty is one of the most commonly performed *functional* as well as *cosmetic* ophthalmic plastic surgical procedures. Involutional skin and structural changes often begin in the periorbital area and they can obstruct the superior visual field. Blepharoplasty is frequently performed to relieve this obstruction. Functional indications for blepharoplasty are documented by means of external photography and visual field testing with and without manual eyelid elevation.

    Patients undergoing blepharoplasty for cosmetic reasons may have different expectations than patients undergoing functional blepharoplasty; thus, a thorough preoperative discussion of the anticipated results is critical to preoperative planning. The surgeon must educate the patient with regard to reasonable postoperative expectations. Cosmetic blepharoplasty is more commonly performed in relatively young patients with less dermatochalasis than is found in the elderly patient presenting with visual field obstruction.

Lower Eyelid

Lower eyelid blepharoplasty is rarely considered functional. The surgery would be considered functional if a patient's excess skin and fat completely covered the spectacle bifocals so the patient was unable to read. For cosmetic lower lid surgery, satisfactory results often require skin rejuvenation with chemical peels or laser resurfacing in addition to surgical alterations of periocular structure. The preoperative discussion should clearly explain the reasonable expectations as well as risks. Patients should understand that aggressive resection of lower eyelid skin and fat may lead to eyelid retraction, ectropion, or a sunken, aged periorbital appearance.

    Physical examination prior to upper blepharoplasty should include the following elements:

- A complete ocular examination including visual acuity testing and documentation
- Visual field testing to demonstrate superior visual field defects if present

- Evaluation of tear secretion or the tear film, which may be carried out through Schirmer testing, tear breakup time, or assessment of the adequacy of the tear meniscus
- Evaluation of the forehead and eyebrows (including brow height and contour) to detect forehead and eyebrow ptosis; the surgeon should make careful observations when the patient's facial and brow musculature is relaxed
- Notation of the position of the upper eyelid crease; the position of the upper eyelid crease varies according to genetic as well as involutional factors: the typical Asian upper eyelid crease is absent or significantly lower than that of the typical occidental eyelid, and the upper eyelid crease is usually 8–9 mm in occidental males and 9–11 mm in occidental females

Preoperative testing for lower blepharoplasty should also include:

- Testing of the elasticity and distractibility of the lower eyelid; the surgeon should be alert to the need for possible horizontal tightening of the lower eyelids as part of the lower blepharoplasty procedure
- Notation and discussion of prominent supraorbital rims, if present; malar hypoplasia or relative exophthalmos may predispose the patient to postoperative scleral show following lower blepharoplasty; burring of the rim is not recommended

Preoperative testing for both upper and lower blepharoplasty should include:

- Assessment of the amount and areas of excess skin, as well as the amount and contours of prolapsed orbital fat, in the upper and lower eyelids
- Evaluation for lagophthalmos; incomplete eyelid closure can lead to postoperative drying and exposure keratitis
- Examination of periorbital bone contours and discussion of findings with the patient
- A detailed discussion of anticipated surgical results as well as possible surgical complications
- Photographic documentation for medicolegal and other purposes.

Jelks GW, Jelks EB. Preoperative evaluation of the blepharoplasty patient. Bypassing the pitfalls. *Clin Plast Surg.* 1993;20:213–223.

Technique

Blepharoplasty begins with a thorough working knowledge of periorbital and eyelid anatomy (discussed in Chapter 9). In addition, just as the brow and glabellar areas affect the upper eyelids, the midfacial structures are influential in the position, tone, contour, and function of the lower eyelid and must be considered in the planning of lower eyelid surgery.

Preoperative planning should include marking excess skin for excision prior to the infiltration of local anesthetic. Often, the surgeon determines the amount of excess skin to be excised by using a pinch technique. For the upper lid, this involves placing one tip of a forceps in the eyelid crease. The other forceps tip is then advanced superiorly until the upper eyelid lashes begin to evert. The excess upper eyelid skin is then allowed to fall between the two tips of the forceps, and the tips are pinched together. The surgeon then uses a surgical marking pen to mark out the parameters of the excess upper eyelid skin. The marking pen is then used to draw out the existing or a new upper eyelid crease as well as the superior border of the planned area of excision. Typically, this marking process results in the delineation of a crescent shape on the upper eyelid. To avoid excessive skin removal, the surgeon usually leaves 20 mm of skin remaining between the inferior border of the brow and the eyelid margin. The surgeon must be careful to avoid aggressive skin resection in the lower lid to avoid lid retraction or ectropion.

Anesthesia for blepharoplasty surgery is typically a combination of local infiltration of anesthetic agents and intravenous administration of sedatives. Often, a rapid-onset, short-duration agent such as lidocaine 1% with epinephrine 1:100,000 is mixed 50–50 with a slower-onset, longer-duration agent such as bupivacaine. A final epinephrine concentration of 1:200,000 is sufficient for maximizing pharmaceutical hemostasis while minimizing the risk of epinephrine toxicity. Injection is best accomplished with sedation before the patient is prepared and draped and prior to surgical scrubbing. This allows enough time for the epinephrine to cause vasoconstriction and thereby reduce the risk of significant perioperative bleeding. Additional local anesthetic and intravenous sedation may be administered intraoperatively if needed.

Upper blepharoplasty

Upper blepharoplasty is begun by incising around the crescent-shaped area marked on the upper eyelid. The skin and underlying orbicularis oculi muscle are usually excised as a single flap in a crescent shape. Surgeons may consider preservation of all or most of the orbicularis oculi muscle in patients with dry eye syndrome.

The orbital septum is incised exposing the underlying preaponeurotic fat pad. The surgeon may remove the fat by gently teasing it forward and excising it with scissors, cautery, or laser. When performed, resection of the preaponeurotic fat pad is carried no deeper than the boundary created by the superior orbital rim. Removal of fat deeper than the rim may result in a hollow superior sulcus. The medial upper eyelid fat pad is typically the most prolapsed and is opened and contoured or excised in a similar manner. However, because the medial palpebral blood vessels overlie the medial upper eyelid fat pads, caution is necessary to avoid significant bleeding in this area. The upper eyelid crease is created by the attachments of the levator aponeurosis to the orbicularis muscle and skin near the upper tarsal border. Aging often results in elevation or loss of the upper eyelid crease. A high, low, or absent eyelid crease can be corrected during blepharoplasty by anchoring the eyelid skin to the levator aponeurosis with deep fixation sutures at the desired position. Alternatively, many surgeons rely on placement of the incision and excision of skin and muscle to manipulate the position of the upper eyelid crease. The upper eyelid skin is closed with a running or subcuticular suture.

Lower blepharoplasty

Lower eyelid blepharoplasty, almost always performed for cosmetic purposes, is most often accomplished through a transconjunctival incision. At times, excess lower eyelid skin may necessitate skin excision through a transcutaneous incision. Skin removal during lower blepharoplasty carries a higher risk of lower eyelid contour abnormalities, retraction, or frank ectropion. Alternatively, excess skin can be tightened without excision through the precise application of laser skin resurfacing techniques or through chemical peeling with exfoliating solutions.

For transconjunctival surgery, preoperative evaluation defines the extent and location of lower eyelid fat prolapse and thus determines the boundaries of surgical excision. The lower eyelid is retracted. The incision is created using a No. 15 blade, a monopolar cautery unit equipped with a Colorado needle, or the CO_2 laser. The incision is begun just medial to the lower eyelid punctum to avoid damage to the lower canaliculus and then courses laterally 2–3 mm below the inferior tarsal border across the length of the eyelid. The incision is carried through the conjunctiva and lower eyelid retractors to gain access to the anterior face of the inferior orbital septum.

Dissection is then carried along the relatively avascular plane of the septum toward the inferior orbital rim. Dissection along the septum is also carried medially and laterally in order to expose the central, medial, and lateral fat compartments. The medial fat compartment is separated from the central fat compartment by the inferior oblique muscle. The surgeon must be aware of the location of this muscle and work carefully around it to avoid damaging it during lower blepharoplasty. The medial fat pad of the lower eyelid, as in the upper eyelid, is paler than the more yellow lateral fat pads. The central fat compartment is separated from the lateral fat compartment by a fascial layer extending off the capsulopalpebral fascia: removal or incision of this fascial barrier may improve access to the lateral fat pad.

After the orbital septum overlying the fat pads has been exposed and opened, the surgeon may carefully and gradually excise the fat while repeatedly checking the external contour of the lower eyelid. Gentle pressure on the globe helps to prolapse the fat forward to improve access and removal. Excision is discontinued when the visible fat remains at or slightly behind the inferior orbital rim when gentle pressure is applied to the globe. Typically, similar volumes of fat are removed from each lower eyelid. Excessive fat removal may give the lower eyelid a hollow appearance. Maintaining maximal hemostasis throughout lower blepharoplasty is critical to the avoidance of vision-threatening complications. The conjunctival incision edges can usually be reapproximated without formal closure with sutures, although absorbable suture closure may occasionally be necessary if the conjunctival edges do not approximate naturally.

Complications

Loss of vision is the most dreaded complication of blepharoplasty. Almost every case of postblepharoplasty visual loss reported has been associated with *lower* blepharoplasty surgery. Although blindness following eyelid surgery is rare, it has been reported to occur at a rate of between 1 in 2000 and 1 in 5000 cases. Such blindness is typically thought to be secondary to postoperative retrobulbar hemorrhage, with the increased intraorbital pressure resulting in ischemia due to compression of the ciliary arteries supplying the optic nerve. Other mechanisms of injury may also be present, however, including excessive, idiopathic constriction of retrobulbar blood vessels in response to epinephrine in the local anesthetic. Orbital hemorrhage may result from injury to the deeper orbital blood vessels or from bleeding from the orbicularis muscle. Risk factors for this complication are thyroid ophthalmopathy and blood dyscrasias (see Chapter 10). Postoperative pressure dressings should be avoided: they increase orbital pressure and obscure underlying problems. Finally, patients should be observed postoperatively to detect possible orbital hemorrhage. Any patient complaining of significant pain, asymmetric swelling, or proptosis following surgery should be evaluated immediately. Visual dimming, darkness, or significant or asymmetric blurred vision following eyelid surgery may also be indicative of orbital hemorrhage and should be assessed and treated immediately.

Visual loss from orbital hemorrhage is an ophthalmologic emergency. When compressive hemorrhage occurs in the orbit, the surgeon may decompress the orbit by opening the surgical wounds, performing lateral canthotomy with cantholysis, and administering high doses of intravenous corticosteroids. Anterior chamber paracentesis has no role in the management of orbital hemorrhage. Additionally, medical glaucoma management is not useful because the increased intra*ocular* pressure reflects increased underlying intra*orbital* pressure. Lack of immediate response to these procedures may necessitate surgical decompression of the orbit with removal of the orbital floor or medial wall.

Diplopia secondary to injury of extraocular muscles is the next most severe complication of blepharoplasty. Diplopia may result from injury to the inferior oblique muscle, the inferior rectus muscle, or the superior oblique muscle. The inferior oblique muscle originates near the anterior lacrimal crest along the infraorbital rim and is anterior in the orbit. It separates and courses across the central and medial lower eyelid fat pads and may be injured during the removal of lower eyelid fatty tissue. The trochlea of the superior oblique muscle also may be injured by deep dissection in orbital fat in the superior nasal aspect of the upper eyelid.

> Jordan DR, Anderson RL, Thiese SM. Avoiding inferior oblique injury during lower blepharoplasty. *Arch Ophthalmol.* 1989;107:1382–1383.

Excessive removal of skin is a serious complication that can lead to lagophthalmos of the upper eyelids as well as cicatricial ectropion or retraction of the lower eyelids (Fig 12-20). Topical lubricants and massage may be helpful for managing mild postoperative lagophthalmos, retraction, or ectropion, all of which may resolve over time without

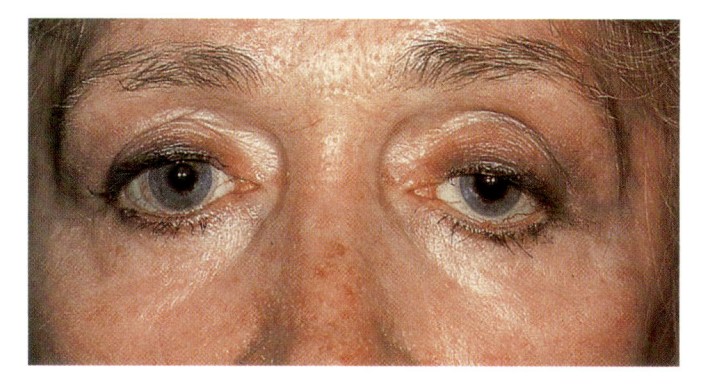

Figure 12-20 Lower eyelid retraction following blepharoplasty.

further intervention. Injectable steroids (triamcinolone acetonide, 10 mg/mL [Kenalog-10]) can be used if a deep cicatrix contributes to the retraction. Severe cases require the use of free skin grafts, lateral canthoplasty, or release of scar tissue or eyelid retractors. Inferior scleral show can also result from septal scarring, orbicularis hematoma, and malar hypoplasia, even when minimal skin has been excised.

> Baylis HI, Long JA, Groth MJ. Transconjunctival lower eyelid blepharoplasty. Technique and complications. *Ophthalmology.* 1989;96:1027–1032.
>
> Baylis HI, Nelson ER, Goldberg RA. Lower eyelid retraction following blepharoplasty. *Ophthal Plast Reconstr Surg.* 1992;8:170–175.
>
> Dailey RA. Upper eyelid blepharoplasty. In: *Focal Points: Clinical Modules for Ophthalmologists.* San Francisco: American Academy of Ophthalmology; 1995: vol 13, no 8.
>
> Dortzbach RK. Lower eyelid blepharoplasty by the anterior approach. Prevention of complications. *Ophthalmology.* 1983;90:223–229.
>
> Lowry JC, Bartley GB. Complications of blepharoplasty [major review]. *Surv Ophthalmol.* 1994;38:327–350.
>
> Neuhaus RW. Complications of blepharoplasty. In: *Focal Points: Clinical Modules for Ophthalmologists.* San Francisco: American Academy of Ophthalmology; 1990: vol 8, no 3.
>
> Ophthalmic Procedures Assessment Committee. *Functional Indications for Upper and Lower Eyelid Blepharoplasty.* San Francisco: American Academy of Ophthalmology; 1994.

Brow Ptosis

Loss of elastic tissues and involutional changes of the forehead skin result in drooping of the forehead and, most noticeably, drooping of the eyebrows. This condition is known as *brow ptosis*. Visually significant brow ptosis may also result from facial nerve palsy. Brow ptosis frequently accompanies dermatochalasis and must be recognized as a factor that contributes to the appearance of aging in the periorbital area. Brow ptosis may become severe enough to affect the superior visual field. The patient often involuntarily attempts to compensate for this condition by chronic use of the frontalis muscle to elevate the eyebrows (Fig 12-21). Such chronic contracture of the frontalis muscle often leads to brow ache, headache, and prominent transverse forehead rhytids.

In most patients, the brow is located above the superior orbital rim. Generally, the female brow is higher and more arched than the typical male brow. The brow is con-

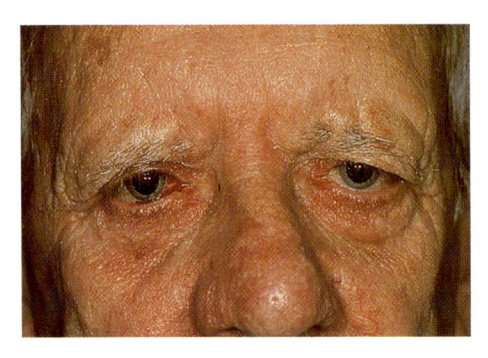

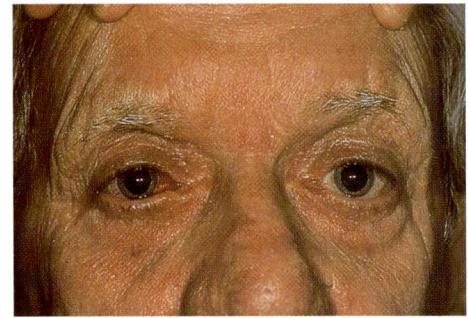

Figure 12-21 Brow ptosis.

sidered ptotic when it falls below the superior orbital rim. Brow ptosis is documented by measuring the distance in millimeters between the central brow and the superior orbital rim.

Treatment of Functional Brow Ptosis

Brow ptosis must be recognized and treated prior to or concomitant with the surgical repair of coexistent dermatochalasis of the eyelids. Because brow elevation results in a reduction of the amount of dermatochalasis present, it should be performed or simulated first when combined with upper blepharoplasty. Aggressive upper blepharoplasty in a patient with concomitant brow ptosis results in further depression of the brow. Functional brow ptosis is generally corrected with browpexy or direct brow lift.

Browpexy

Browpexy is performed through an upper eyelid blepharoplasty incision for mild to moderate brow ptosis. The sub-brow tissues are resuspended with sutures to the frontal bone periosteum above the orbital rim as part of a blepharoplasty.

> McCord CD, Doxanas MT. Browplasty and browpexy: an adjunct to blepharoplasty. *Plast Reconstr Surg.* 1990;86:248–254.

Direct eyebrow elevation

The eyebrows can be elevated with incisions placed at the upper edge of the eyebrow. This procedure is useful for men and women with lateral eyebrow ptosis. When direct eyebrow elevation is used across the entire brow, it may result in an arch that is unacceptable in men. A conspicuous scar may occur, especially above the medial portion of the eyebrow when the entire brow is lifted.

> Kerth JD, Toriumi DM. Management of the aging forehead. *Arch Otolaryngol Head Neck Surg.* 1990;116:1137–1142.

Cosmetic Facial Surgery

Most ophthalmic plastic surgeons think that effective treatment of cosmetic and reconstructive upper eyelid problems must include consideration of eyebrow and forehead surgery. Likewise, effective lower eyelid cosmetic and reconstructive surgery must include consideration of midface and cheek surgery. Consequently, most ophthalmic plastic surgical fellowship programs in the United States include training in facial cosmetic and reconstructive surgery. It is important that any eyelid surgeon understand the surgical procedures discussed below. The performance of these procedures, however, generally requires special training, experience, and expertise.

The human face is an essential component of human communication. The aging face may communicate tiredness, depression, anger, or fear in an otherwise well-rested, well-adjusted, fully functioning person. To understand the problems and solutions of facial plastic surgery as they relate to communication and human beauty, the patient and surgeon must appreciate that our perception of the face and its communicative ability is based on the relative appearance and position of its parts in an additive fashion. The face is composed of smaller cosmetic units such as the forehead, eyelids, cheek, nose, lips, and neck. As we age, one or more of these cosmetic units undergo changes that lead to facial imbalance, disharmony, and ultimately miscommunication. If a single subunit has aged out of proportion to the rest of the face, as in dermatochalasis, a bilateral upper blepharoplasty produces a nice result. On the other hand, if the patient has concomitant aging changes of the mid and lower face and neck yet only undergoes lower eyelid blepharoplasty, the result will be far from satisfactory and will perpetuate further facial miscommunication, chronologic facial imbalance, and perceptual confusion.

Pathogenesis of the Aging Face

Factors that lead to involutional facial changes can be divided into two categories: intrinsic and extrinsic. *Intrinsic aging* refers to changes that occur as a result of chronologic aging. *Extrinsic aging* results from environmental factors such as cigarette smoke, ultraviolet radiation, wind, and gravity.

The facial contour and appearance is derived from soft tissue draped over underlying bone. The soft tissue component is composed of skin, subcutaneous fat, muscle, deeper fat pads, and fascial layers. The underlying structural element is composed of bone, cartilage, and teeth.

As the face ages, the soft tissue component moves inferiorly and the bone component loses mass, leaving relatively more soft tissue to hang from its attachments to the bone. Loss of subcutaneous fat, skin atrophy, and descent of facial fat pads compound this sagging face phenomenon. Around the eyes, the lateral brow typically descends more than the medial brow, leading to temporal hooding. The orbital septum stretches, bulges, or dehisces, allowing fat to move forward. In the lower lid, midface descent produces the skeletonization of the infraorbital rim and increases the prominence of the orbital fat. This has been described as a *double convexity deformity*. This also contributes to the increased prominence of the nasolabial fold. Sagging of the platysma muscle in the neck posterior to the mandibular ligament gives rise to jowling. The *turkey gobbler defect* in the neck is the result of redundant skin and separated medial borders of the platysma muscle at the midline.

Physical Examination of the Aging Face

Much of the surgeon's appraisal of the aging face can be obtained through close observation of the patient during the introduction and history phase of the initial meeting. From the top, so to speak, the surgeon should observe the hairstyle and thickness, the presence of bangs, the height of the hairline, frontalis use, brow position, facial skin texture and quality, presence and location of rhytids, telangiectasias, pigmentary dyschromia, and expressive furrows. In addition, eyelid skin and fat should be assessed along with margin position relative to the pupil and cornea, presence or absence of horizontal lower lid laxity, midface position, presence of jowling, accumulation of subcutaneous fat in the neck, and chin position. Any nasal deformities and tip descent and broadening, as well as thinning of the lips, should be noted. A side view of the neck is particularly helpful in determining the extent of aging. Preoperative photographs are necessary for use as a reference in the operating room, for assessment of postoperative results, and for medicolegal use.

Facial Rejuvenation Surgery (Beyond Blepharoplasty)

Cosmetics, chemical peels, microdermabrasion, and laser resurfacing may be used to treat involutional and actinic facial skin changes. These relatively superficial procedures may precede or be combined with other surgical procedures that reposition deeper structures. Although upper and lower eyelid surgery have been discussed earlier in this chapter, it is important to remember that the upper eyelid appearance is inextricably linked to the position of the eyebrow. The same applies to the lower eyelid and midface as well as lower face and neck. Subunits of the facial cosmetic superstructure cannot be viewed or manipulated individually but must be addressed in the context of the entire face and neck.

Laser Skin Resurfacing

Laser skin resurfacing, a technology popularized in the early 1990s, is designed to reduce wrinkles and enhance the texture and appearance of the facial and periorbital skin. A variety of lasers have been developed to perform laser resurfacing, but the carbon dioxide (CO_2) laser is the most widely used. Although the CO_2 laser had other applications for many years, its usefulness in skin resurfacing was originally limited because the laser caused peripheral thermal damage, resulting in scarring. However, by the early 1990s, the development of the ultrapulsed CO_2 laser allowed ablative skin resurfacing without the secondary thermal damage and scarring. The ultrapulsed laser is designed to deliver small pulses of high-energy laser to the skin. Pauses between the pulses allow cooling of the tissues in the treated area, minimizing the risk of secondary thermal damage. Although other skin resurfacing techniques, such as chemical peeling and dermabrasion, have been used for many years, CO_2 laser resurfacing has gained popularity due in part to the predictability and accuracy of the laser. The surgeon is able to reliably judge the appropriate treatment depth and endpoint while using the CO_2 laser.

Superpulsed CO_2 laser resurfacing has been shown to be useful in the treatment of involutional and actinic facial skin changes, scars (including acne scarring), and exophytic skin lesions. The erbium laser can also be used for ablative skin resurfacing. These laser techniques have been applied primarily to facial skin because of the high density of pilosebaceous units in this region (the facial skin contains about 40 times more pilosebaceous units than the skin of the neck). Application of this technology in areas of lower pilosebaceous unit density, especially the neck, is not recommended because of an unacceptably high risk of scarring.

Laser resurfacing has also been shown to be a useful adjunct to blepharoplasty, particularly lower blepharoplasty. The skin-shrinking, collagen-tightening effect of the CO_2 laser often allows the surgeon to avoid an external incision and skin removal. Accordingly, this may reduce the incidence of common complications of lower blepharoplasty such as eyelid retraction, ectropion, lagophthalmos, or exposure keratitis. Many CO_2 laser units have interchangeable hand pieces that concentrate the laser energy and allow the laser to be used as a cutting instrument, or a type of scalpel. The laser scalpel can be beneficial to the ophthalmic surgeon because, when used appropriately, it allows nearly bloodless surgery in many patients and may reduce postoperative edema, ecchymosis, and healing time.

Safe and effective laser resurfacing requires special training. Additional understanding of skin, skin anatomy, laser physics, and perioperative care is crucial to a successful outcome. Ophthalmologists who receive training in intraocular laser use tend to feel comfortable with other laser modalities as well. Laser skin resurfacing complications may include a variety of ophthalmologic problems including lagophthalmos, exposure keratitis, corneal injury, and lower eyelid retraction. Patient selection is critical for successful laser skin resurfacing. Patients with reasonable expectations and goals who are educated preoperatively by the physician or staff are best suited to this procedure. Patients with a fair complexion and generally healthy, well-hydrated skin are ideal candidates. Patients with greater degrees of skin pigmentation can be safely treated, but additional care and caution is necessary. The darker the skin pigmentation, the greater the risk of postoperative inflammatory hyperpigmentation. Most surgeons treat all patients, but especially those with Fitzpatrick skin type III or IV, with a preoperative melanocyte-suppressing bleaching agent such as hydroquinone for 4–8 weeks. Treatment of deeply pigmented skin types, Fitzpatrick type V or VI, carries a high risk of significant, prolonged hyperpigmentation and should be approached with caution. Laser resurfacing is contraindicated in patients who have used isotretinoin (Accutane) within the past 12 months because reepithelialization is inhibited. Other contraindications include inappropriate, unrealistic expectations; collagen vascular disease such as active systemic lupus erythematosus; and significant uncorrected lower eyelid laxity.

Most surgeons treat patients preoperatively with suppressing doses of anti-viral agents as prophylaxis against outbreaks of herpes simplex virus on the laser-resurfaced skin. Herpes simplex virus infection after laser resurfacing may lead to irreversible scarring. Antiviral prophylaxis should begin 1–2 days before the procedure and continue for 10–14 days after surgery. Antibiotic prophylaxis such as cephazolin or ciprofloxacin is generally used.

The details of the technique of laser resurfacing are beyond the scope of this book. Generally, however, laser energy is applied to facial skin at power levels sufficient to cause ablation of the skin without significant attendant thermal effect. The first laser application to the area, commonly called the *first pass,* vaporizes the dead surface epithelium. Because live virus has been cultured from a laser plume, it is important to remove laser-generated smoke with a vacuum system. After each pass, the resultant debris is gently wiped away with a saline-moistened gauze pad. Additional passes are then used to tighten or ablate underlying collagen in order to retexture and recontour the skin. Treatment is continued until the surgeon notes a chamois color, the endpoint. Different facial areas require different levels of power and numbers of passes to reach optimal effect. Generally, thicker and more damaged skin requires more laser energy. In contrast, eyelid skin is among the thinnest in the body and requires gentle treatment if complications are to be avoided.

Patients require much reassurance following laser resurfacing, especially until regrowth of the epithelium is complete. Many patients experience erythema of the treated skin for weeks to months following this surgery and should be warned of this possibility preoperatively. Makeup can be applied to the treated skin after reepithelialization is complete, usually about 10–14 days postoperatively.

Goldbaum AM, Woog JJ. The CO_2 laser in oculoplastic surgery. *Surv Ophthalmol.* 1997; 42:255–267.

Sullivan SA, Dailey RA. Complications of laser resurfacing and their management. *Ophthal Plast Reconstr Surg.* 2000;16:417–426.

Cosmetic Uses of Botulinum Toxin

The initial use of botulinum toxin in patients with blepharospasm and hemifacial spasm led to the observation that botulinum toxin reduces or eliminates some facial wrinkles. Use of botulinum toxin (Botox Cosmetic) for the treatment of upper facial wrinkles has become widespread and was approved by the FDA in 2002 for use in the glabellar area to reduce or eliminate wrinkles. The areas that are most amenable to this treatment are the glabella, forehead, lateral canthus (crow's feet), perioral rhytids, and platysmal bands. The amount and location of botox injection in the forehead and platysmal bands varies significantly and should be individualized.

Botulinum toxin has also been used in the temporary treatment of cosmetic eyebrow ptosis when injected into the depressors of the eyebrow. Onset of action, peak effect, and duration of effect are the same as those noted earlier for botulinum toxin. Complications of botulinum toxin injections for cosmetic purposes are identical to those listed for blepharospasm.

Upper Face Rejuvenation (Brow and Forehead Lift)

Many surgical options are available to the surgeon, but our discussion includes two methods commonly used in cosmetic surgery: standard endoscopic brow lift and the pretrichial endoscopic approach.

Endoscopic brow and forehead lift (standard approach)

Endoscopic techniques allow the surgeon to raise the brow and rejuvenate the forehead (foreheadplasty) through small incisions about 1 cm behind the hairline (Fig 12-22A). An endoscope protected by a hooded sleeve is attached through a fiberoptic light cord to a bright light source. A camera is also attached to the endoscope and is connected in turn to a video monitor. Dissection is accomplished with an endoscopic periosteal elevator, sharp scissors, suction, and monopolar cautery.

Typically, one 2 cm incision is placed just posterior to the hairline in the midline. Two parasagittal incisions are also placed behind the hairline about 5 cm lateral to the midline incision. Each of these incisions then is carried down to bone. Subperiosteal dissection is initially performed without the endoscope. A central subperiosteal space or *optical pocket* is developed posteriorly to the occiput and anteriorly to 1–2 cm above the superior orbital rim. This allows insertion of the hooded endoscope to complete the dissection in the area of the orbital rim. The supraorbital and supratrochlear neurovascular bundles are visualized and avoided. To eliminate glabellar lines, the corrugator and procerus muscles are stripped or removed altogether. The central subperiosteal pocket is used to release periosteum along the superior rim, and the temporal pockets allow release of periosteum along the lateral brow. Temporally, incisions are placed 2–3 cm behind and parallel to the hairline in the temporal fossa. Blunt dissection is carried down to the deep temporalis fascia. An ellipse of scalp is excised, and dissection is begun under direct

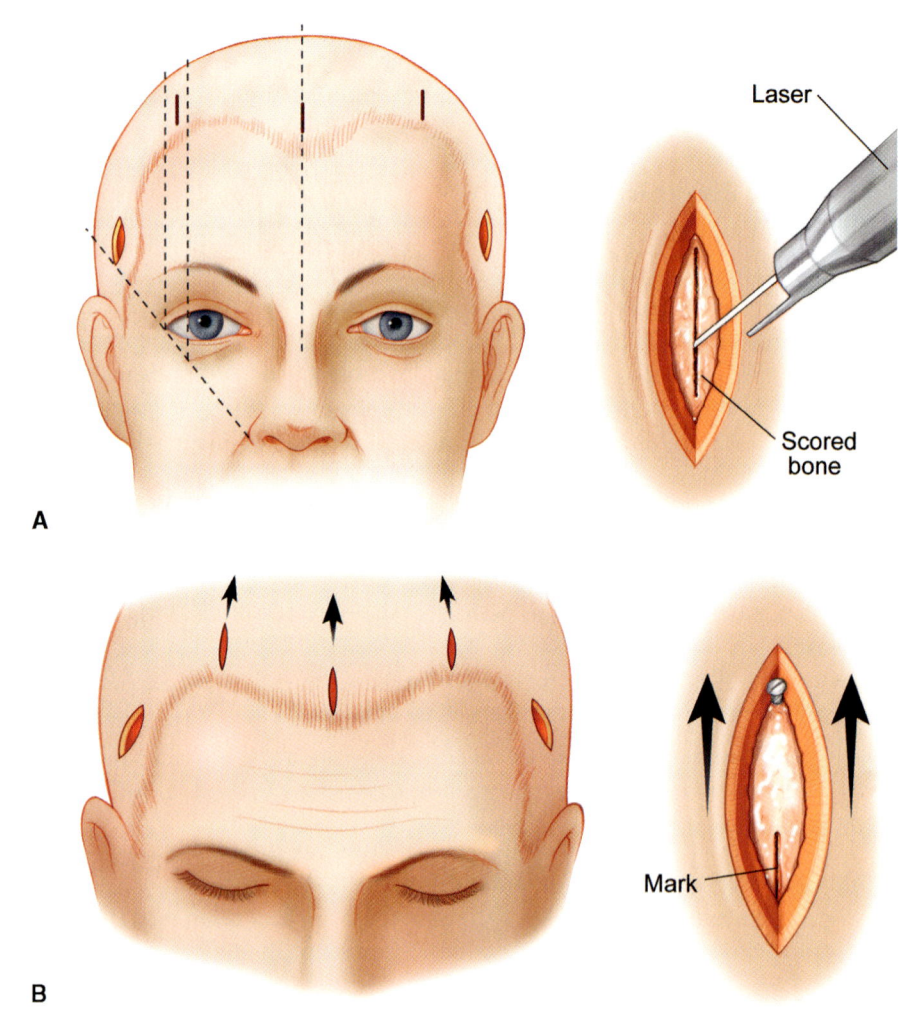

Figure 12-22 Standard endoscopic browlift. **A,** CO$_2$ laser is used for incision of scalp and scoring of bone. **B,** The scalp is retracted posteriorly and the fixation screw is placed at the posterior aspect of the incision. *(Illustrations by Christine Gralapp.)*

visualization along the deep temporalis fascia. This pocket, deep to the temporoparietal fascia, is enlarged under endoscopic guidance. Dissection along the deep temporalis fascia spares the frontal branch of the facial nerve in the overlying temporoparietal fascia. The central and temporal pockets are joined by releasing the conjoint fascia, which is firmly adherent tissue along the temporal lines.

Elevation, fixation, and closure are the final steps. Fixation points are based on the preoperative brow position. Paracentral elevation increases the arch of the brow; central elevation lifts the glabella and medial brows. Holes in the skull are drilled with an appropriate-sized bit. Fixation screws anchor the periosteum to its new position (Fig 12-22B). The temporoparietal fascia is sutured to the deep temporalis fascia, providing temporal brow elevation. The wounds are closed with surgical staples.

Daniel RK, Tirkanits B. Endoscopic forehead lift: an operative technique. *Plast Reconstr Surg.* 1996;98:1148–1157.

Putterman AM. *Cosmetic Oculoplastic Plastic Surgery.* 3rd ed. Philadelphia: WB Saunders; 1999.

Endoscopic brow lift (pretrichial approach)

The pretrichial approach is used in patients whose hairline is to be raised above 70 mm or in those worried about developing a high hairline. Access occurs through a pretrichial incision instead of the small skin incisions with the standard approach. Periosteal release is performed endoscopically through incisions in the galea, frontalis muscle, and periosteum. An appropriate amount of forehead skin is resected, and the underlying frontalis and galea are plicated with a subsequent layered closure.

Midface Rejuvenation (Suborbicularis Oculi Fat/Midface Lift)

The entire midface should be evaluated in a patient presenting for lower eyelid blepharoplasty. With age, cheek tissue descends and orbital fat herniates, creating the double-convexity deformity. Varying degrees of suborbicularis oculi fat (SOOF) and midface elevation combined with conservative transconjunctival fat removal or redistribution restores youthful anterior projection of the midface, rendering a single smooth contour to the lower eyelid and midface region. A lower lid approach (infraciliary or transconjunctival) or a combined oral mucosal and temporal endoscopic approach may be used. These techniques of midfacial elevation allow the lower eyelid/midface unit to be fully addressed as part of facial rejuvenation.

SOOF lift (preperiosteal)

SOOF lifts are indicated for cosmetic midface rejuvenation as well as correction of mildly or moderately retracted or ectropic lower lids when anterior lamellar skin shortage is the main problem. In many of these cases, a full-thickness skin graft can be avoided. The elevation can occur in the subperiosteal or preperiosteal plane.

The midface is accessed through a transconjunctival or subciliary incision. One approach uses a conjunctival incision (with lateral canthotomy) immediately deep to the inferior tarsal border with dissection down to just below the inferior orbital rim. The orbit is not entered unless orbital fat is to be manipulated. The SOOF is visualized on the anterior maxillary surface (Fig 12-23). This fat is darker yellow and tougher in consistency than orbital fat. An incision is made between the periosteum and SOOF for the entire width of the infraorbital rim. Dissection continues inferiorly in the preperiosteal plane. The SOOF is elevated and secured to the arcus marginalis. The lateral canthal region is reformed and sutured to the lateral orbital rim. The transconjunctival wound can be left open.

Hoenig JA, Shorr N, Shorr J. The suborbicularis oculi fat in aesthetic and reconstructive surgery. *Int Ophthalmol Clin.* 1997;37:179–191.

Midface lift (subperiosteal)

A subperiosteal midface lift is done in cases of more severe retraction of the lower lid. This lift is also commonly combined with brow lift or lower face lift and can be done

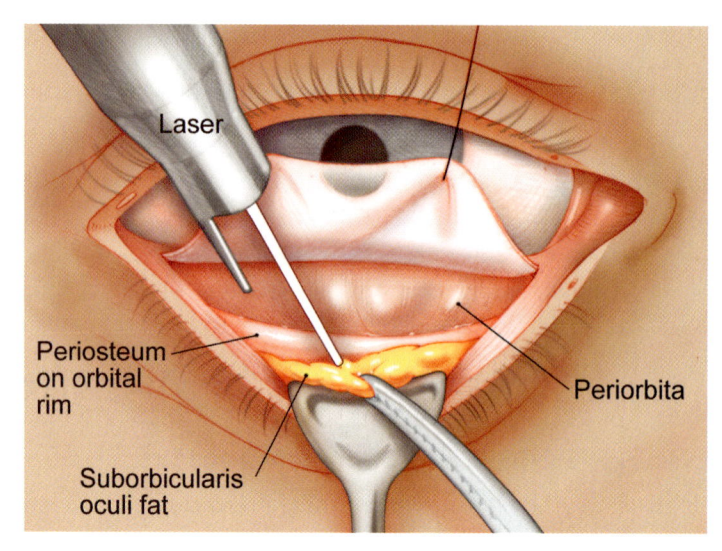

Figure 12-23 Preperiosteal approach to suborbicularis oculi fat (SOOF) lift. *(Illustration by Christine Gralapp.)*

without a lateral canthal incision. The subperiosteal midface can be accessed from the lateral canthus or a superior gingival sulcus incision to avoid a visible scar at the lateral canthus.

The anterior maxillary surface is approached as discussed above for the SOOF lift. In cosmetic cases, access is typically through a temporal scalp incision and gingival sulcus incision. A transconjunctival incision is also used and, in this case, the periosteum is incised 3–4 mm inferior to the orbital rim, leaving a rim of periosteum from which the cheek SOOF and periosteum will be suspended. A periosteal elevator is used to lift the periosteum from the maxilla and medial zygoma. The infraorbital neurovascular bundle is visualized and spared. Dissection extends to the piriform aperture medially, the superior alveolar ridge inferiorly, and the anterior border of the masseter muscle laterally. The periosteum is released with electrocautery or digital blunt dissection. The endpoint is a well-mobilized midface. The cheek is secured to the arcus marginalis medially and the intermediate temporalis fascia laterally. This multivector lift corrects the infraorbital depression secondary to SOOF descent and softens the nasolabial fold.

Endoscopic midface lift (subperiosteal)

The endoscopic technique is used when significant elevation is needed and the patient has redundant forehead and mid-facial skin. There are three major steps. First, a temporal pocket is created as for standard endoscopic brow lifts (Fig 12-24A). Second, the midface is mobilized by subperiosteal dissection via either transconjunctival or superior gingival sulcus oral mucosal incision. The third step is elevation and suspension of the midface to the deep temporalis fascia with sutures passed through the temporal pocket (Fig 12-24B). The oral incision, if used, is closed with 4-0 chromic gut, with the remaining incisions closed as previously described.

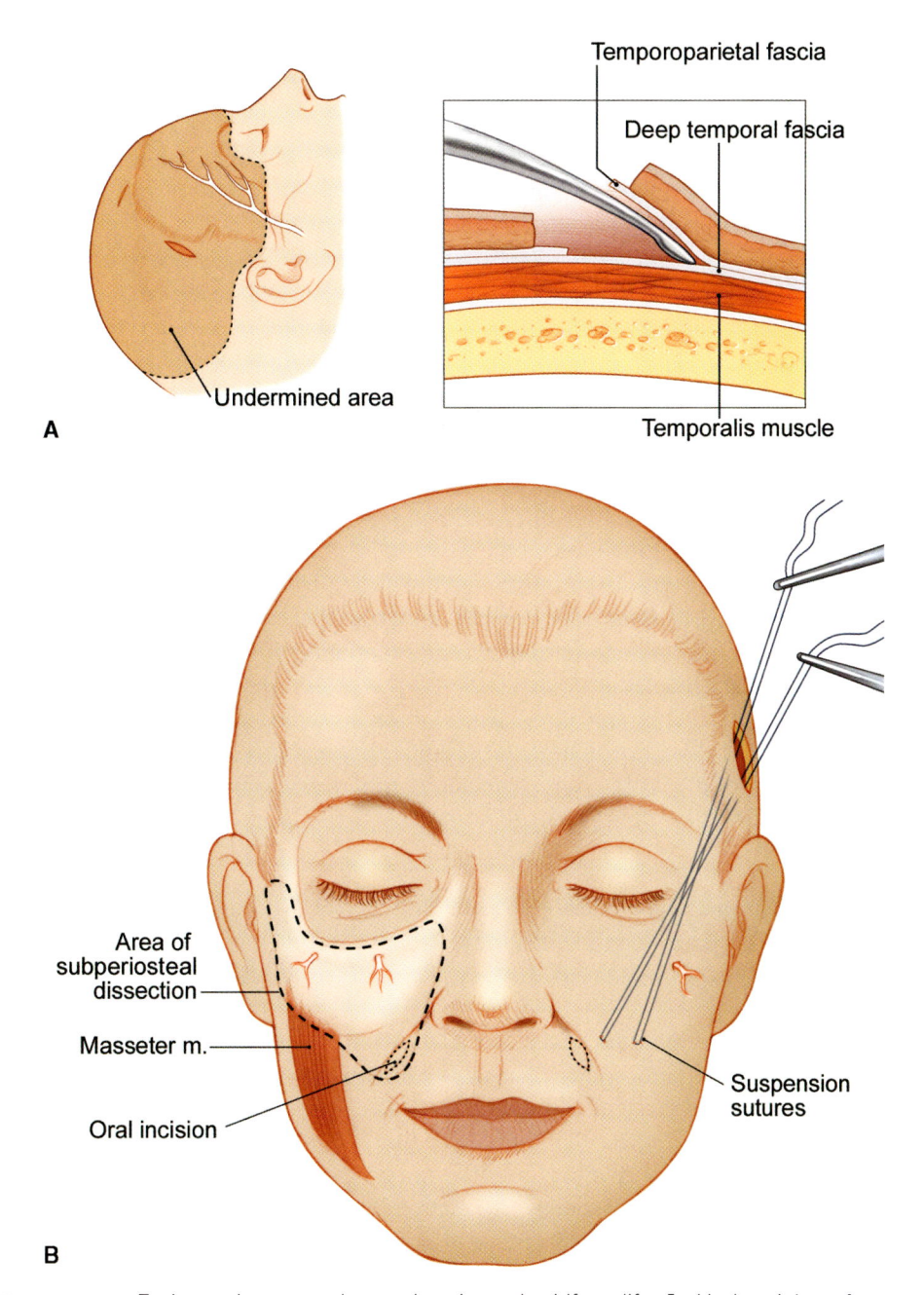

CHAPTER 12: Periocular Malpositions and Involutional Changes • 243

Figure 12-24 Endoscopic approach to subperiosteal midface lift. **A,** Undermining of temporoparietal fascia. **B,** Midface subperiosteal dissection and suture fixation. *(Illustrations by Christine Gralapp.)*

Lower Face and Neck Rejuvenation

During preoperative evaluation, the entire face and neck should be considered as a single cosmetic unit. Correction of the cosmetic subunits of the upper and midface without the lower face and neck can create a chronologically out-of-balance appearance that is unacceptable to many patients. At the very least, these concerns must be discussed with the patient preoperatively along with surgical options.

Rejuvenation of the aging face requires a multitude of techniques. Peels, laser resurfacing, dermabrasion, liposculpting, and various other laser treatments can all augment the results following surgical intervention or even preclude incisional intervention.

Rhytidectomy

Credit for the first cosmetic full facelift is generally given to Lexer, who performed the procedure in 1916. Today, the most common procedures include the classic (subcutaneous) rhytidectomy, the subcutaneous rhytidectomy with the superficial musculoaponeurotic system (SMAS), and the deep plane rhytidectomy. The classic rhytidectomy was the procedure of choice throughout the majority of the 1970s. The anatomic work of Mitz and Peyronie and the surgical approach of Skoog led surgeons to mobilize and secure the deeper SMAS layer, allowing better skin support and more lasting results. Rhytidectomies typically include surgical management of the neck including liposuction with or without platysmaplasty.

The three rhytidectomy procedures briefly discussed below differ mainly in the location and extent of dissection. The more superficial procedures are generally safer but are less likely to produce lasting improvement. The more extensive procedures are more dangerous (ie, facial nerve injury) but are more likely to produce dramatic, longer-lasting improvement.

Classic (subcutaneous) rhytidectomy The standard facelift incisions are marked. A pretragal incision is made in men in the groove; a posttragal incision is generally used in women. The submental incision, if used, is placed 2 mm posterior to the submental crease.

Subcutaneous undermining of the skin is then initiated first with a blade and then with scissors. The more medial dissection can be visualized with direct illumination from a fiberoptic retractor or surgeon's headlight. Once this dissection is finished, attention is turned to the other side, where the same procedure is performed. The skin is then redraped in a posterosuperior manner, and skin resection is initiated. Fixation sutures are placed, but there should be essentially no traction on the flap, particularly the postauricular portion, as it is the most susceptible to necrosis.

Complications of this technique are directly related to the extent of subcutaneous undermining. These complications are hematoma, seroma, skin necrosis, hair loss, paresthesias, motor deficits, incisional scarring, asymmetry, and contour irregularities. Hematoma is the leading facelift complication, but patient dissatisfaction is the most common problem facing the facial surgeon postoperatively.

Subcutaneous rhytidectomy with SMAS The subcutaneous rhytidectomy with SMAS differs from the classic rhytidectomy in that the SMAS is mobilized in some fashion along

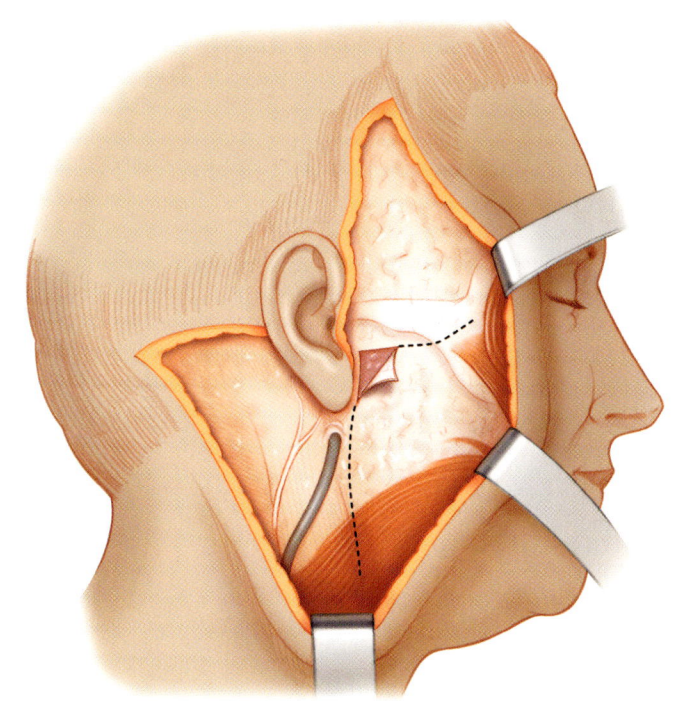

Figure 12-25 Subcutaneous rhytidectomy with superficial musculoaponeurotic system (SMAS). *(Illustration by Christine Gralapp.)*

with subcutaneous dissection (Fig 12-25). Mobilization of the SMAS allows more skin to be repositioned with deep support for a more natural, less surgical appearance. Improvement of jowling and the appearance of the jaw line are greatly enhanced.

Deep plane rhytidectomy The deep plane rhytidectomy also involves mobilization of the SMAS. The extent of SMAS dissection is greater than with the combined technique, but subcutaneous dissection over the SMAS is less. Dissection is extended to the mandible for greater mobilization. The edge of the SMAS flap is attached to the firm preauricular tissues (Fig 12-26). The lateral platysma in the neck is plicated, and excess skin is resected and closed without tension. Although the deep plane approach is considered the most surgically demanding, troublesome subcutaneous hematomas occur less frequently.

Neck liposuction

Stab incisions or *adits* are made just posterior to the earlobe on each side and just anterior to the central submental crease. Microcannulas allow fat removal (Fig 12-27). A layer of fat is left on the dermis, and the liposuction cannula openings are always oriented away from the dermis to avoid injury to the vascular plexus deep to the dermis. In addition to abnormalities in skin quality, damage in this area can lead to unsightly scarring of the dermis of the underlying neck musculature. The adits are left open, and a compression bandage is worn for 1 week.

246 • Orbit, Eyelids, and Lacrimal System

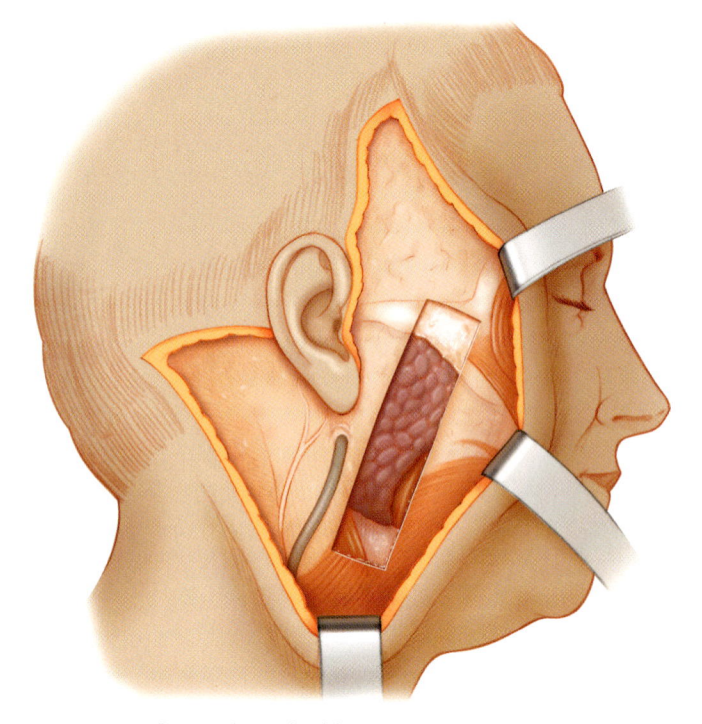

Figure 12-26 Deep plane rhytidectomy. *(Illustration by Christine Gralapp.)*

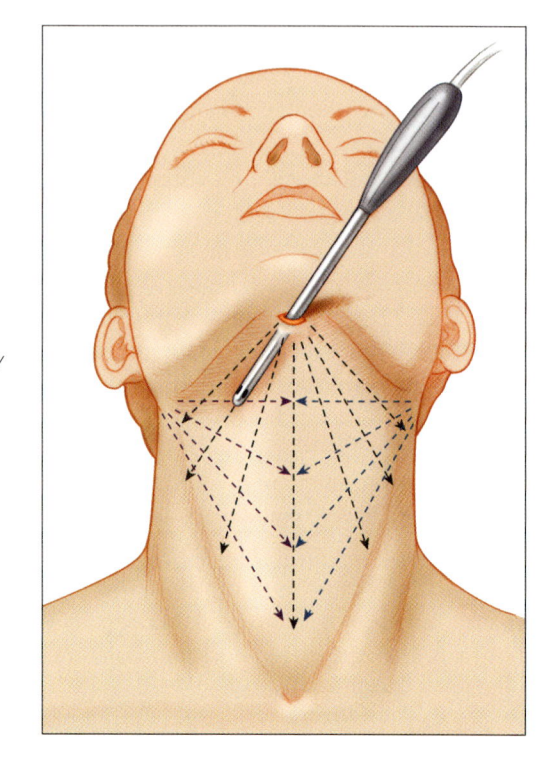

Figure 12-27 Neck liposuction. *(Illustration by Christine Gralapp.)*

CHAPTER 12: Periocular Malpositions and Involutional Changes • 247

Platysmaplasty

Platysmaplasty is performed to correct troublesome platysmal bands. A subcutaneous dissection is carried out in the preplatysmal plane centrally under the chin to the level of the thyroid cartilage (Fig 12-28A). As part of a rhytidectomy, lateral platysmal undermining and suspension may be performed. Midline platysma resection (Fig 12-28B) and reconstruction (Fig 12-28C) is performed if midline neck support is needed. A drain and a light compression dressing are placed. Postoperatively, the cervicomental angle is more acute, yielding a more youthful look.

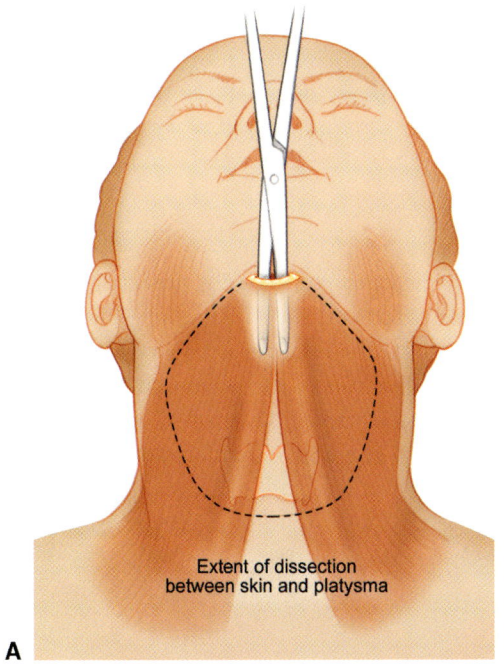

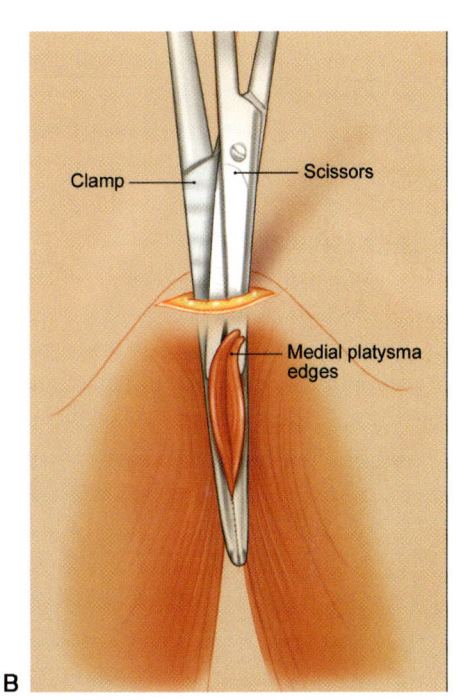

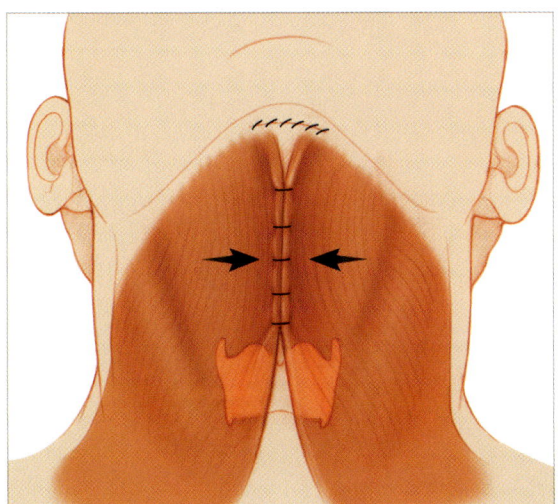

Figure 12-28 Cervicoplasty. **A,** Undermining of the skin. **B,** Resection of medial platysma. **C,** Platysmaplasty. *(Illustrations by Christine Gralapp.)*

Baker DC. Minimal incision rhytidectomy (short scar face lift) with lateral SMASectomy: evolution and application. *Aesthetic Surg J.* 2001;21:14–26.

Baker TJ, Stuzin JM. Personal technique of face lifting. *Plast Reconstr Surg.* 1997;100:502–508.

Baylis HI, Goldberg RA, Shorr N. The deep plane facelift: a 20 year evolution of technique. *Ophthalmology.* 2000;107:490–495.

Dailey RA, Jones LT. Rejuvenation of the aging face. In: *Focal Points: Clinical Modules for Ophthalmologists.* San Francisco: American Academy of Ophthalmology; 2003: vol 21, no 11.

Kamer FM, Frankel AS. Deep plane face-lift for improvement of the lateral oral groove. *Facial Plast Surg Clin North Am.* 1997;5:23–28.

Kamer FM, Halsey W. The two-layer rhytidectomy. *Arch Otolaryngol.* 1981;107:450–453.

Klein JA. *Tumescent Technique: Tumescent Anesthesia and Microcannular Liposuction.* St. Louis: Mosby; 2000.

Rees TD. The classic operation. In: Rees TD, LaTrenta GS, eds. *Aesthetic Plastic Surgery.* 2nd ed. Philadelphia: WB Saunders; 1994:683–707.

Conclusions

The periocular area, where most comprehensive ophthalmologists work, is part of a larger anatomic superstructure called the face. The primary function of this composite entity is communication; changes that occur through aging, disease, or surgery alter the message. If a single subunit is changed without consideration of the other subunits, facial miscommunication, chronologic facial imbalance, and perceptual confusion can result. It is therefore incumbent on the ophthalmic facial surgeon to understand the aging process, anatomy, and available surgical techniques prior to embarking on surgery that changes any portion of the face. Discussion of these issues with the patient preoperatively helps to avoid unhappy patients postoperatively.

PART III

Lacrimal System

Introduction

The lacrimal system consists of two components: the main and accessory glands and their secretions and the lacrimal excretory outflow system. The symptom of overflow tearing, or *epiphora*, is often the reason a patient seeks treatment from an ophthalmologist. In evaluating this complaint, the physician needs a firm understanding of the basic tenets of lacrimal anatomy, physiology, and pathology in order to make the correct diagnosis and to plan rational therapy. Two key questions need to be answered:

- Is epiphora secondary to outflow anomalies, or is there increased (reflex) lacrimal secretion secondary to an ocular surface abnormality such as keratitis (sicca), trichiasis, ocular surface anomalies, or allergy or other environmental factors?
- If the lacrimal system is not draining normally, where is the anomaly and what is the cause?

CHAPTER 13

Anatomy and Physiology

Normal Anatomy

Secretory Apparatus

The main lacrimal gland is an exocrine gland located in the superior lateral quadrant of the orbit within the lacrimal gland fossa (Fig 13-1). Embryologic development of the lateral horn of the levator aponeurosis dents the lacrimal gland and partially divides it into orbital and palpebral lobes. The superior transverse ligament (Whitnall's ligament) inserts at the division of the two lobes, and some fibers project onto the lateral orbital tubercle. Developmental abnormalities of the levator muscle and aponeurosis may occur, and prolapse is evident in many cases of congenital ptosis.

The 8 to 12 major lacrimal ducts empty into the superior cul-de-sac approximately 5 mm above the lateral tarsal border after passing through the retroaponeurotic space, Müller's muscle, and the conjunctiva. The two to six ducts from the orbital portion run through and join the ducts of the palpebral lobe. Therefore, removal of or damage to the palpebral portion of the gland can seriously reduce secretion from the entire gland.

The ophthalmic branch of cranial nerve V (trigeminal nerve), is the *afferent* pathway in the reflex tear arc. Stimulation of receptors in the fifth nerve distribution activates tear production from the lacrimal gland. The *efferent* pathway is more complicated. Parasympathetic fibers leave cranial nerve VII in the greater superficial petrosal nerve and pass to the sphenopalatine ganglion. From there, they are thought to enter the lacrimal gland via the superior branch of the zygomatic nerve, through an anastomosis between the zygomaticotemporal nerve and the lacrimal nerve. Sympathetic pathways are still not completely understood.

The accessory exocrine glands of Krause and Wolfring are located in the superior fornix and above the superior border of the tarsus, respectively. Aqueous lacrimal secretion is divided into basal low-level secretion and reflex secretion. The tear film composition is as follows:

- Goblet cells within the conjunctiva provide the inner layer of the tear film by secreting mucin, which allows for even distribution of the tear film over the ocular surface.
- The main and accessory lacrimal gland secretions form the intermediate aqueous layer of the tear film.
- Meibomian glands produce the oily outer layer of the tear film, which reduces the evaporation of the underlying aqueous layer.

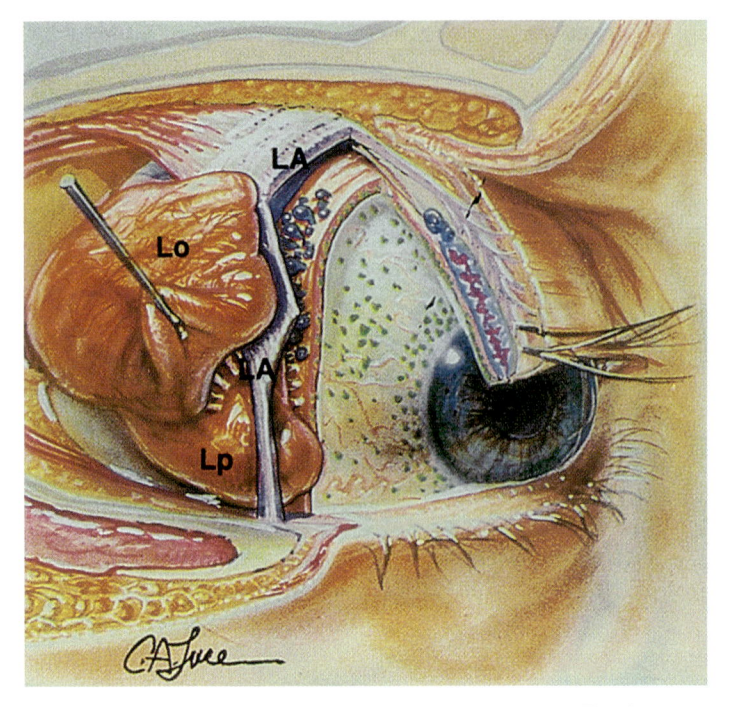

Figure 13-1 Relationship of lacrimal gland to lateral levator horns. The levator palpebrae superioris muscle (LA) divides the lacrimal gland into two lobes. The orbital lobe of the lacrimal gland (Lo) is considerably larger than the palpebral lobe (Lp). *(Reproduced by permission from Zide BM, Jelks GW, eds.* Surgical Anatomy of the Orbit. *New York: Raven; 1985:35. Illustration by Craig A. Luce.)*

Excretory Apparatus

The superior and inferior puncta that provide the entrance to the lacrimal excretory system (Fig 13-2) should be found slightly inverted against the globe in the tear lake. Each punctum expands into its respective ampulla, which is 2 mm in length and oriented perpendicular to the eyelid margin.

The canaliculi are each 8–12 mm long. In approximately 90% of patients, the canaliculi combine to form a single common canaliculus that enters the lateral wall of the tear sac. A fold of mucosa, called the *valve of Rosenmüller*, has traditionally been described as the structure that prevents tear reflux from the sac back into the canaliculi with operation of the tear pump (see under Physiology, below). More recent studies suggest that the common canaliculus consistently bends from a posterior to an anterior direction behind the medial canthal tendon before entering the lacrimal sac at an acute angle. This bend may act as the so-called valve of Rosenmüller in blocking reflux from the sac to the canaliculus when the lacrimal sac gets distended. With total nasolacrimal duct obstruction, the retained mucoid or purulent contents of the sac may cause lacrimal sac distension. External massage may cause the contents to reflux through an incompetent valve of Rosenmüller and through the canalicular system onto the surface of the eye. However, when reflux is not possible, mucus and purulent material accumulate under pressure in the sac, with resultant pain.

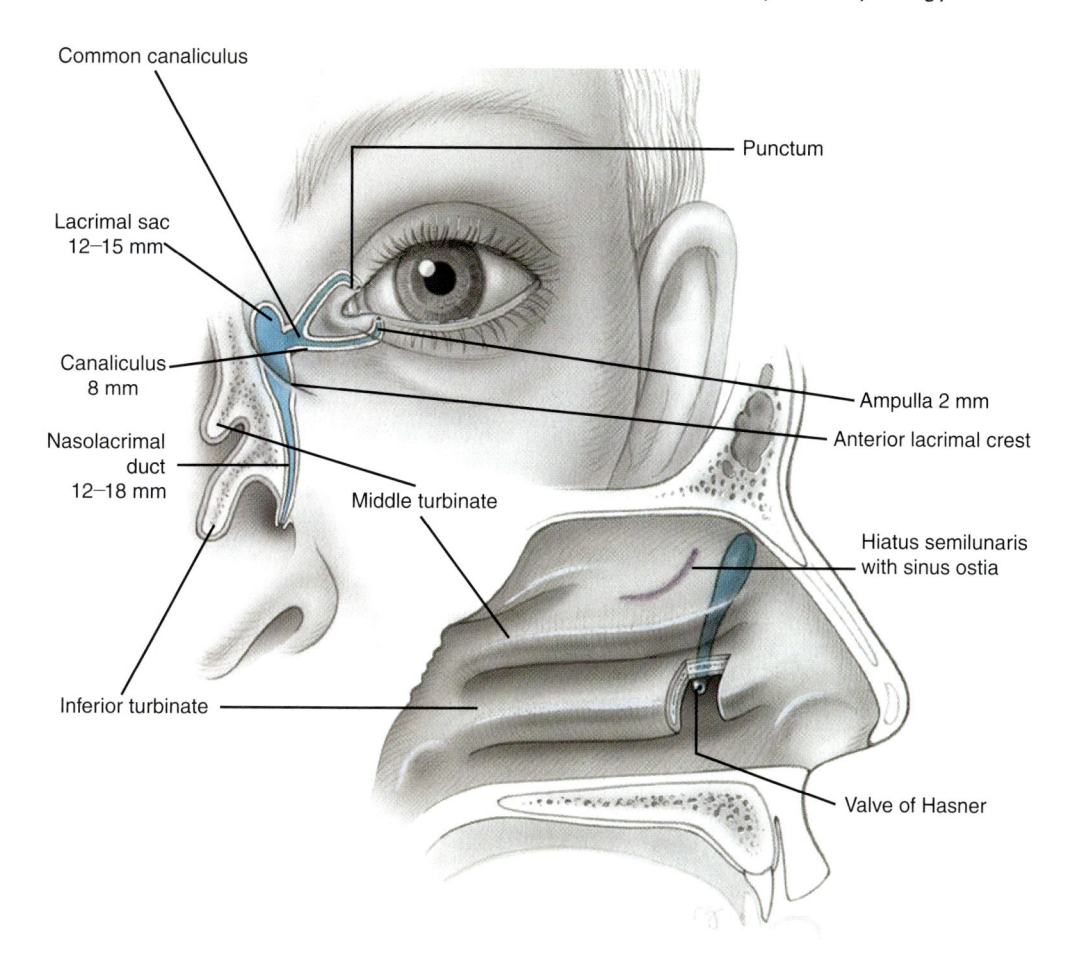

Figure 13-2 Normal anatomy of the lacrimal excretory system. Measurements are for adults. (Illustration by Christine Gralapp.)

The lacrimal sac lies between the anterior and posterior crura of the medial canthal tendon, within the lacrimal sac fossa. The dome of the sac, which extends above the medial canthal tendon, is covered by tough fibers. In cases of lacrimal-cutaneous fistulas, these fibers generally cause the fistula to exit below the medial canthal tendon; further, they cause most sac distensions due to infection to extend below the medial canthal tendon. Medial to the sac is the middle meatus of the nose and sometimes anterior ethmoid cells, separated by the thin lacrimal bone and the thicker frontal process of the maxilla.

The medial canthal tendon is a complex structure composed of superficial and deep heads of the pretarsal orbicularis muscle. The superficial head attaches to the anterior lacrimal crest; the deep head (Horner's muscle) attaches to the posterior lacrimal crest (Fig 13-3). The angular artery and vein lie 7–8 mm medial to the medial canthal angle and anastomose with the vascular systems of the face and orbit.

Figure 13-3 Details of medial canthal insertions of the orbicularis muscle in the lower eyelid. *1*, muscle of Riolan; *2*, Horner's muscle; *3*, lacrimal sac; *4*, superior head of pretarsal portion; *5*, superior head of preseptal portion; *6*, superficial head of orbital portion. *(Reproduced by permission from Dutton JJ. Atlas of Ophthalmic Surgery. St Louis: Mosby; 1992:9.)*

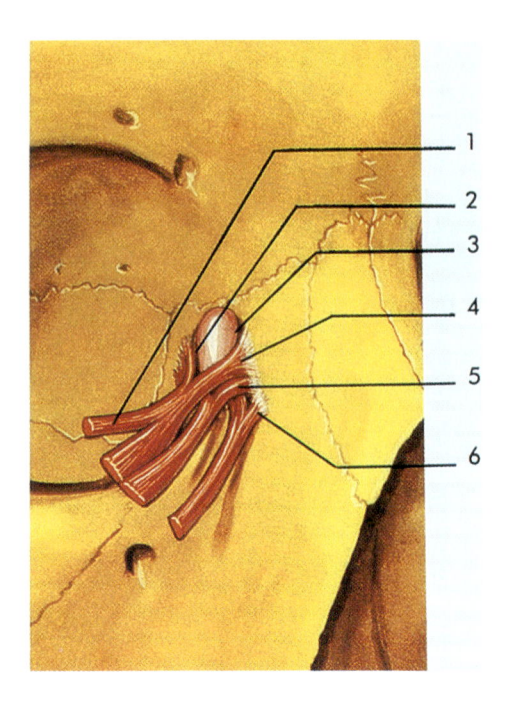

The upper segment of the nasolacrimal canal curves generally in an inferior and slightly lateral and posterior direction. The nasolacrimal duct measures approximately 12 mm in length. The distal portion bends medially in an irregular J-shape in many neonates, but it tends to straighten out with growth. The distal portion extends into the middle meatus before penetrating the nasal mucosa, forming the meatal portion of the duct, and then opening into the nose through an ostium under the inferior turbinate that is usually partially covered by a mucosal fold (the valve of Hasner) (see Fig 13-2). The configuration of the ostium varies, but it is located fairly anteriorly in the inferior nasal meatus, approximately 2.5 cm posterior to the naris.

Physiology

Evaporation accounts for approximately 10% of tear elimination in the young and for 20% or more in older adults. Most of the tear flow is actively pumped from the tear lake by the actions of the orbicularis muscle. The Jones description of the lacrimal pump was accepted for years; later physiologic studies suggested a better explanation. In the tear pump described by Rosengren-Doane (Fig 13-4), the contraction of the orbicularis provides the motive power. The contraction is thought to produce positive pressure in the tear sac, forcing tears into the nose. As the eyelids open and move laterally, negative pressure is produced in the sac and contained by the valve of Hasner. When the eyelids are fully opened, the puncta finally pop open and the negative pressure draws tears into the ampullae and canaliculi.

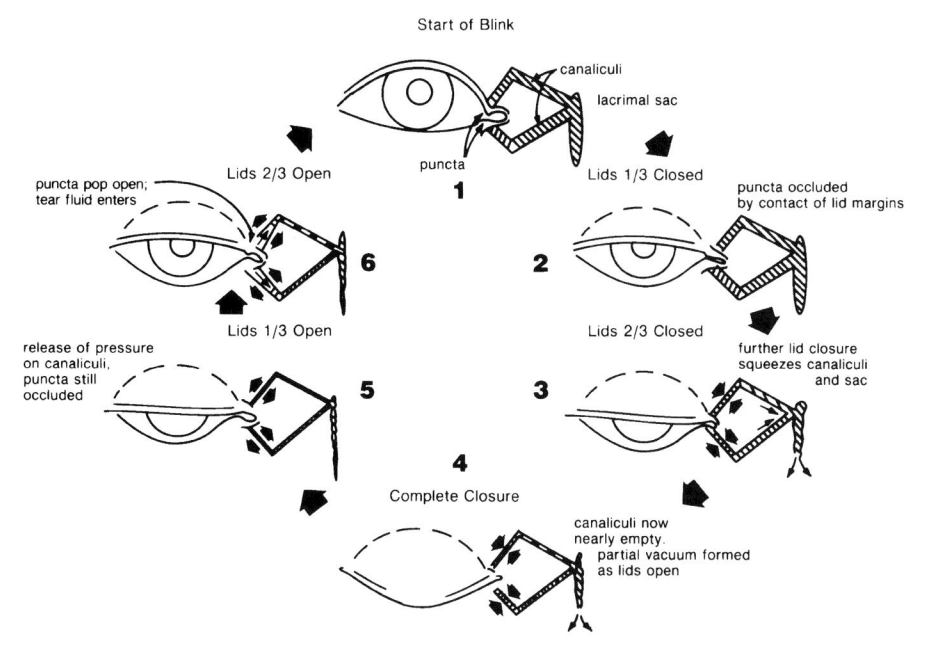

Figure 13-4 Mechanism of lacrimal drainage (Rosengren-Doane). Clockwise from top: *1,* At the start of the blink, the lacrimal drainage passages already contain tear fluid that has entered following the previous blink. *2,* As upper eyelid descends, the papillae containing the punctal openings elevate from the medial lid margin. By the time the upper eyelid has descended halfway, the papillae forcefully meet the opposing lid margin, effectively occluding the puncta and preventing fluid regurgitation. *3,* The remaining portion of lid closure acts to squeeze the canaliculi and sac through the action of the orbicularis oculi, forcing out the contained fluid via the nasolacrimal duct. *4,* At complete eyelid closure, the system is compressed and largely empty of fluid. *5,* At the beginning of the opening phase of a blink, the puncta are still occluded, and valving action at the inner end of canaliculi (and perhaps in the nasolacrimal duct) acts to prevent reentry of fluid or air. Compressive action ends and elastic walls of passages try to expand to their normal shape. This elastic force causes a partial vacuum or suction to form within the canaliculi and sac. *6,* Suction force holding punctal region of eyelid margin together is released when eyelid separation is sufficient, about two thirds fully open. The punctal papillae suddenly pop apart at this point, opening the canaliculi for fluid entry, which occurs during the first few seconds after the blink. *(After Doane MG. Blinking and the mechanics of the lacrimal drainage system.* Ophthalmology. *1981;88:850.)*

Developmental Abnormalities

The embryonic anlage of the lacrimal excretory system begins as a cord of ectodermal cells between the area of the medial canthus and the nasal cavity. Cavitation of the canaliculi and ducts normally occurs to form the lumen. The duct is the last portion of the system to canalize, usually around the time of birth. Obstruction of the nasolacrimal duct at the distal end (the valve of Hasner) is present in approximately 50% of infants at birth. Patency usually occurs spontaneously within the first few months of life. Excessive tearing may not immediately be obvious, as lacrimation does not begin until 6 weeks. Anomalies of the puncta and canaliculi include membrane occlusion of the punctum, complete absence, stenosis, and duplication. Close evaluation with magnification may reveal a punctum with membrane occlusion in patients who were initially thought to have complete punctal agenesis.

A congenital lacrimal–cutaneous fistula from an otherwise normal canalicular system or lacrimal sac may cause tears to drain to the skin surface in the medial canthal area (Fig 13-5).

Major facial cleft deformities can pass through or be adjacent to the nasolacrimal drainage pathways and produce outflow disorders (Fig 13-6).

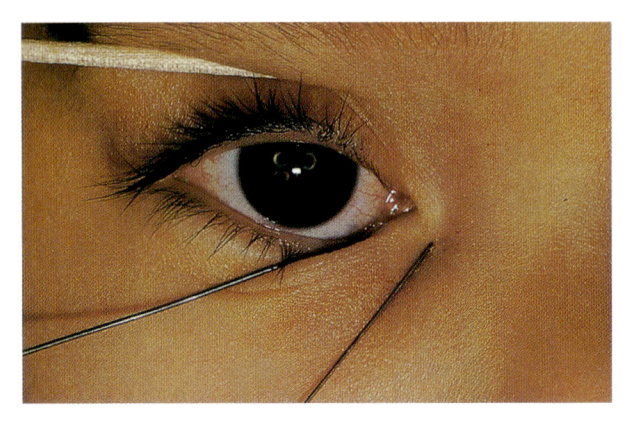

Figure 13-5 Congenital lacrimal–cutaneous fistula draining to the skin surface.

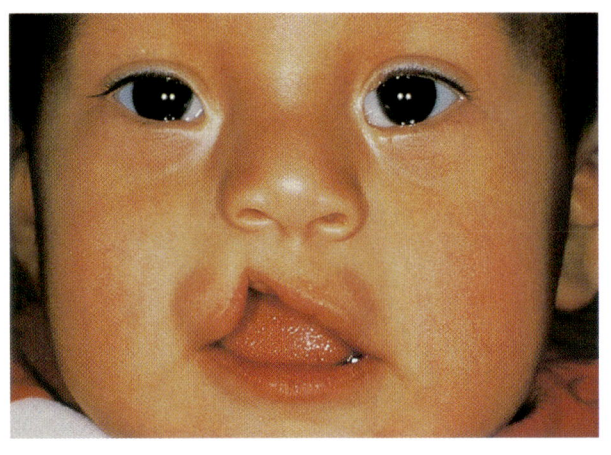

Figure 13-6 Cleft lip and palate with abnormal medial canthal angles and tearing as a result of hypoplasia of nasolacrimal ducts.

CHAPTER 14

Evaluation and Management of the Tearing Patient

Because of differing pathophysiology, congenital and acquired lacrimal abnormalities require different evaluation and management.

Congenital Tearing

Evaluation

The evaluation of congenital tearing is straightforward in most cases: the patient's parents give a history of tearing or mucopurulent discharge (or both) beginning at birth or shortly thereafter. In rare cases, distension of the sac is present at birth, suggesting a congenital dacryocele. Otherwise, distinction should be made among the following characteristics:

- Constant tearing with minimal mucopurulence, which suggests an upper system block caused by punctal or canalicular dysgenesis
- Constant tearing with frequent mucopurulence and matting of the lashes, which suggests complete obstruction of the nasolacrimal duct
- Intermittent tearing with mucopurulence, which suggests intermittent obstruction of the nasolacrimal duct, most likely the result of impaction of a swollen inferior nasal turbinate associated with an upper respiratory tract infection

Office examination includes inspection of the eyelid margins for open puncta and evaluation for extrinsic causes of reflex hypersecretion secondary to ocular surface irritation. These causes may include infectious conjunctivitis, epiblepharon with secondary trichiasis, or congenital glaucoma. Inspection of the medial canthal region for a distended lacrimal sac, inflammation, or congenital defects such as a medial encephalocele is important. However, the single most important maneuver is digital pressure over the tear sac. A dome-shaped distension of the sac suggests congenital obstruction. If mucoid reflux is present, complete obstruction at the level of the nasolacrimal duct becomes the working diagnosis.

260 • Orbit, Eyelids, and Lacrimal System

Management

Dacryocystocele

A dilated lacrimal sac at birth presenting in the absence of inflammatory signs may indicate a congenital dacryocystocele or mucocele (Fig 14-1). This condition occurs when the nasolacrimal duct is obstructed and amniotic fluid or mucus (elaborated by lacrimal sac goblet cells) is trapped in the tear sac. A congenital dacryocystocele often extends

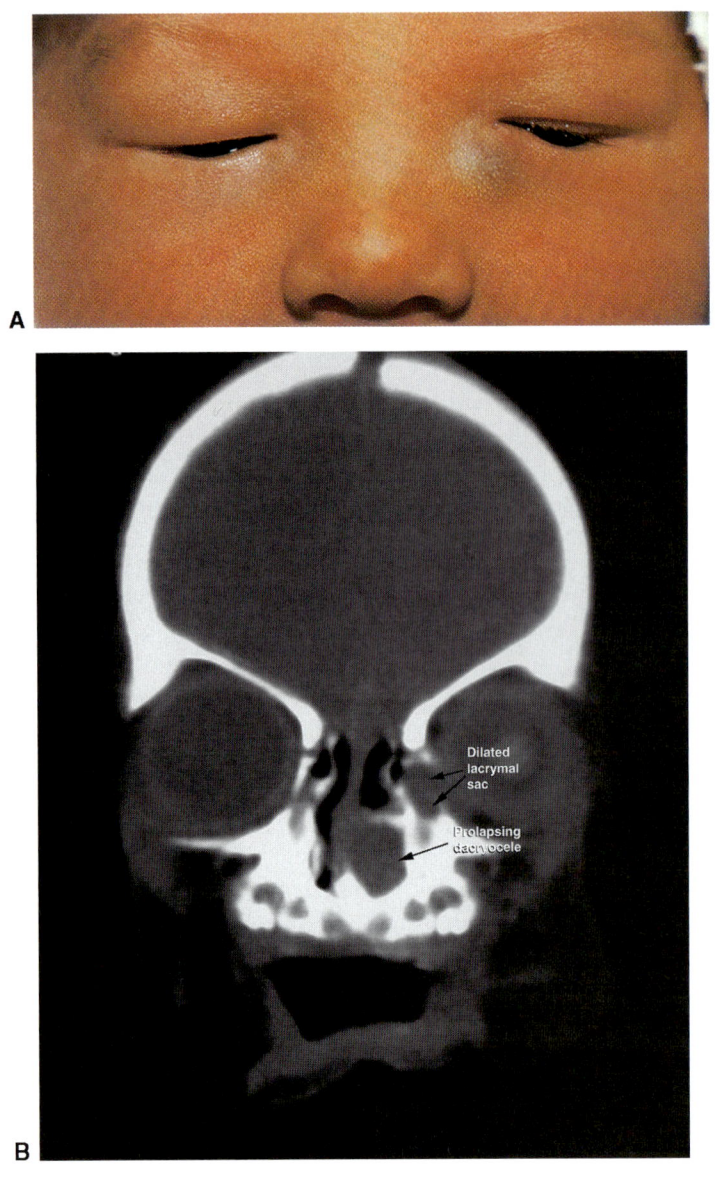

Figure 14-1 A, Left congenital dacryocystocele 1 week postpartum. **B,** CT scan of a congenital dacryocele. *(Photographs courtesy of Pierre Arcand, MD, University of Montreal.)*

inferiorly under the inferior turbinate, where it can be observed during nasal examination. The dacryocystocele is initially sterile and may respond to conservative management with topical antibiotics and massage. If there is no response in 1–2 weeks or if infection develops, probing of the tear system is needed. Urgent treatment may be necessary in the neonate if the condition is bilateral and nasal prolapse of the sac significant, causing nasal and, therefore, partial breathing obstruction. Probing or marsupialization of the prolapsing distended duct with nasal endoscopy is often necessary in these difficult cases. Congenital swelling above the medial canthal tendon, especially in the midline, also may indicate a meningoencephalocele, hemangioma, or other tumor. Proper imaging with CT and MRI become mandatory to confirm these more complex diagnoses.

> Grin TR, Mertz JS, Stass-Isern M. Congenital nasolacrimal duct cysts in dacryocystocele. *Ophthalmology*. 1991;98:1238–1242.
> Mansour AM, Cheng KP, Mumma JV, et al. Congenital dacryocele: a collaborative review. *Ophthalmology*. 1991;98:1744–1751.
> Paysse EA, Coats DK, Bernstein JM, et al. Management and complications of congenital dacryocele with concurrent intranasal mucocele. *J AAPOS*. 2000;4:46–53.

Congenital nasolacrimal obstruction

Congenital obstruction of the lacrimal drainage system, which is usually caused by a membranous block of the valve of Hasner covering the nasal end of the nasolacrimal duct, may be present in up to 50% of newborn infants. Such an obstruction may become clinically evident in only 2%–6% of full-term infants at 3–4 weeks of age, and approximately one third of the patients have bilateral involvement. Most obstructions open spontaneously within 4–6 weeks after birth. Conservative management with topical antibiotics and properly performed Crigler massage (as illustrated in Kushner, cited below) are appropriate during the first 6 months of age.

> Kushner BJ. Congenital nasolacrimal system obstruction. *Arch Ophthalmol*. 1982;100:597–600.

Approximately 90% of all congenital nasolacrimal duct obstructions resolve in the first year of life. Opinions differ regarding the optimal age for probing and how long conservative management should be continued. In the majority of infants with clinical symptoms at 6 months, obstructions spontaneously clear by 1 year without any surgical treatment. Reports vary as to whether delay in probing past 13 months of age may be associated with a decreased success rate. Probing is still used as the primary procedure in the older child with congenital nasolacrimal duct obstruction. The risks and benefits of both medical and surgical approaches prior to this age should be explained clearly to the parents to assist their informed decision on the matter.

> Kassoff J, Meyer DR. Early office-based vs late hospital-based nasolacrimal duct probing. A clinical decision analysis. *Arch Ophthalmol*. 1995;113:1168–1171.
> Katowitz JA, Welsh MG. Timing of initial probing and irrigation in congenital nasolacrimal duct obstruction. *Ophthalmology*. 1987;94:698–705.
> Kushner BJ. Early office-based vs late hospital-based nasolacrimal duct probing [editorial]. *Arch Ophthalmol*. 1995;113:1103–1104.
> Sturrock SM, MacEwen CJ, Young JDH. Long term results after probing for congenital nasolacrimal duct obstruction. *Br J Ophthalmol*. 1994;78:892–894.

Prior to probing, during the period of observation and massage, the chronic use of topical antibiotics may be needed to suppress chronic mucoid discharge with matting of the lashes. Use of topical antibiotics should be limited to minimal frequency and duration until the lacrimal duct spontaneously opens or probing is performed.

In some instances of congenital nasolacrimal duct obstruction, an acute dacryocystitis may manifest as an acutely inflamed lacrimal sac with associated adjacent eyelid cellulitis. This possibility should be discussed with the parents so that treatment with systemic antibiotics can be started promptly. If a lacrimal sac abscess develops despite treatment, surgical drainage may be necessary. Following resolution of the infectious process, elective probing should not be delayed to prevent recurrence of the dacryocystitis.

Most surgeons prefer to use general anesthesia for elective probing procedures. Occasionally, office restraining techniques can be used for very young patients or for decompressing an enlarged, infected lacrimal sac. However, recent pediatric studies indicate that pain may be a significant consideration that should not be ignored, even in an infant.

Irrigation and probing Irrigation alone is inadequate to confirm a patent lacrimal drainage system. However, after probing, irrigation should be performed to confirm an open and functioning lacrimal drainage system.

Probing is a delicate surgical maneuver that is facilitated by immobilizing the patient and shrinking the nasal mucosa with oxymetazoline hydrochloride (Afrin). Cocaine should be avoided in children because of possible cardiac toxicity. When probing, the physician should recall that the upper system begins at each punctum with a 2 mm vertical segment (ampulla) followed by an 8 mm horizontal segment (canaliculus). Punctal dilation is needed to safely introduce a small Bowman probe (usually size 00). The surgeon initially inserts the probe into the punctum and ampulla perpendicular to the eyelid margin and then advances it down the canalicular system toward the medial canthal tendon while maintaining lateral traction with the opposite hand. (Manual lateral traction of the eyelid straightens the canaliculus and decreases the chance of damage to the canalicular mucosa or creation of a false passage.) Resistance of passage of the probe along with medial movement of the eyelid soft tissue, causing wrinkling of the overlying skin, may signify a canalicular atresia. Bunching of the soft tissues in front of the probe tip as it is advanced toward the medial canthal tendon, creating a kink of the canaliculus, can also cause canalicular atresia. In that case, withdrawing the probe and maintaining lateral horizontal traction while reprobing eliminates canalicular kinking (Fig 14-2). If the probe advances successfully through the common canalicular system and across the lacrimal sac, the medial wall of the lacrimal sac and adjacent lacrimal bone will be encountered, resulting in a tactile hard stop.

The probe is rotated superiorly against the brow until it lies over the supraorbital notch at the superior orbital rim and then directed posteriorly and slightly laterally as it is advanced down the nasolacrimal duct. If significant resistance is encountered at any point during the probing procedure, the probe should be withdrawn and the procedure attempted again. The distance from the punctum to the level of the inferior meatus in the infant is approximately 20 mm. Direct visualization of the probe tip is usually possible with the use of a nasal speculum and a fiberoptic headlight or endoscope along the lateral

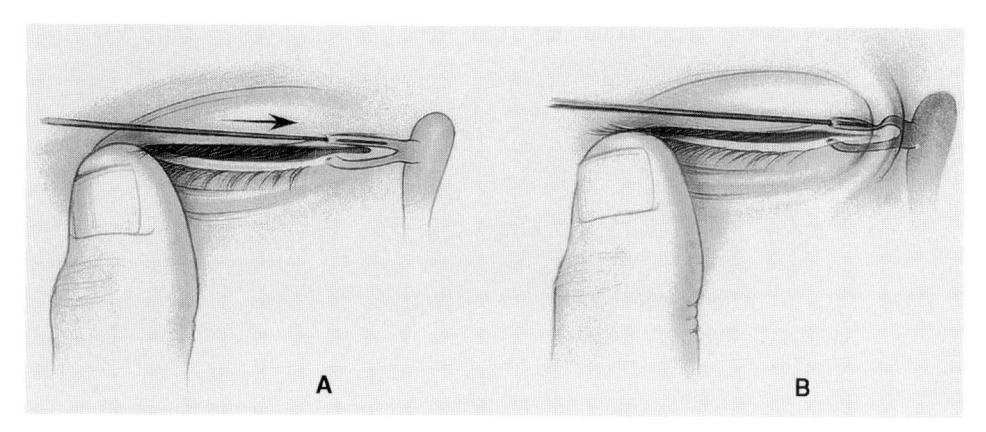

Figure 14-2 A, Bowman probe in right upper horizontal canaliculus. **B,** Attempted advancement of Bowman probe at site of canalicular atresia produces wrinkling of skin over the medial canthus. *(Illustration by Christine Gralapp.)*

wall of the nose approximately 20–25 mm posterior to the naris. Probe rotation may facilitate visualization because the probe tip enters the inferior nasal meatus against the lateral nasal wall.

Once the probe is withdrawn, patency of the duct can be confirmed by irrigation with saline mixed with fluorescein. (Forceful irrigation is considered essential by many clinicians to confirm patency and as a therapeutic method to further stretch open the distal end of the duct. This is especially important if the duct does not follow a linear course and an unknown false passage was present on probing). The fluorescein can be retrieved from the inferior meatus with a transparent suction catheter (Fig 14-3).

A single lacrimal probing is successful in opening a congenital nasolacrimal obstruction in 90% of patients who are 13 months old or younger. In adults, irrigation and probing are limited to the canalicular system for diagnostic purposes only to confirm the site of obstruction. Probing of the nasolacrimal duct in the latter is potentially traumatic and rarely effective in permanently relieving an obstruction. Merely puncturing the sometimes extensive scar tissue of the nasolacrimal duct will only lead to contraction.

Turbinate infracture If the inferior turbinate seems to be impacted on the nasolacrimal duct and inferior meatus at the time of probing and irrigation, medial infracturing of the inferior turbinate should be performed. This condition should be suspected in patients whose symptoms appear primarily related to upper respiratory infections, when swelling of the mucosa over the turbinate may cause intermittent obstruction of the inferior meatus. The blunt end of a Freer elevator is placed within the inferior meatus along the lateral surface of the inferior turbinate. The inferior turbinate is then rotated medially and superiorly toward the septum (Fig 14-4). Fracturing the turbinate at its base significantly enlarges the inferior meatus and permits direct visualization of the lacrimal probe tip.

Silicone intubation Silicone intubation is indicated for children who have recurrent epiphora following nasolacrimal system probing and irrigation or for older children when

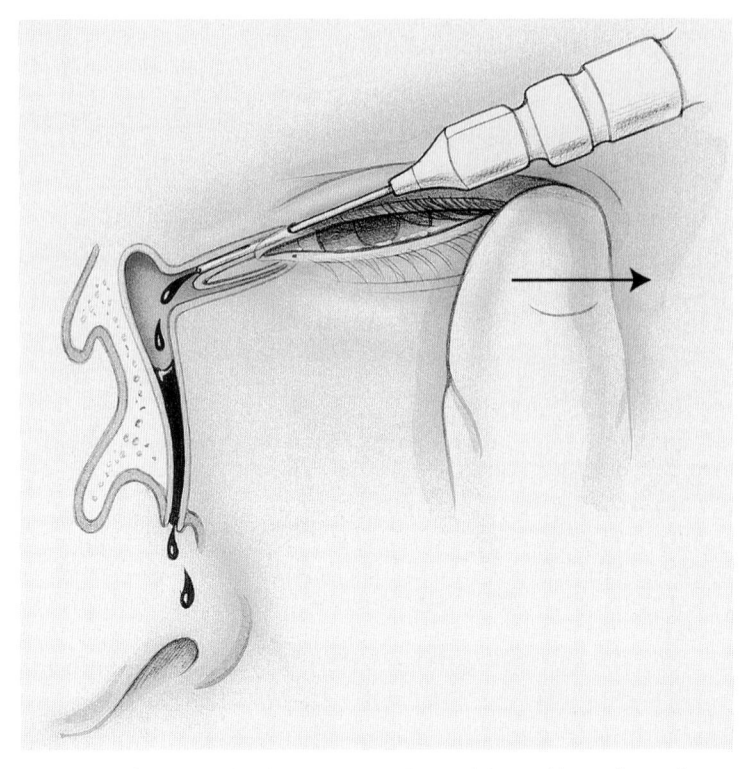

Figure 14-3 Irrigation of the nasolacrimal system. Dye is injected from the syringe, and patency of the system is confirmed by suctioning the dye from the inferior meatus of the nose. *(Illustration by Christine Gralapp.)*

initial probing reveals significant stenosis or scarring. Intubation is also useful for upper system abnormalities such as canalicular stenosis and agenesis of the puncta or ampullae. However, the segment of canalicular stenosis must be small for this technique to be successful.

Many techniques and types of intubation sets have been described (Fig 14-5). Keys to success include shrinkage of the nasal mucosa with a topical vasoconstrictor and adequate lighting with a fiberoptic headlight. In more difficult cases, a rigid endoscope can be used and turbinate infracture is sometimes performed. The silicone tubing can be secured by a simple square knot that allows removal of the tube through the canalicular system in a retrograde fashion. Alternately, the silicone stent may be directly sutured to the lateral wall of the nose, or the limbs of silicone stent can be passed through either a silicone band or sponge in the inferior meatus of the nose.

Balloon dacryoplasty Balloon catheter dilation of the nasolacrimal canal has recently been used successfully in congenital nasolacrimal obstruction. A collapsed balloon catheter is placed in a manner similar to probing and inflated inside the duct at different levels. Although early results seem promising, the role of this modality has not been defined because the necessary catheter equipment is expensive and because simple probing has a high success rate. Thus, balloon dacryoplasty is now generally limited to difficult

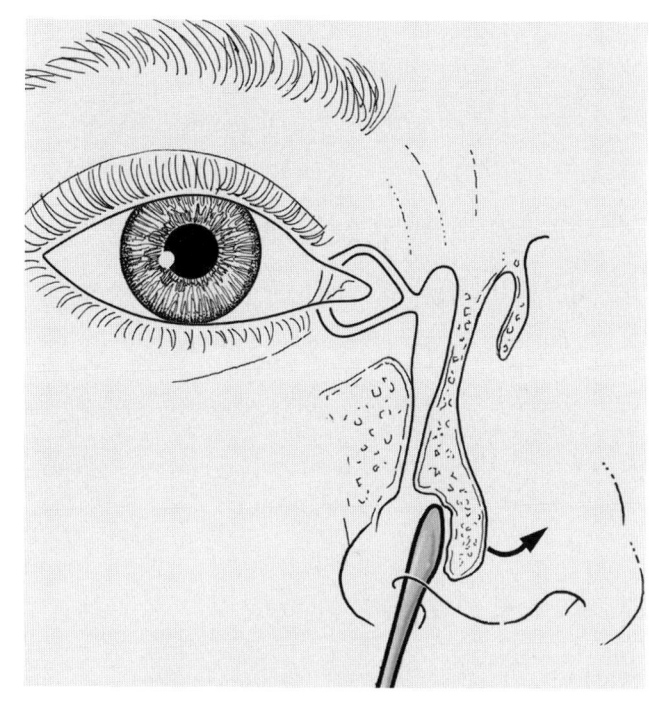

CHAPTER 14: Evaluation and Management of the Tearing Patient • 265

Figure 14-4 Infracture of inferior turbinate. A periosteal elevator is slipped into the inferior meatus and, using the lateral wall of the nose as a fulcrum, the elevator is pushed medially, fracturing the turbinate easily and creating a larger space for the exit of tears from the nasolacrimal duct. *(From Nerad JA. The Requisites in Ophthalmology: Oculoplastic Surgery. Philadelphia: Mosby; 2001:229.)*

cases or probing failures. Balloon dacryoplasty is also being evaluated in the treatment of adult partial dacryostenosis.

Punctal agenesis and dysgenesis

The medial eyelid margin should be carefully inspected for the presence of the elevated lacrimal papillae. In rare cases, a thin membrane, which can be easily punctured with a sharp probe or dilator, occludes the intact punctum. The remainder of the system is usually open upon irrigation testing. If the punctum is absent, the surgeon may cut down through the eyelid margin in the expected area of the lateral canaliculus or perform retrograde probing through an open lacrimal sac with direct visualization of the common canalicular opening into the lacrimal sac (common internal punctum). However, punctal agenesis is usually associated with the absence of underlying canalicular tissue. Occasionally, these maneuvers reveal the presence of a relatively mature canalicular system with a patent nasolacrimal sac and duct. In this case, silicone intubation may be performed. Symptomatic patients with a single punctum frequently require surgery to relieve nasolacrimal rather than canalicular obstruction. Complete absence of the punctum and canalicular system requires a conjunctivodacryocystorhinostomy (CJDCR) when the patient is old enough to allow manipulation and care of the Jones tube (CJDCR is discussed later in this chapter under Acquired Tearing).

266 • Orbit, Eyelids, and Lacrimal System

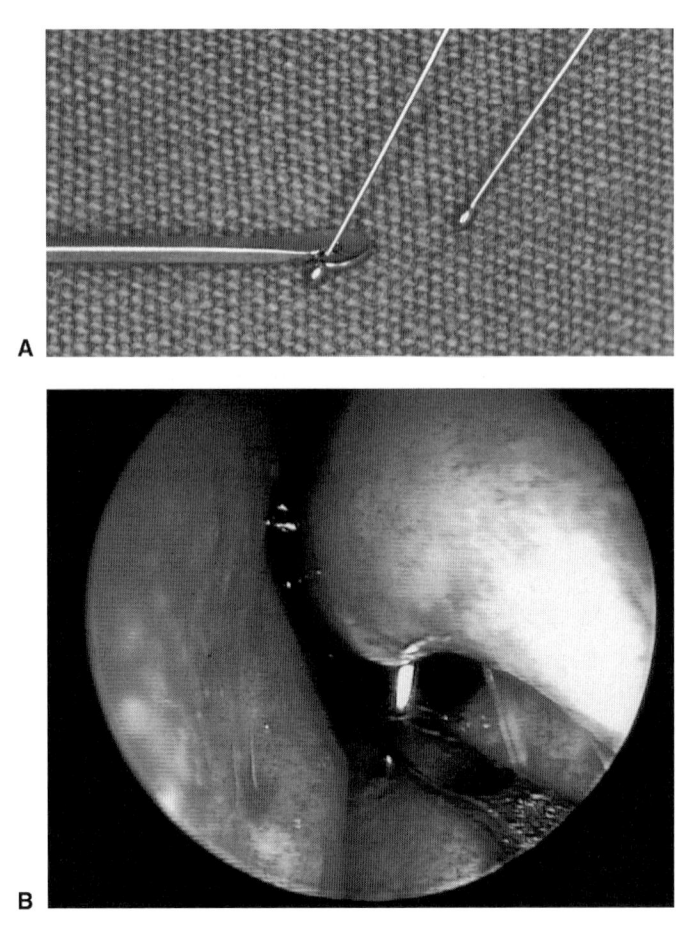

Figure 14-5 Crawford hook. **A,** Hook engaging "olive tip" of stent. **B,** Intranasal view of engaged hook retrieving the stent. *(Reproduced with permission from Nerad JA. The Requisites in Ophthalmology: Oculoplastic Surgery. Philadelphia: Mosby; 2001:233.)*

Lyons CJ, Rosser PM, Welham RA. The management of punctal agenesis. *Ophthalmology*. 1993;100:1851–1855.

Dacryocystorhinostomy Dacryocystorhinostomy (DCR) is usually reserved for children who have persistent epiphora following silicone intubation or for patients with extensive developmental abnormalities of the nasolacrimal drainage system that prevent probing or silicone intubation. The details of DCR are discussed later in this chapter under Acquired Tearing.

Congenital lacrimal–cutaneous fistulas

These fistulas are frequently asymptomatic or associated with a minimal amount of tears exiting from the cutaneous fistula infranasal to the medial canthal angle (see Fig 13-5). Approximately one third of patients have an underlying nasolacrimal duct obstruction, wherein chronic mucoid discharge from the affected nasolacrimal sac may be present. In symptomatic patients, direct surgical excision of the epithelium-lined fistulous tract with direct suture closure is indicated. In patients with underlying nasolacrimal duct obstruction and chronic dacryocystitis, silicone intubation without DCR is indicated.

> Birchansky LD, Nerad JA, Kersten RC, et al. Management of congenital lacrimal sac fistula. *Arch Ophthalmol.* 1990;108:388–390.

Acquired Tearing

Evaluation

The cause of tearing can be related to one of these two large groups:

- Hypersecretion of tears (lacrimation)
- Impairment of drainage (epiphora)

Assessment

History

The following items help guide the examiner in the assessment of the patient with tearing:

- Unilateral versus bilateral
- Subjective ocular surface discomfort
- Constant versus intermittent
- With or without period of remission
- Presence of allergy
- Use of topical medications
- Probing as a child
- Sinus disease or surgery, midfacial trauma, or a nasal fracture
- Previous episodes of lacrimal sac inflammation
- History of ocular surface infections
- Clear tears versus tears with discharge or blood (blood in the tear meniscus may indicate an intrinsic malignancy)

Examination

Systematic examination helps to pinpoint the cause of tearing. Inspection and evaluation of the ocular surface may reveal an inadequate tear meniscus, protein precipitates in the tear film, and a rapid tear breakup time; these signs suggest that the ocular symptoms may be related to an abnormal tear film with secondary ocular surface irritation and mucoid discharge rather than true epiphora. Mechanical irritation of the cornea—as seen, for example, in trichiasis or entropion—may be present. Exposure keratitis from incomplete blinking may also be a cause of reflex epiphora. Evaluation of lid laxity, by direct palpation and by resistance to forced closure, may uncover an incipient ectropion or explain a poor lacrimal pump function. Punctal stenosis, eversion, or frank ectropion can be present. Slit-lamp examination during the blink cycle may be needed to determine whether the punctum is properly positioned in the lake of tears. Sometimes, eyelid or conjunctival abnormalities such as concretion, cyst, chalazion, molluscum, or others may also cause tearing.

Palpation with pressure on a distended lacrimal sac may cause reflux of mucoid or mucopurulent material through the canalicular system if the common canaliculus and valve of Rosenmüller are patent (Fig 14-6). This reflux confirms complete nasolacrimal duct obstruction, and no further diagnostic tests are needed if a lacrimal sac tumor is not suspected. Routine nasal examination may uncover an unsuspected cause for the epiphora such as an intranasal tumor, turbinate impaction, chronic allergic rhinitis, or polyposis. These conditions may occlude the nasal end of the nasolacrimal duct.

Diagnostic tests

The clinical evaluation of the lacrimal drainage system was originally outlined by Lester Jones in the form of a dye disappearance test followed by a Jones I and Jones II test. By using this sequence (with modifications) as a guide, the physician can frequently condense diagnostic testing into a streamlined process compatible with a busy office practice.

The *dye disappearance test (DDT)* is useful for assessing the presence or absence of adequate lacrimal outflow, especially in unilateral cases. It is especially useful in children, in whom lacrimal irrigation is impossible without anesthesia or deep sedation. Fluorescein is instilled in the conjunctival fornices of each eye using a drop of sterile 2% fluorescein solution or a moistened fluorescein strip. The tear film is observed, preferably with the cobalt blue filter of the slit lamp (Fig 14-7). Persistence of significant dye and especially asymmetric clearance of the dye from the tear meniscus over a 5-minute period indicates a relative obstruction on the side retaining the dye. If the DDT result is normal, severe lacrimal drainage dysfunction is highly unlikely. However, intermittent causes of tearing such as allergy, dacryolith, or nasal polyp disease cannot be ruled out.

The Jones I and Jones II tests have historically been described in the evaluation of epiphora. Table 14-1 shows the results obtained with both types of tests. Like the DDT, the *Jones I test,* or *primary dye test,* investigates lacrimal outflow under normal physiologic conditions. Fluorescein (2%) is instilled into the conjunctival fornices and recovered in the inferior nasal meatus by passing a cotton-tipped wire applicator into the region of the ostium of the nasolacrimal duct at 2 and 5 minutes. However, this test is tedious to perform properly and gives an abnormal result in up to one third of normal patients; thus, it is not used frequently.

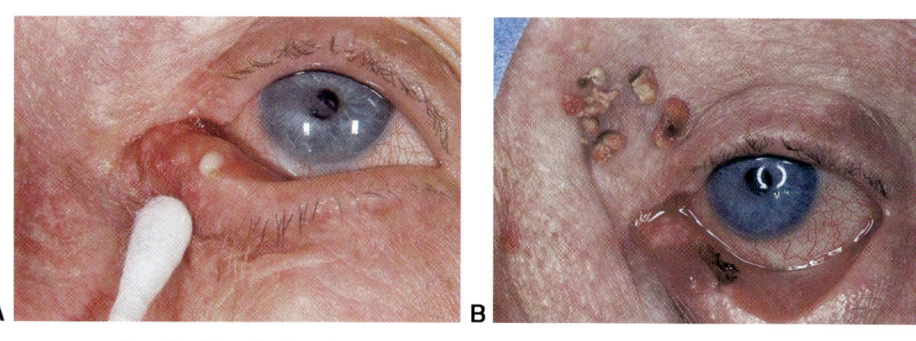

Figure 14-6 Canaliculitis. **A,** Pouting punctum expressing purulent material. **B,** Several small stones curetted from canaliculitis. *(Photographs courtesy of Jeffrey A. Nerad, MD.)*

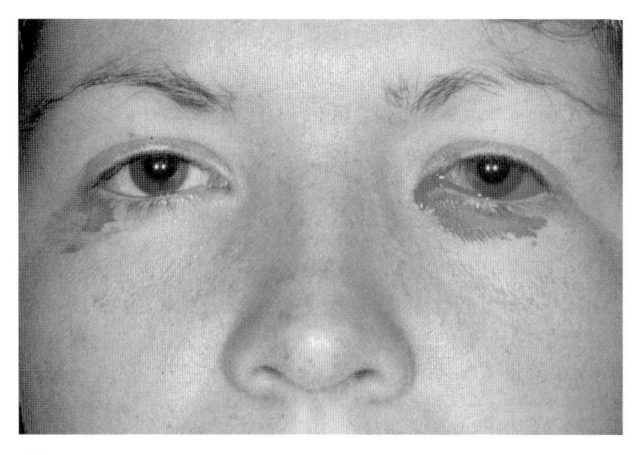

CHAPTER 14: Evaluation and Management of the Tearing Patient • 269

Figure 14-7 Dye disappearance test. *(Reproduced with permission from Nerad JA. The Requisites in Ophthalmology: Oculoplastic Surgery. Philadelphia: Mosby; 2001:219.)*

Table 14-1 Results of Primary and Secondary Jones Tests

Result	Interpretations
Jones I	
+	Patent system, probably normal physiologic function
−	False negative *or* physiologic dysfunction, anatomic obstruction
Jones II	
+ Dye in nose	Partial block at lower sac or duct
− Saline in nose	Punctal or canalicular stenosis
− Regurgitation at opposite punctum with dye	Complete nasolacrimal dust obstruction
− Regurgitation at opposite punctum without dye	Complete common canaliculus obstruction
− Regurgitation at same punctum with dye	Complete common canaliculus obstruction

(Modified from Stewart WB, ed. *Surgery of the Eyelid, Orbit, and Lacrimal System.* Ophthalmology Monograph 8, vol 3. San Francisco: American Academy of Ophthalmology; 1995:261.)

Tucker NA, Codere F. The effect of fluorescein volume on lacrimal outflow transit time. *Ophthal Plast Reconstr Surg.* 1994;10:256–259.

Wright MM, Bersani TA, Frueh BR, et al. Efficacy of the primary dye test. *Ophthalmology.* 1989;96:481–483.

The nonphysiologic *Jones II test* determines the presence or absence of fluorescein in the irrigating saline fluid retrieved from the nose. The residual fluorescein is flushed from the conjunctival sac following an unsuccessful Jones I test. The patient's head is tilted forward, and irrigation is performed with clear saline. Because of technical difficulties in retrieving the irrigating fluid from the internal aspect of the nose, a formal Jones II test is infrequently performed and has limited clinical usefulness.

Hagele JE, Guzek JP, Shavlik GW. Lacrimal testing: age as a factor in Jones testing. *Ophthalmology*. 1994;101:612–617.

Most clinicians proceed with simpler modifications that have better clinical value and are more reproducible. *Lacrimal drainage system irrigation* (Table 14-2) is most frequently performed immediately after a DDT to determine the level of lacrimal drainage system occlusion. After installation of topical anesthesia, the lower eyelid punctum is dilated and any punctal stenosis noted. The irrigating cannula is placed into the canalicular system. Lateral traction of the lower eyelid is maintained to prevent canalicular kinking and difficulty in advancing the irrigating cannula (see Fig 14-2). Canalicular stenosis or occlusion should be noted and confirmed by subsequent diagnostic probing. Once the blunt-tipped 23-gauge irrigating cannula has been advanced into the horizontal canaliculus, clear saline is injected and the results noted. Careful observation and interpretation determine the area of obstruction without additional testing.

Difficulty advancing the irrigating cannula and an inability to irrigate fluid suggest total canalicular obstruction. However, kinking of the canaliculus over the irrigating cannula tip should be ruled out by withdrawing the cannula, reinserting it, and attempting irrigation again. If saline can be irrigated successfully but refluxes either around the irrigating cannula shaft or in a retrograde fashion through the upper canalicular system, and if no distension of the lacrimal sac is noted with palpation, the diagnosis is complete blockage of the common canaliculus at the common internal punctum (Fig 14-8). Subsequent probing determines whether the common canalicular stenosis is total or can be dilated. If mucoid material or fluorescein refluxes through the opposite canaliculus with possible palpable lacrimal sac distension, then the diagnosis is complete nasolacrimal duct obstruction. If saline irrigation is not associated with canalicular reflux or fluid passing down the nasolacrimal duct, then inflation of the lacrimal sac with significant

Table 14-2 Lacrimal Drainage System Irrigation

Result	Anatomic Interpretation
Difficulty advancing cannula Inability to irrigate	Complete canalicular obstruction
Difficulty advancing cannula Reflux of clear saline through canalicular system	Complete common canalicular obstruction
Easy cannula placement Mucoid reflux through canalicular system	Complete nasolacrimal duct obstruction
Easy cannula placement Irrigation with nasolacrimal sac distension No reflux or fluid into nose	Complete nasolacrimal duct obstruction
Easy cannula placement Combination of reflux and saline into the nose	Partial nasolacrimal duct stenosis Possible complete functional obstruction under normal physiologic conditions
Easy cannula placement Successful irrigation into the nose	Patent nasolacrimal duct Possible functional obstruction Repeat evaluation for secondary irritative hypersecretion

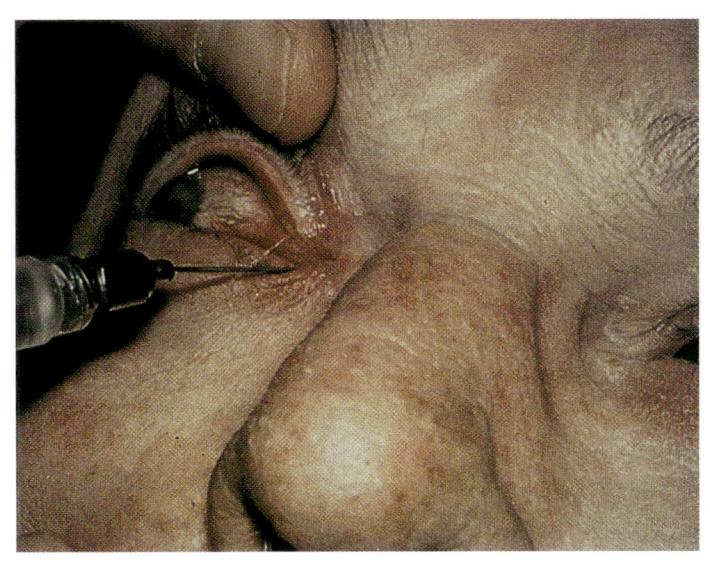

CHAPTER 14: Evaluation and Management of the Tearing Patient • 271

Figure 14-8 Reflux from opposite canaliculus caused by common canalicular obstruction.

patient discomfort will occur. This result confirms a complete nasolacrimal duct obstruction with a patent valve of Rosenmüller preventing reflux through the canalicular system.

A combination of saline reflux through the opposite canaliculus and saline irrigation through the nasolacrimal duct into the nose may indicate a partial nasolacrimal duct stenosis but not total occlusion.

If saline irrigation passes freely into the nose with no reflux through the canalicular system, a patent nasolacrimal drainage system is present. However, it is important to note that even though this irrigation is successful under a nonphysiologic condition of increased hydrostatic pressure on the irrigating saline, a *functional* obstruction may still be present secondary to a valve or flap of mucosal tissue that blocks outflow. A dacryolith may also impair tear flow without causing blockage to irrigation.

Diagnostic probing of the upper system (puncta, canaliculi, lacrimal sac) is useful in confirming the level of obstruction. In adults, this procedure can easily be performed with topical anesthesia. A small probe (0000) should be used initially to detect any canalicular obstruction. If an obstruction is encountered, the distance is measured by clamping the probe at the punctum before withdrawal. A large probe may be useful to determine the extent of a partial obstruction, but the probe should not be forced through any area of resistance. Diagnostic probing of the nasolacrimal duct has no place in adults because obstruction of the nasolacrimal duct can be determined by other means. Although therapeutic probing of infants is a useful and largely successful procedure, it rarely produces lasting patency when attempted in adults.

Nasal endoscopy has become more commonly available and can be helpful in the evaluation of the nasal and turbinate anatomy and disease processes in selected cases. More recently, advances in endoscopic equipment have allowed for direct visualization of the lacrimal passages.

Pifaretti JM. [Endoscopy of the lacrimal ducts]. *Klin Monatsblat Augenheilk.* 1998;212: 259–260.

Scintigraphy, using gamma ray–emitting radionuclides such as technetium-99, can be used to evaluate the physiologic flow of tears when functional blockage is difficult to differentiate from eyelid problems or other causes (Fig 14-9). This physiologic test gives fewer false-positive results than the conventional Jones I test. A drop of radionuclide tracer technetium-99m in saline or technetium sulfur colloid is instilled in the conjunctival cul-de-sac followed by imaging of the lacrimal system with a gammagram. Scintigraphy is useful in patients who show contradictory or inconsistent results with lacrimal drainage system irrigation but have a strong history of epiphora. Because the test is performed under normal physiologic conditions, a functional obstruction can be determined more accurately. Radiation exposure to the lens is much less than with dacryocystography, and the test is easily performed and noninvasive. However, dacryoscintigraphy does not provide the fine anatomic detail as visualized with contrast dacryocystography.

Contrast dacryocystography can add useful information by radiologically defining the lacrimal sac anatomy. Radiopaque dye is injected into the canalicular systems on one or both sides and is simultaneously followed by immediate imaging. Films taken at 10 minutes show any delay in drainage. This information is especially helpful in determining the level of blockage, checking the extent of lacrimal sac maldevelopment, or detecting tumor, but it is not helpful in determining lacrimal drainage physiology. Computerized digital subtraction allows better imaging of the lacrimal system by removing the images of the surrounding bones (Fig 14-10).

Computed tomography (CT) is useful for assessing lacrimal obstruction following craniofacial injury, in congenital craniofacial deformities, or when lacrimal sac neoplasia is suspected. Particular attention must be given to preoperative identification of any abnormal position of the cribriform plate to avoid a possible cerebrospinal fluid leak at the time of surgery. CT is also often used in evaluating concomitant sinus or nasal disease that may contribute to excess tearing.

Guzek JP, Ching AS, Hoang T-A, et al. Clinical and radiologic lacrimal testing in patients with epiphora.*Ophthalmology.* 1997;104:1875–1881.

Pseudoepiphora evaluation

In the absence of a clear obstruction to the tear flow, other causes for tearing must be considered, especially if the problem is intermittent. *Epiphora* is defined as overflow tearing. Some patients perceive that their eyes have too many tears without exhibiting frank epiphora. These sensations are often caused by other ocular or eyelid abnormalities. For example, patients with dry eye may perceive foreign body sensation or increased mucous production as excess tearing but in reality do not exhibit true overflow of tears over the lid margin or down the cheek. In assessing pseudoepiphora, the ophthalmologist should consider the following points.

Tear meniscus The size of the lacrimal lake as well as the presence of precipitated proteins and stringy mucus may indicate an abnormal tear film.

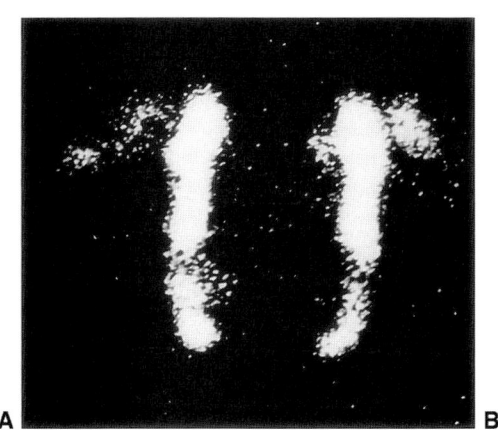

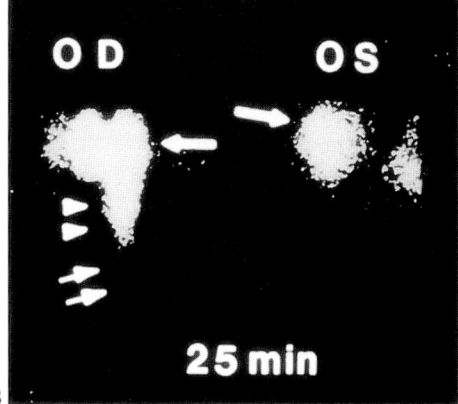

CHAPTER 14: Evaluation and Management of the Tearing Patient • 273

Figure 14-9 **A,** Normal lacrimal scintigraphy. **B,** Total nasolacrimal duct obstruction on the left (OS) with partial obstruction on the right (OD). *Arrows* = lacrimal sac. *(Images courtesy of Robert C. Kersten, MD.)*

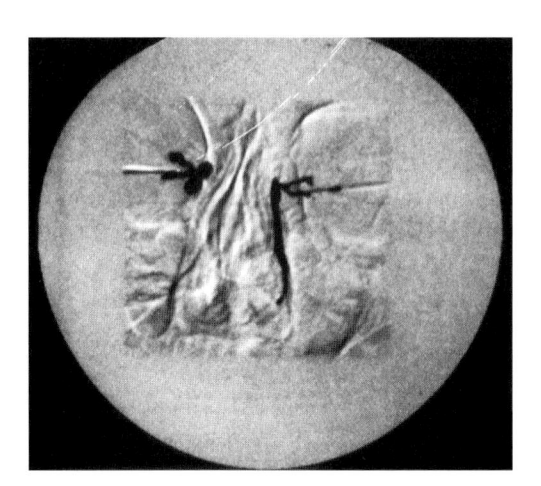

Figure 14-10 Computerized digital subtraction dacryocystogram in a patient with unilateral epiphora after facial trauma. Right lacrimal sac is dilated, and obstruction is visible at the sac–duct junction. The left side shows lacrimal system of normal caliber. *(Reproduced by permission from Stewart WB, ed. Surgery of the Eyelid, Orbit, and Lacrimal System. Ophthalmology Monograph 8. San Francisco: American Academy of Ophthalmology; 1995;3:262.)*

Tear breakup time The mucin layer of the tear film helps spread the other layers evenly over the corneal surface. This can be observed best after fluorescein has been placed in the conjunctival cul-de-sac. The patient is asked to open the eyes and refrain from blinking. The normal time before breakup should be at least 15 seconds. Tear breakup in a rapid range (10 seconds or less) may indicate poor function of the mucin layer despite a sufficient amount of tears. Tear breakup testing is affected by instillation of topical anesthetics or holding the eyelids open and should be done before instillation of any eyedrops.

Corneal and conjunctival epithelium evaluation A rose bengal strip in the tear lake detects subtle ocular surface abnormalities by staining devitalized conjunctival and corneal epithelium. Fluorescein staining in the inferior third of the cornea indicates more severe tear film malfunction because fluorescein can contact and stain the underlying collagen of Bowman's layer only if the tight junctions within the epithelium have been broken.

Schirmer I This test measures tear secretion. A strip of filter paper is placed without anesthetic in the cul-de-sac for 5 minutes, and the amount of wetting is recorded. The normal amount is approximately 15 mm. Hypersecretion is considered when the filter strip is rapidly inundated with tears. However, excess secretion may occur in response to the irritation from the measuring strips themselves. Serial testing should be performed to confirm this assumption. Some clinicians prefer the basic Schirmer test, measured after installation of a topical anesthetic drop, as more useful in determining tear production deficiency. However, the significance of this test is unclear because recent studies have shown that virtually all tearing is reflexive.

See also BCSC Section 8, *External Disease and Cornea*, for further discussion of tear film abnormalities.

Management

The treatment of acquired abnormalities differs according to the location of the obstruction and whether it involves the puncta, the canaliculi, the lacrimal sac, or the nasolacrimal duct.

Upper System Abnormalities

Punctal conditions

A single functioning punctum and canaliculus for each eye may be sufficient to drain tears and keep the patient from tearing. A functionally significant punctal stenosis may be treated by dilation and punctoplasty, ampullotomy (snip procedure), or silicone intubation or a similar stent procedure if simpler procedures fail.

In cases of epiphora secondary to punctal malposition, the anatomic abnormality must be corrected. Medial ectropion repair by resection of a horizontal ellipse of conjunctival and subconjunctival connective tissue below the punctum with reapposition of the edges rotates the punctum inward into the tear lake. A lacrimal probe in the canaliculus during surgery helps prevent canalicular damage. This procedure may be combined with a horizontal eyelid-tightening or shortening of the lateral canthal tendon if horizontal eyelid laxity is also present. Frequently, punctal stenosis coexists and may require a punctoplasty.

In cases of severe dry eye syndrome with chronic foreign body sensation and mucoid discharge secondary to ocular surface irritation, punctal occlusion may be necessary. Dissolvable collagen plugs are often inserted into the puncta as a diagnostic trial. Subjective or objective improvement for a few days indicates candidacy for permanent blockage. Plastic punctal plugs are often used and usually well tolerated and do not lead to the surgical difficulty, irreversibility, or discomfort of punctal or canalicular surgery. However, plug extrusion, pyogenic granuloma, canaliculitis, and dacryocystitis secondary to displacement of plugs into the canaliculus or sac have been reported.

Alternatively, puncta may be permanently closed by means of surgical ampullectomy, thermal obliteration of the punctal lumen, or more complex procedures. Although the argon laser can be used for thermal punctal occlusion, it offers no advantage over conventional cautery techniques in most patients and is often less effective.

CHAPTER 14: Evaluation and Management of the Tearing Patient • 275

Canalicular obstruction

Obstruction can occur within either the upper or lower canaliculus or in the common canaliculus. Diagnostic canalicular probing may uncover a total canalicular obstruction, and subsequent irrigation may be unsuccessful. However, a partial canalicular obstruction may be discovered during lacrimal system irrigation with partial fluid flow into the nose and partial reflux. The clinician should keep in mind that what appears to be a partial canalicular obstruction may sometimes be a total functional occlusion resulting from weakness of the lacrimal pump or inability of tears to pass through the partial obstruction under normal physiologic conditions without external hydrostatic pressure.

Total common canalicular obstruction is characterized by flow from the lower to the upper canaliculus with no flow into the lacrimal sac during lacrimal system irrigation. The lacrimal probe enters only approximately 8 mm from the punctum and then encounters a tactile soft stop because the probe cannot be advanced beyond the total common canalicular obstruction. In normal conditions, a hard stop would be reached when the probe successfully passes through the open canalicular system into the lumen of the lacrimal sac and finally encounters the medial lacrimal sac and lacrimal bone. When common canalicular obstruction is present, lacrimal system irrigation results in a high-velocity reflux from the adjacent canaliculus (see Fig 14-8). Causes of acquired canalicular obstruction include trauma, toxic medications (5-fluorouracil, idoxuridine, phospholine iodide, eserine), viral infections (vaccinia, herpes simplex), or autoimmune disorders (such as pemphigoid or Stevens-Johnson syndrome).

With symptomatic canalicular constriction but not occlusion, silicone intubation of the nasolacrimal drainage system may be helpful. If a limited area of total occlusion is discovered near the punctum, the occluded canaliculus can be resected and the cut ends of the canaliculus anastomosed over a silicone tube stent in an attempt to establish lacrimal drainage. If obstruction is total at the common canaliculus, *canaliculodacryocystorhinostomy* may be performed. In this procedure, the area of total common canalicular obstruction is removed and the remaining patent canalicular system is directly anastomosed to the lacrimal sac mucosa. Use of a silicone tube as a stent for the reconstructed canalicular system is an important part of this type of reconstruction. Because the failure rate of canalicular resection surgery for total obstruction is significant, Jones tube placement is a surgical alternative.

Conjunctivodacryocystorhinostomy (CJDCR) When both upper and lower canaliculi are severely obstructed (>4 mm), a CJDCR may be required. This procedure is a complete bypass of the lacrimal drainage system. CJDCR is indicated when the canalicular system is too stenotic or obstructed to be used in the reconstruction of the tear outflow apparatus or when the lacrimal pump cannot be made functional. A Pyrex tube (Jones tube) is placed through an opening created at the inferior half of the caruncle and then through an osteotomy site into the middle nasal meatus. The tube is inclined slightly inferiorly, and the bony osteotomy corresponds to that created in a DCR. The ocular end of the tube must be situated in the tear lake, whereas the nasal end must clear the anterior end of the middle turbinate. Different lengths of these tubes should be available at the time of surgery to obtain a tube that emerges clearly in the nose without abutting the nasal septum.

Postoperative care and complications, including obstruction of the tube with mucus or tear salts and extrusion or migration of the tube, can be troublesome. Forced inspiration with the mouth and nose manually closed creates significant airflow through the tube into the nasal airway and usually clears mucous debris and prevents obstruction. Patients should be instructed to perform this maneuver daily. They should also be informed that loss of the tube, even if only for a few days, may cause significant closure of the soft tissue tract of the Jones tube. Periodic Jones tube removal and cleaning in the office, followed by immediate replacement, may be needed. Jones tubes themselves often cause chronic foreign body sensation and mucous production and may incite pyogenic granuloma formation. Despite these drawbacks, many patients with otherwise intractable epiphora are helped by this procedure.

Rosen N, Ashkenazi I, Rosner M. Patient dissatisfaction after functionally successful conjunctivodacryocystorhinostomy with Jones tube. *Am J Ophthalmol.* 1994;117:636–642.

Canalicular infection or inflammation

Canaliculitis may be caused by a variety of bacterial, viral, chlamydial, or mycotic organisms. However, the most common cause is *Actinomyces israelii*. This bacterium is a filamentous gram-positive rod. The patient presents with unexplained persistent weeping, sometimes accompanied by a follicular conjunctivitis around the medial canthus. An erythematous, dilated, and pouting punctum, a grating sensation with probing, and reflux of purulent discharge on milking the canaliculus with cotton-tipped applicators help make the diagnosis (Fig 14-11). Treatment consists of warm compresses, appropriate antibiotics, and curettage combined with canaliculotomy to remove the concretions. The canaliculotomy, which also confirms the diagnosis, should be limited to the horizontal canaliculus and approached from the conjunctival surface of the eyelid. The incision is left open to heal by second intention and does not require silicone intubation. Some surgeons "paint" the canaliculus with povidone-iodine (Betadine) or use specially formulated penicillin-fortified drops perioperatively. In recurrent cases, canaliculotomy combined with silicone intubation is frequently successful.

Canalicular trauma

Traumatic injury to the canalicular system frequently occurs when sudden lateral traction on the upper or lower eyelid causes avulsion of the medial canthal tendon and associated canaliculus. The avulsion injury often appears trivial on superficial inspection, but de-

Figure 14-11 Canaliculitis. *(Photograph courtesy of Roger Dailey, MD.)*

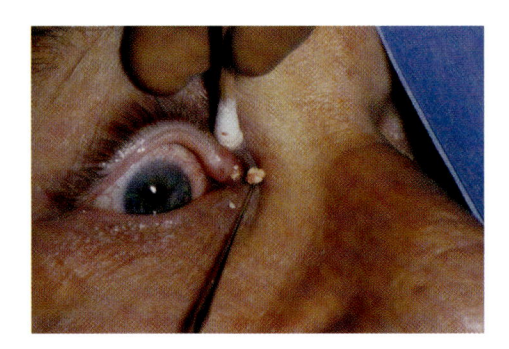

tailed examination of the area shows the true extent of the avulsion. Diagnostic canalicular irrigation and probing may be helpful in an adult but frequently is impossible in a child.

Locating the severed ends of the canalicular system can be frustrating, but the controlled conditions of an operating room—including the use of general anesthesia and magnification with optimal illumination—facilitates the search. The lacerated canaliculus often appears as a pouting gray structure surrounded by the red orbicularis muscle. A thorough understanding of the medial canthal anatomy guides the surgeon to the appropriate area to begin exploration for the medial end of the severed canaliculus. Laterally, the canaliculus is located near the eyelid margin, but for lacerations close to the lacrimal sac, the canaliculus is deep to the anterior limb of the medial canthal tendon. Irrigation of air, fluorescein, yellow viscoelastic, through an intact adjacent canaliculus may be helpful, but methylene blue is not recommended because it stains the entire operative field. In difficult cases, the careful use of a smooth-tipped pigtail probe may be helpful to identify the medial cut end. The probe is introduced through the opposite, uninvolved puncta, through the common canaliculus, and then through the medial cut end.

Complete silicone intubation of the injured canaliculus, normal adjacent canaliculus, lacrimal sac, and nasolacrimal duct prevents postoperative canalicular strictures and facilitates the soft tissue reconstruction of the medial canthal tendon and eyelid avulsion. Single canalicular stenting through the injured canalicular system may be useful in certain cases but may also be associated with decreased surgical success. Delays in surgery for 24–48 hours is acceptable in this well-vascularized area. Direct anastomosis of the cut canaliculus over the silicone tube can be accomplished with closure of the pericanalicular tissues using fine absorbable or nonabsorbable sutures. Recent studies have shown that direct suturing of the canalicular ends is not necessary. Intubation with careful suturing of the surrounding tissue is as effective.

>   Kersten RC, Kulwin DR. "One-stitch" canalicular repair. A simplified approach for repair of canalicular laceration. *Ophthalmology.* 1996;103:785–789.

The silicone tube stent may remain in place for 3–12 months, depending on the severity of the injury as long as the stent is well-tolerated without eyelid inflammation, erosion of the punctum, or canalicular slitting.

Because some patients who have only one functioning canaliculus may be asymptomatic, some authors consider the repair of an isolated single canalicular laceration to be optional. However, it is much easier to perform a primary repair than a secondary reconstruction if the single remaining canaliculus proves inadequate to prevent symptomatic epiphora.

>   Reifler DM. Management of canalicular laceration. *Surv Ophthalmol.* 1991;36:113–132.
>   Wulc AE, Arterberry JR. The pathogenesis of canalicular laceration. *Ophthalmology.* 1991; 98:1243–1249.

Neoplasms

When neoplasms are present in the medial canthal area, complete resection may also include removal of the puncta and canaliculi. Complete tumor excision must be ascertained by histopathologic examination of excised tissue before connection of the lacrimal drainage system with another body cavity, eg, the middle meatus, is considered. When only these structures are involved, the canaliculi may be marsupialized with or without silicone intubation. However, reconstructive procedures including DCR or CJDCR should be delayed for 5 or more years following the excision of invasive tumors because recurrence and subsequent increased morbidity or mortality must be considered.

Lower System Abnormalities

Nasolacrimal obstructions

The intraosseous portion of the nasolacrimal duct may become obstructed as a result of naso-orbital trauma, chronic sinus disease, dacryocystitis, or involutional stenosis. *Involutional stenosis* is probably the most common cause of nasolacrimal duct obstruction in older persons, affecting women twice as frequently as men. Although the inciting event in this process is unknown, clinicopathologic study suggests that compression of the lumen of the nasolacrimal duct by inflammatory infiltrates and edema precedes any development of clinical dacryocystitis. *Granulomatous disease,* including sarcoidosis, Wegener granulomatosis, and lethal midline granuloma, may also lead to nasolacrimal duct obstruction.

> Bartley GB. Acquired lacrimal drainage obstruction: an etiologic classification system, case reports, and a review of the literature, parts 1–3. *Ophthal Plast Reconstr Surg.* 1992;8:237–249 and 1993;9:11–26.
>
> Linberg JV, McCormick SA. Primary acquired nasolacrimal duct obstruction. A clinicopathologic report and biopsy technique. *Ophthalmology.* 1986;93:1055–1063.
>
> Tucker N, Chow D, Stockl F, et al. Clinically suspected primary acquired nasolacrimal duct obstruction. Clinicopathologic review of 150 patients. *Ophthalmology.* 1997;104:1882–1886.

Persistent stenosis of the nasolacrimal duct with symptomatic epiphora sometimes responds to surgical silicone intubation of the entire lacrimal drainage system. This procedure should be performed only if the tubes can be passed easily. In complete nasolacrimal duct obstruction, silicone intubation alone is not effective and a DCR should be considered.

Dacryocystitis

Acute dacryocystitis has various causes. However, the common factor is complete nasolacrimal duct obstruction that prevents normal drainage from the lacrimal sac into the nose. Chronic tear stasis and retention lead to secondary infection with bacteria. Clinical findings include edema and erythema below the medial canthal tendon with distension of the lacrimal sac (Fig 14-12). The degree of pain varies. Complications may include mucocele formation in the lacrimal sac, chronic conjunctivitis, and orbital cellulitis in untreated or inadequately treated cases.

The following are guidelines for treating acute dacryocystitis:

- Avoid irrigation or probing of the canalicular system until the infection subsides.
- Diagnostic or therapeutic probing of the nasolacrimal duct is not indicated in adults with acute dacryocystitis.

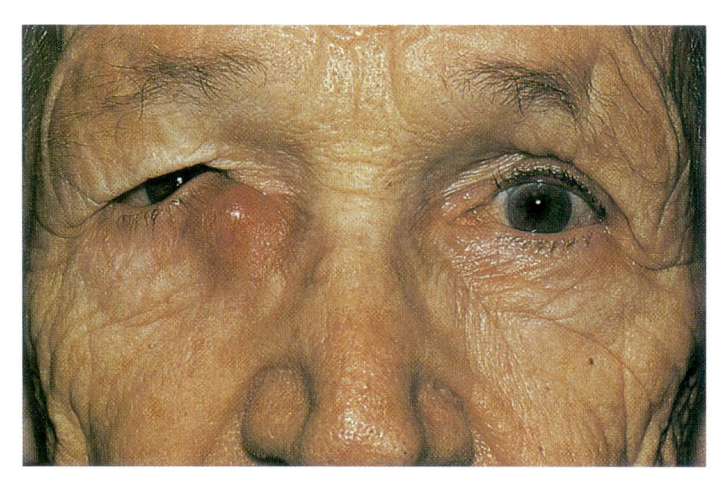

Figure 14-12 Acute dacryocystitis with cellulitis.

- Warm compresses should be applied to the affected area.
- Topical antibiotics are of limited value when stasis is present.
- Oral antibiotics are of value in most infections. Gram-positive bacteria are the most common cause of acute dacryocystitis, but gram-negative organisms should be suspected in patients who are diabetic, immunocompromised, or residing in a nursing home.
- Parenteral antibiotics are necessary for severe cases, especially if cellulitis is present.
- Aspiration of the lacrimal sac may be performed if a pyocele-mucocele is localized and pointing. Information regarding appropriate systemic antibiotic therapy may be obtained from smears and cultures of the aspirate material.
- A localized abscess involving the lacrimal sac and adjacent eyelid soft tissues requires incision and drainage. The incised abscess is packed open and allowed to heal by second intention.

Dacryocystitis, indicating total nasolacrimal duct obstruction, necessitates a DCR in most cases because of inevitable persistent epiphora and recurrent infection. In general, such surgery is deferred until resolution of the acute inflammation. Some patients, however, continue to have a subacute infection until definitive drainage surgery is performed.

Chronic dacryocystitis results in distension of the lacrimal sac. Massage of the lacrimal sac may reflux mucoid material through the canalicular system onto the surface of the eye. Diagnostic probing and irrigation should be confined to the upper system in adults, because probing of the nasolacrimal duct does not achieve permanent patency in adults. If a tumor is not suspected, no further diagnostic evaluation is indicated to confirm the diagnosis of a total nasolacrimal duct obstruction. Chronic dacryocystitis needs to be surgically resolved prior to elective intraocular surgery.

Dacryocystorhinostomy If the patient has an episode of acute dacryocystitis, chronic mucoid reflux from a distended lacrimal sac, or bothersome epiphora, and if evaluation has confirmed the site of obstruction in the nasolacrimal duct, a DCR may be indicated.

280 • Orbit, Eyelids, and Lacrimal System

The operation creates an anastomosis between the lacrimal sac and the nasal cavity through a bony ostium (Fig 14-13). Intraoperative hemostasis can be enhanced by preoperative injection of lidocaine with epinephrine into the medial canthal soft tissues and internal nasal packing with vasoconstrictive agents (oxymetazoline hydrochloride or cocaine).

External DCR (Fig 14-14) remains the preferred procedure of most ophthalmic lacrimal surgeons, with success rates usually above 90%. Surgery can be performed on most adults with local anesthetic infiltration combined with anesthetic and vasoconstrictive nasal packing under monitored anesthesia care. The skin incision should be made so as to avoid the angular blood vessels and prevent bowstring contractures leading to epicanthal folds. The osteotomy adjacent to the medial wall of the lacrimal sac can be created with a rongeur, trephine, or drill. A large osteotomy site facilitates the formation of posterior and anterior mucosal flaps from both the lacrimal sac and the nasal mucosa. Suturing of the corresponding posterior flaps and anterior flaps is common. Simultaneous silicone intubation of the canalicular system may be needed, especially in patients who have common canalicular stenosis or common internal punctum stenosis where the common canaliculus enters the lacrimal sac. A biopsy with frozen-section examination should be considered if abnormal tissue is found. Many surgeons routinely perform a biopsy of the excised lacrimal sac.

External DCR is successful in the large majority of patients. Failure may be caused by fibrosis and occlusion of the rhinostomy site, common canalicular obstruction, or inappropriate placement or size of the bony ostium. Success also is influenced by surgical approach, preoperative active dacryocystitis, trauma, postoperative soft tissue infection, silicone tube complication, and many other factors. Repeated DCR by any approach has a lower success rate.

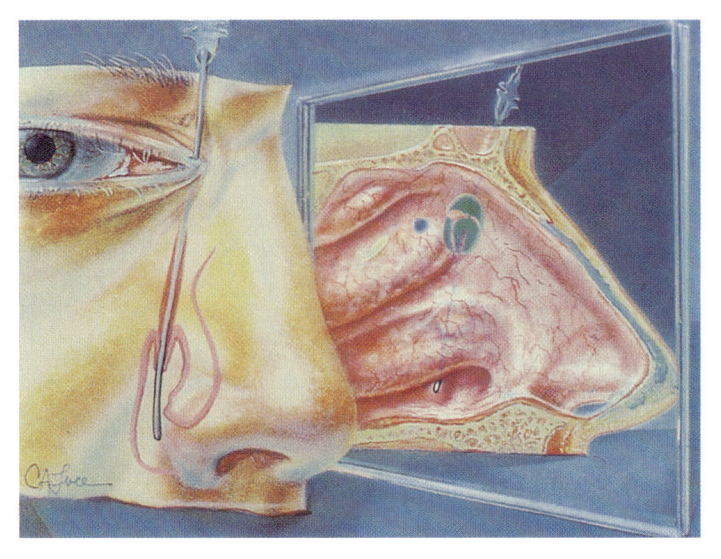

Figure 14-13 The origin of the middle turbinate corresponds well to the location of the lacrimal fossa *(green)*. *(Reproduced by permission from Zide BM, Jelks GW, eds. Surgical Anatomy of the Orbit. New York: Raven; 1985:39. Illustration by Craig A. Luce.)*

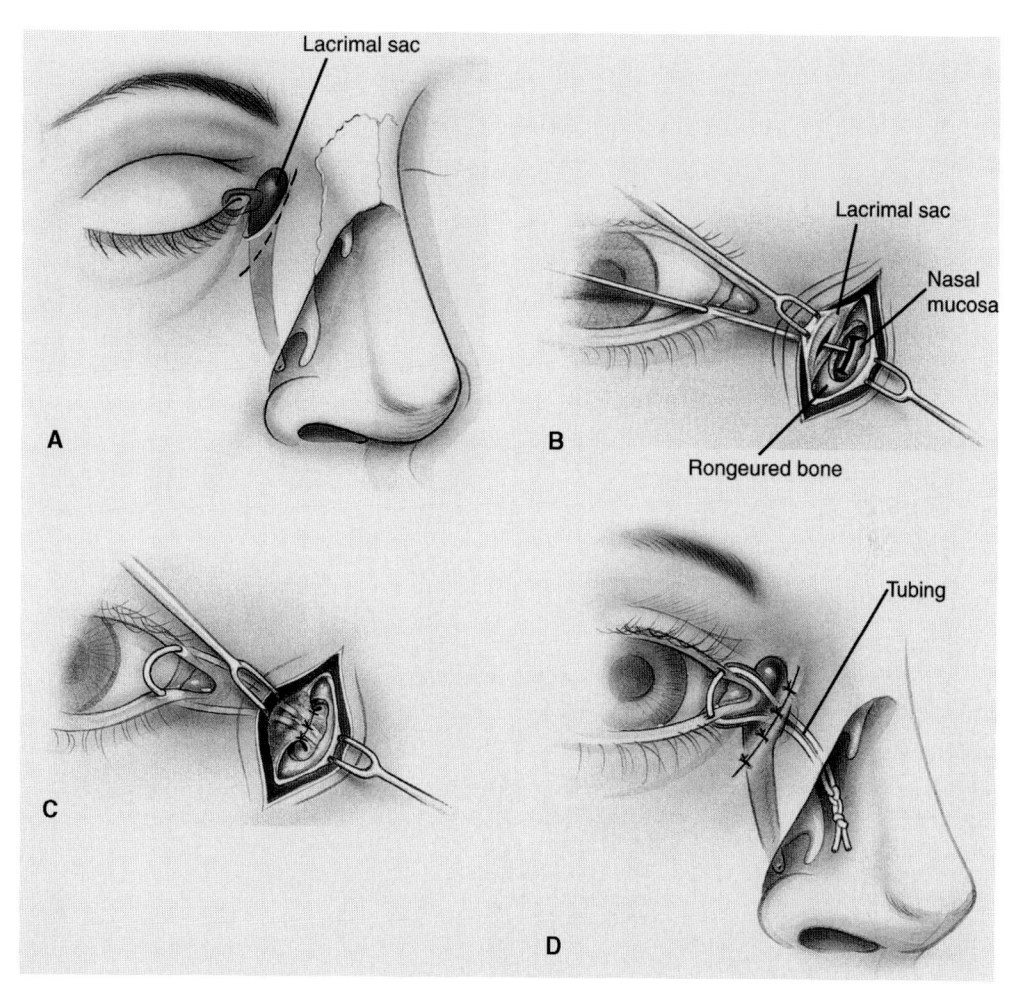

CHAPTER 14: Evaluation and Management of the Tearing Patient • 281

Figure 14-14 External dacryocystorhinostomy. **A,** Incision is marked 10 mm from the medial canthus, starting just above the medial canthal tendon and extending inferiorly. **B,** Bone from the lacrimal fossa and anterior lacrimal crest has been resected. Flaps have been fashioned in the nasal mucosa. A lacrimal probe extends through an incision in the lacrimal sac. **C,** Anterior lacrimal sac flap is sutured to the anterior nasal mucosal flap after a silicone tube is placed. **D,** Final position of the silicone tube following closure of the skin incision. *(Illustration by Christine Gralapp.)*

Tarbet KJ, Custer PL. External dacryocystorhinostomy: surgical success, patient satisfaction, and economic cost. *Ophthalmology.* 1995;102:1065–1070.

Walland MJ, Rose GE. Factors affecting the success rate of open lacrimal surgery. *Br J Ophthalmol.* 1994;78:888–891.

Transnasal laser DCR (Fig 14-15) has attracted much interest, but most surgeons find that the results are not as good as with the external approach. In addition, this procedure requires expensive equipment and difficult exposure. *Endocanalicular laser DCR* has shown promise in some investigations, but long-term results remain varied.

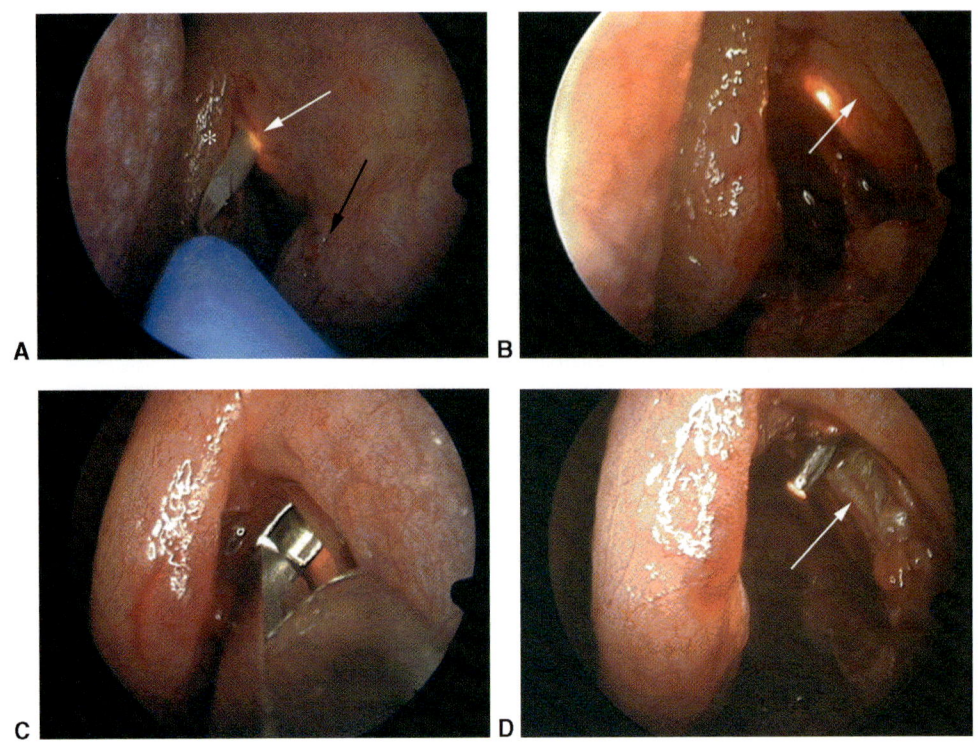

Figure 14-15 Endoscopic laser dacryocystorhinostomy. **A,** Posterior incision behind the intracanalicular transilluminator *(white arrow)*, above the inferior turbinate *(black arrow)*, and just anterior to the insertion of the middle turbinate *(*)*. **B,** Frontal process of the maxilla after nasal mucosal removal *(white arrow)*. **C,** Removal of frontal process of the maxilla with Kerrison rongeurs. **D,** Lacrimal sac has been opened *(white arrow)* and the transilluminator can be seen in the nose. *(Photographs courtesy of François Codére, MD.)*

Interest has been growing in *endoscopic nasal DCR* using endoscopic nasal instrumentation developed in ear, nose, and throat surgery.

Careful selection of patients with an adequate normal nasal cavity is crucial for success. The nasal passage is prepared with topical vasoconstrictors and packing with infiltration of the nasal mucosa with epinephrine. A fine fiberoptic probe can be used to transilluminate the lacrimal sac and help the surgeon identify the thin lacrimal bone.

The surgery consists of removing a nasal mucosal flap over the area corresponding to the nasolacrimal sac and duct. An osteotomy is performed to remove the frontal process of the maxilla and the lacrimal bone covering the lacrimal sac. Often, the uncinate process also has to be removed to allow proper exposure or the superior aspect of the lacrimal passage. The lacrimal sac is then opened and the medial wall of the sac is removed, allowing marsupialization of the sac into the nose. Bicanalicular intubation is usually performed at the end of the procedure. Techniques to preserve the lacrimal and nasal mucosa have been proposed to enhance the predictability of this procedure.

Tsirbas A, Wormald PJ. Endonasal dacryocystorhinostomy with mucosal flaps. *Am J Ophthalmol*. 2003;135:76–83.

Postoperative care consists of office cleaning of nasal debris over the following weeks, and some surgeons recommend daily washing of the nostril for the same period.

A recent report by the American Academy of Ophthalmology suggests that endonasal DCR may be a viable alternative to external DCR in selected patients. Some studies have suggested a lower success rate for the former, but other studies have yielded comparable results. The main advantage to endonasal DCR is the absence of a skin incision and a shorter rehabilitation with less discomfort. On the other hand, expensive equipment and a steep learning curve are known drawbacks.

Mitomycin C, a potent antiproliferative alkylating agent, has been used in a few cases in which external and intranasal DCR failed. Further studies are necessary to better understand the role of mitomycin C in preventing fibrosis at the osteotomy site and increasing the osteotomy size in primary procedures as well as this agent's effect on normal healing and the long-term benefits and risks in lacrimal surgery. *Balloon catheters* are also being evaluated for their usefulness in enlarging contracted osteotomy sites as well as in primary DCRs.

> Bartley GB. The pros and cons of laser dacryocystorhinostomy. *Am J Ophthalmol.* 1994; 117:103–106.
>
> Gonnering RS, Lyon DB, Fisher JC. Endoscopic laser-assisted lacrimal surgery. *Am J Ophthalmol.* 1991;111:152–157.
>
> Massaro BM, Gonnering RS, Harris GJ. Endonasal laser dacryocystorhinostomy. A new approach to nasolacrimal duct obstruction. *Arch Ophthalmol.* 1990;108:1172–1176.
>
> Tsirbas A, Wormald PJ. Endonasal dacryocystorhinostomy with mucosal flaps. Paper presented at: RANZO 33rd Annual Meeting; 2002; Adelaide, Australia.
>
> Woog JJ, Kennedy RH, Custer PL, et al. Endonasal dacryocystorhinostomy: a report by the American Academy of Ophthalmology. *Ophthalmology.* 2001;108:2369–2377.

Dacryoliths

Dacryoliths (shed epithelial cells, amorphous debris, and lipids with or without calcium) or cast formation within the lacrimal sac can also produce obstruction, or they may result from preexisting obstruction. Infection with *Actinomyces israelii* or *Candida* species or long-term administration of topical medications such as epinephrine can lead to the formation of such a cast.

Acute impaction of a dacryolith in the nasolacrimal duct can produce acute noninfectious dacryocystic retention. Severe, painful, lacrimal colic with a minimally enlarged noninflamed sac is present. Dacryocystography is helpful in the diagnosis of this condition. Mechanical removal of the impacted dacryolith, usually along with a DCR, is necessary to relieve symptoms.

> Baratz KH, Bartley GB, Campbell RJ, et al. An eyelash nidus for dacryoliths of the lacrimal excretory and secretory systems. *Am J Ophthalmol.* 1991;111:624–627.
>
> Hawes MJ. The dacryolithiasis syndrome. *Ophthal Plast Reconstr Surg.* 1988;4:87–90.

Neoplasms

Lacrimal sac tumors are rare and usually present clinically as a mass located above the medial canthal tendon that is associated with epiphora or chronic dacryocystitis. Dacryocystitis associated with tumor may differ from simple nasolacrimal duct obstruction in that the irrigation fluid may pass into the nose, and blood may reflux from the punctum when a tumor is present. Tumors may produce skin ulceration with telangiectasia over the lacrimal sac and may cause regional lymphadenopathy. Dacryocystography is useful to outline uneven, mottled densities in the dilated lacrimal sac. CT may also reveal bone erosion and invasion of the orbit or sinuses.

> Madreperla SA, Green WR, Daniel R, et al. Human papillomavirus in primary epithelial tumors of the lacrimal sac. *Ophthalmology.* 1993;100:569–573.
>
> Pe'er JJ, Stefanyszyn M, Hidayat AA. Nonepithelial tumors of the lacrimal sac. *Am J Ophthalmol.* 1994;118:650–658.

Skin tumors, such as basal cell carcinoma, squamous cell carcinoma, and sebaceous adenocarcinoma, may involve the medial canthal region. Unless they invade the lacrimal system or cause pressure in the area or malposition of the eyelids, these tumors should not cause a malfunction of the lacrimal drainage system. Secondary involvement of the nasolacrimal sac may also arise from tumors of the nasal mucosa, such as a squamous cell carcinoma or inverted papillomatosis.

Histologically, approximately 45% of lacrimal sac tumors are benign and 55% are malignant. Squamous cell papillomas and carcinomas are the most common tumors of the sac. Many papillomas initially grow in an inverted pattern into the lacrimal sac wall and, consequently, are often incompletely excised. With recurrence, malignant degeneration may occur.

Treatment of benign lacrimal sac tumors commonly requires *dacryocystectomy.* Malignancies may require dacryocystectomy combined with a lateral rhinotomy, performed by an otolaryngologist. *Exenteration,* including bone removal in the medial canthal area, is necessary if bone and the soft tissues of the orbit are involved by a malignant epithelial tumor. *Radiation* is useful in treating lymphomatous lesions or as an adjunctive therapy in extensive epithelial lesions. The recurrence rate for invasive squamous and transitional cell carcinoma of the lacrimal sac is approximately 50%, with 50% of those being fatal.

After therapy and freedom from recurrence for up to 5 years, the patient may undergo a DCR or CJDCR to relieve the troublesome epiphora.

Trauma

The lacrimal sac and nasolacrimal duct may be injured by direct laceration or by naso-orbital fracture. Injuries of the lacrimal sac or nasolacrimal duct may also occur during rhinoplasty or endoscopic sinus surgery when the physiologic maxillary sinus ostium is being enlarged anteriorly. Early treatment by fracture reduction and soft tissue repair of the lacrimal sac and nasolacrimal duct is indicated, with silicone intubation of the entire lacrimal drainage system. Late treatment for persistent epiphora may require DCR.

> Neuhaus RW. Orbital complications secondary to endoscopic sinus surgery. *Ophthalmology.* 1990;97:1512–1518.

Basic Texts

Orbit, Eyelids, and Lacrimal System

Baker SR, Swanson NA. *Local Flaps in Facial Reconstruction.* St Louis: Mosby; 1995.

Bron AJ, Tripathi RC, Tripathi BJ. *Wolff's Anatomy of the Eye and Orbit.* 8th ed. Philadelphia: Lippincott-Raven; 1998.

Collin JRO, ed. *A Manual of Systematic Eye Surgery.* New York: Churchill Livingstone; 1989.

Dutton JJ. *Atlas of Clinical and Surgical Orbital Anatomy.* Philadelphia: Saunders; 1994.

Dutton JJ, Byrne SF, Proia AD. *Diagnostic Atlas of Orbital Diseases.* Philadelphia: Saunders; 2000.

Henderson JW, Campbell RJ, Farrow GM, et al. *Orbital Tumors.* New York: Raven; 1994.

Hurwitz JJ, ed. *The Lacrimal System.* Philadelphia: Lippincott-Raven; 1996.

Lemke BN, Della Rocca RC, eds. *Surgery of the Eyelids and Orbit: An Anatomical Approach.* East Norwalk, CT: Appleton & Lange; 1990.

Linberg JV, ed. *Lacrimal Surgery.* Contemporary Issues in Ophthalmology, 5. New York: Churchill Livingstone; 1988.

McCord CD, Tanenbaum M, Nunery WR, eds. *Oculoplastic Surgery.* 3rd ed. New York: Lippincott Williams & Wilkins; 1995.

Nerad JA. *The Requisites in Ophthalmology: Oculoplastic Surgery.* Philadelphia: Mosby; 2001.

Nesi FA, Lisman RD, Levine RM, eds. *Smith's Ophthalmic Plastic and Reconstructive Surgery.* 2nd ed. St Louis: Mosby; 1998.

Putterman AM. *Cosmetic Oculoplastic Surgery: Eyelid, Forehead, and Facial Techniques.* 3rd ed. Philadelphia: Saunders; 1999.

Rootman J, ed. *Diseases of the Orbit: A Multidisciplinary Approach.* 2nd ed. Philadelphia: Lippincott Williams & Wilkins; 2003.

Rootman J, Stewart B, Goldberg RA, eds. *Orbital Surgery: A Conceptual Approach.* New York: Lippincott Williams & Wilkins; 1995.

Shields JA, Shields CL. *Atlas of Eyelid and Conjunctival Tumors.* New York: Lippincott Williams & Wilkins; 1999.

Shields JA, Shields CL. *Atlas of Orbital Tumors.* New York: Lippincott Williams & Wilkins; 1999.

Spencer WH, ed. *Ophthalmic Pathology: An Atlas and Textbook.* 4th ed. Philadelphia: Saunders; 1996.

Zide BM, Jelks GW, eds. *Surgical Anatomy of the Orbit.* New York: Raven; 1985.

Related Academy Materials

Focal Points: Clinical Modules for Ophthalmologists

Alford MA. Management of trichiasis (Module 4, 2001).
Bartley GB. Periorbital animal bites (Module 3, 1992).
Biesman BS. Lasers in periorbital surgery (Module 7, 2000).
Boynton JR. Management of cicatricial entropion, trichiasis, and distichiasis (Module 12, 1993).
Cockerham KP, Kennerdel JS. Thyroid-associated orbitopathy (Module 1, 1997).
Dailey RA. Upper eyelid blepharoplasty (Module 8, 1995).
Dresner SC. Ophthalmic management of facial nerve paralysis (Module 4, 2000).
Gossman MD. Management of eyelid trauma (Module 10, 1996).
Howard GR. Management of acquired ptosis (Module 8, 1999).
Lauer SA. Ectropion and entropion (Module 10, 1994).
Lemke BN. Management of thyroid eyelid retraction (Module 6, 1991).
Lyon DB. Evaluation of the tearing adult patient (Module 9, 2002).
Meyer DR. Congenital ptosis (Module 2, 2001).
Nelson CC, Oestreicher J. Eyelid trauma (Module 10, 1991).
Nerad JA, Carter KD. The anophthalmic socket (Module 8, 1992).
Patel BCK, Anderson RL. Essential blepharospasm and related diseases (Module 5, 2000).
Rubin PAD, Bilyk JR, Shore JW. Management of orbital trauma: fractures, hemorrhage, and traumatic optic neuropathy (Module 7, 1994).
Spinelli HM, Riou J. Aesthetic surgery of the lower eyelid (Module 7, 1995).
Steinkuller PG. Orbital cellulitis (Module 11, 1991).
Wiggs EO, Popham JK. Evaluation and surgery of the lacrimal drainage system in adults (Module 12, 1995).

Publications

Jordan DR, Anderson RA. *Surgical Anatomy of the Ocular Adnexa: A Clinical Approach* (Ophthalmology Monograph 9, 1996).
Lane SS, Skuta GL, eds. *ProVision: Preferred Responses in Ophthalmology*, Series 3 (Self-Assessment Program, 1999).
Skuta GL, ed. *ProVision: Preferred Responses in Ophthalmology*, Series 2 (Self-Assessment Program, 1996).
Stewart WB, ed. *Surgery of the Eyelid, Orbit, and Lacrimal System* (Ophthalmology Monograph 8). Vol 1, 1993; vol 2, 1994; vol 3, 1995.

Multimedia

Nerad JA, Carter KD, Kersten RC, et al. *LEO Clinical Update Course on Orbit and Ophthalmic Plastic Surgery* (CD-ROM, 2003).

Continuing Ophthalmic Video Education

Bergin DJ. *Management and Surgery of Congenital and Acquired Ptosis* (1990).
Wesley RE. *Ectropion and Entropion Repair of the Lower Lid* (1989).
Wojno TH. *Cosmetic Blepharoplasty* (1996).

Preferred Practice Patterns

Preferred Practice Patterns Committee, Cornea/External Disease Panel. *Dry Eye Syndrome* (1998).

Ophthalmic Technology Assessments

Ophthalmic Technology Assessment Committee. *Endonasal Dacryocystorhinostomy* (2002).
Ophthalmic Technology Assessment Committee. *Functional Indications for Upper and Lower Eyelid Blepharoplasty* (1995).
Ophthalmic Technology Assessment Committee. *Laser Blepharoplasty and Skin Resurfacing* (1998).
Ophthalmic Technology Assessment Committee. *Punctal Occlusion for the Dry Eye* (1996).

To order any of these materials, please call the Academy's Customer Service number at (415) 561-8540, or order online at www.aao.org.

Credit Reporting Form

Basic and Clinical Science Course, 2004–2005
Section 7

The American Academy of Ophthalmology is accredited by the Accreditation Council for Continuing Medical Education to provide continuing medical education for physicians.

The American Academy of Ophthalmology designates this educational activity for a maximum of 30 category 1 credits toward the AMA Physician's Recognition Award. Each physician should claim only those hours of credit that he/she actually spent in the activity.

The American Medical Association has determined that non-US licensed physicians who participate in this CME activity are eligible for AMA PRA category 1 credit.

If you wish to claim continuing medical education credit for your study of this section, you may claim your credit online or fill in the required forms and mail or fax them to the Academy.

To use the forms:

1. Complete the study questions and mark your answers on the Section Completion Form.
2. Complete the Section Evaluation.
3. Fill in and sign the statement below.
4. Return this page and the required forms by mail or fax to the CME Registrar (see below).

To claim credit online:

1. Log on to the Academy website (www.aao.org).
2. Go to Education Resource Center; click on CME Central.
3. Follow the instructions.

Important: These completed forms or the online claim must be received at the Academy within 3 years of purchase.

I hereby certify that I have spent _____ (up to 30) hours of study on the curriculum of this section and that I have completed the Study Questions.

Signature: _____

Date

Name: _____

Address: _____

City and State: _____ Zip: _____

Telephone: (_____) _____ Academy Member ID# _____
        area code

Please return completed forms to: **Or you may fax them to:** 415-561-8557
American Academy of Ophthalmology
P.O. Box 7424
San Francisco, CA 94120-7424
Attn: CME Registrar, Clinical Education

2004–2005
Section Completion Form

Basic and Clinical Science Course

Answer Sheet for Section 7

Question	Answer	Question	Answer
1	a b c d e	24	a b c d e
2	a b c d	25	a b c d e
3	a b c d	26	a b c d e
4	a b c d	27	a b c d
5	a b c d	28	a b c d e
6	a b c d e	29	a b c d e
7	a b c d e	30	a b c d e
8	a b c d e	31	a b c d e
9	a b c d e	32	a b c d e
10	a b c d	33	a b c d e
11	a b c d e	34	a b c d e
12	a b c d	35	a b c d e
13	a b c d	36	a b c d e
14	a b c d	37	a b c d e
15	a b c d e	38	a b c d e
16	a b c d e	39	a b c d e
17	a b c d	40	a b c d e
18	a b c d e	41	a b c d
19	a b c d	42	a b c d
20	a b c d e	43	a b c d
21	a b c d e	44	a b c d
22	a b c d e	45	a b c d
23	a b c d e		

Credit Reporting Form • 291

Section Evaluation

Please complete this CME questionnaire.

1. To what degree will you use knowledge from BCSC Section 7 in your practice?
   - ☐ Regularly
   - ☐ Sometimes
   - ☐ Rarely

2. Please review the stated objectives for BCSC Section 7. How effective was the material at meeting those objectives?
   - ☐ All objectives were met.
   - ☐ Most objectives were met.
   - ☐ Some objectives were met.
   - ☐ Few or no objectives were met.

3. To what degree is BCSC Section 7 likely to have a positive impact on health outcomes of your patients?
   - ☐ Extremely likely
   - ☐ Highly likely
   - ☐ Somewhat likely
   - ☐ Not at all likely

4. After you review the stated objectives for BCSC Section 7, please let us know of any additional knowledge, skills, or information useful to your practice that were acquired but were not included in the objectives. [Optional]

5. Was BCSC Section 7 free of commercial bias?
   - ☐ Yes
   - ☐ No

6. If you selected "No" in the previous question, please comment. [Optional]

7. Please tell us what might improve the applicability of BCSC to your practice. [Optional]

Study Questions

Although a concerted effort has been made to avoid ambiguity and redundancy in these questions, the authors recognize that differences of opinion may occur regarding the "best" answer. The discussions are provided to demonstrate the rationale used to derive the answer. They may also be helpful in confirming that your approach to the problem was correct or, if necessary, in fixing the principle in your memory. Where relevant, additional references are given.

1. This nerve to an extraocular muscle does not pass through the muscle cone on entering the orbit
   a. CN III
   b. CN IV
   c. CN V
   d. CN VI
   e. CN VII

2. Which is true regarding orbital anatomy?
   a. The lacrimal gland fossa is located within the lateral orbital wall.
   b. The optic canal is located within the greater wing of the sphenoid bone.
   c. The medial wall of the optic canal is formed by the lateral wall of the sphenoid sinus.
   d. The nerve to the inferior rectus muscle travels anteriorly along the medial aspect of the muscle and innervates the muscle on its posterior surface.

3. The five major branches of the facial nerve include the temporal, buccal, marginal mandibular, cervical, and
   a. Temporal parietal
   b. Zygomatic
   c. Infraorbital
   d. Zygomaticofacial

4. What structure is deep to the plane of the facial nerve branches in the lower face?
   a. Masseter muscle
   b. Parotidomasseteric fascia
   c. Deep temporal fascia
   d. Parotid gland

5. The superior transverse ligament is also referred to as
   a. Lockwood's ligament
   b. Sommerring's ligament
   c. The ROOF
   d. Whitnall's ligament

6. Compared to CT scanning, MRI scanning provides better
   a. View of bone and calcium
   b. View of the orbital apex and orbitocranial junction
   c. Elimination of motion artificact
   d. Comfort for claustrophobic patients
   e. Safety to patients with prosthetic implants

7. In patients with a facial nerve paralysis, all of the following characteristics may be present *except:*
   a. Eyebrow ptosis
   b. Blepharoptosis
   c. Lower eyelid ectropion
   d. Epiphora
   e. Ocular exposure symptoms

8. A 1-year-old presents with a round, well-demarcated mass at the superotemporal rim. The lesion has been present since birth. The most likely diagnosis is
   a. Rhabdomyosarcoma
   b. Neurofibroma
   c. Dermoid cyst
   d. Capillary hemangioma
   e. Metastatic Ewing sarcoma

9. A 65-year-old woman presents with a progressively enlarging mass in the right inferior orbit. Distraction of the lower eyelid reveals a "salmon patch" appearance to the fornix. The most likely diagnosis is
   a. Reactive lymphoid hyperplasia
   b. Lymphoma
   c. Sebaceous carcinoma
   d. Melanoma
   e. Apocrine hidrocystoma

10. Which of the following signs is most likely to be present in a patient with Graves ophthalmopathy?
    a. Exophthalmos
    b. External ophthalmoplegia
    c. Eyelid retraction
    d. Optic neuropathy

11. Subperiosteal abscess of the orbit in adults is more likely than in children to
    a. Drain spontaneously
    b. Respond to single antibiotic therapy
    c. Be polymicrobial
    d. Arise from the ethmoid sinus
    e. Arise from acute sinusitis

12. In exploring upper eyelid trauma with a full-thickness laceration involving the eyelid margin, the physician must be aware of the order in which the anatomical structures are normally encountered. The correct order is

    a. Skin, preaponeurotic fat, septum, orbicularis muscle, levator aponeurosis, Müller's muscle, conjunctiva

    b. Skin, orbicularis muscle, preaponeurotic fat, Müller's muscle, levator aponeurosis, conjunctiva

    c. Skin, preaponeurotic fat, orbicularis muscle, septum, levator aponeurosis, Müller's muscle, conjunctiva

    d. Skin, orbicularis muscle, septum, preaponeurotic fat, levator aponeurosis, Müller's muscle, conjunctiva

13. Which of the following statements about the relationship of Graves ophthalmopathy with thyroid status is true?

    a. Ophthalmopathy resolves after hyperthyroidism is adequately treated.

    b. Ophthalmopathy generally develops prior to the diagnosis of thyroid dysfunction.

    c. Serum thyroid-stimulating hormone level is a good marker for the intensity of ophthalmopathy.

    d. Ophthalmopathy may develop even though a patient is euthyroid.

14. Congenital Horner syndrome is associated with miosis, ptosis, anhidrosis, and

    a. Chemosis

    b. Jaw-winking

    c. Lagophthalmos

    d. Iris hypopigmentation

15. The most common location for orbital lymphoma is

    a. The extraocular muscles

    b. Retro-orbital fat

    c. Lacrimal fossa

    d. Orbital apex

    e. Orbital floor

16. Biopsy of an orbital mass is read as "reactive lymphoid hyperplasia." The appropriate treatment is

    a. Systemic steroids

    b. Radiation with a dose of 1500–2000 cGy

    c. Systemic chemotherapy

    d. Complete surgical excision

    e. Cryotherapy

17. All of the following are true regarding orbital cellulitis, *except:*
    a. Most cases are associated with an underlying sinusitis.
    b. Infections in children tend to be single organism.
    c. Subperiosteal abscesses, especially in children, require drainage.
    d. After initiation of appropriate antibiotic therapy a subperiosteal abscess may enlarge before responding.

18. A 20-year-old man is struck over the right eye, and radiography shows a fracture of the right orbital floor. Forced traction testing is equivocal because of poor cooperation. Four days after injury, 3 mm of right exophthalmos is present, and movements of the eye are restricted in upgaze, downgaze, and horizontal gaze. Treatment at that time should be
    a. Conjunctival incision through the inferior fornix, with examination of the fracture
    b. Caldwell-Luc incision and packing of the maxillary sinus
    c. Skin incision over the inferior orbital rim and covering of the fracture defect with a plastic plate
    d. Skin incision beneath the eyelashes and covering of the fracture defect with a plastic plate
    e. None of the above

19. Which of the following features is most likely to be found on an orbital CT scan of a patient with Graves ophthalmopathy?
    a. An increased amount of orbital fat in the presence of normal-sized extraocular muscles
    b. Diffuse, fusiform enlargement of the extraocular muscle belly and tendon
    c. Pressure erosion of the lateral orbital rim from enlarged muscles
    d. Chronic ethmoid and maxillary sinusitis

20. The most important determinant in selecting a corrective procedure for any type of ptosis is
    a. Vertical height of the palpebral fissure
    b. Age of the patient
    c. Amount of levator function
    d. Duration of the ptosis
    e. Position of the upper eyelid margin relative to the corneal limbus

21. A 70-year-old woman has 4 mm of right upper eyelid ptosis and 1 mm of left upper eyelid retraction. She has a high eyelid crease in the right upper eyelid with normal levator function of both upper eyelids. The treatment of choice is
    a. A moderated internal tarsoconjunctival resection (Fasanella-Servat operation) on the right upper eyelid
    b. A moderate levator recession of the left upper eyelid
    c. A levator aponeurosis advancement on the right upper eyelid
    d. A posterior-approach, standard müllerectomy on the right upper eyelid
    e. A frontalis muscle suspension on the right upper eyelid using a silicone rod to allow postoperative adjustment

22. Risk factors for developing basal cell carcinoma include all of the following *except:*
    a. History of smoking
    b. Excessive sun exposure in the first two decades of life
    c. Brown irides
    d. Blond hair
    e. Celtic ancestry

23. In the evaluation of a child with unilateral exophthalmos, which assumption is correct?
    a. Cavernous hemangiomas are among the most common benign orbital tumors in children.
    b. Thyroid ophthalmopathy is the most common cause of unilateral exophthalmos among children.
    c. Neurofibroma is the malignant tumor that most commonly produces exophthalmos among children.
    d. Optic nerve meningiomas are more common than gliomas in children.
    e. None of the above.

24. Neurofibromatosis type 1 is associated with all of the following *except:*
    a. Skin lesions known as adenoma sebaceum
    b. Café-au-lait skin lesions
    c. Plexiform neurofibromas in the eyelids
    d. Optic nerve glioma
    e. Cutaneous neurofibromas

25. Essential blepharospasm is usually characterized by all of the following *except:*
    a. Unilaterality
    b. Age of onset usually over 50 years
    c. Visual incapacitation
    d. Obscure etiology
    e. Involuntary spasms of the orbicularis muscle

26. Entropion repair of the lower eyelid may utilize any of the following techniques *except:*
    a. Lower eyelid retractor advancement
    b. Lateral canthal tightening
    c. Taping of the eyelid
    d. Mucous membrane grafting to the posterior eyelid
    e. Skin grafting

27. All of the following are true regarding invasive aspergillus infections of the orbit *except:*
    a. Bone destruction is not seen.
    b. Corticosteroids may produce an initial clinical improvement.
    c. An adjacent sinusitis is usually present.
    d. Septate branching hyphae of uniform width are seen histologically.

28. A 40-year-old woman presents with a progressively enlarging clear cystic mass along the eyelid margin. The most likely diagnosis is
    a. Epidermal inclusion cyst
    b. Apocrine hidrocystoma
    c. Syringoma
    d. Trichofolliculoma
    e. Basal cell carcinoma

29. A 3-year-old girl was bitten by her pet dog. A 6-mm-wide block of upper eyelid margin is hanging by a thread of tissue. This block of tissue left a defect in the upper eyelid approximately the same size as the tissue itself. The best treatment would be to
    a. Send the block of tissue to pathology and repair the defect by approximating the two margins
    b. Send the block of tissue to pathology and repair the defect by making a lateral canthotomy so that the skin edges can be approximated
    c. Repair the eyelid by sewing the block of tissue into its normal anatomic position
    d. Send the tissue to pathology and repair the defect by a transfer of tissue from the lower eyelid
    e. Keep the tissue under refrigeration for later use if necessary and close the defect by approximation of the wound edges and lateral canthotomy

30. A 74-year-old woman presents with a 2-year history of a painless, progressively enlarging mass in the central aspect of the upper eyelid. This has resulted in distortion of the eyelid margin and loss of eyelashes. The most likely diagnosis is
    a. Sebaceous gland carcinoma
    b. Squamous cell carcinoma
    c. Amelanotic melanoma
    d. Basal cell carcinoma
    e. Dermal nevus

31. The majority of orbital lymphomas
    a. Are polyclonal proliferations
    b. Are T-cell tumors
    c. Are systemic at presentation
    d. Are well differentiated
    e. Involve both orbits

32. Which of the following statements about the levator palpebrae muscle and its aponeurosis is false?
    a. Levator muscle fibers are sparse in most cases of congenital ptosis.
    b. The orbital (deep) and palpebral (superficial) portions of the lacrimal gland are separated by the aponeurosis.
    c. The orbital septum fuses with the aponeurosis in the upper eyelid.
    d. Whitnall's ligament is a check ligament of the muscle.
    e. None of the above

33. Six hours after a bilateral blepharoplasty, the patient complains of sudden pain near the right eye. The dressings are removed and the right eyelids are tense and ecchymotic. The first step would be to
    a. Open the wound to release a possible retrobulbar hemorrhage
    b. Consider the possibility of a cavernous sinus thrombosis and check corneal sensation
    c. Measure visual acuity and check pupillary responses
    d. Begin treatment with ice packs
    e. Begin treatment with warm compresses

34. A 75-year-old woman complains of tearing and discharge. Irrigation of the lower canaliculus produces mucopurulent reflux. All of the following are true *except:*
    a. Jones testing will not reveal dye in the nose.
    b. There is probably a common canalicular block.
    c. The condition is not likely to resolve with a course of antibiotics.
    d. The most likely diagnosis is a lacrimal duct obstruction.
    e. The correct treatment is dacryocystorhinostomy.

35. A 14-month-old child has had tearing and discharge from the right eye since birth. Which of the following statements is true?
    a. Dye disappearance testing is likely to show no asymmetry.
    b. This condition is likely to resolve spontaneously.
    c. The appropriate treatment is nasolacrimal duct probing.
    d. Punctal abnormalities are likely to be the cause.
    e. Jones I and Jones II tests are necessary to make the diagnosis.

36. Blepharophimosis is generally associated with all of the following *except:*
    a. Ptosis
    b. Epicanthus inversus
    c. Distichiasis
    d. Ectropion
    e. Telecanthus

37. A 30-year-old man received a knife wound involving the right upper eyelid 1 hour before your examination. The patient is awake and alert. A 15-mm-long laceration is present 12 mm above the lash line. The patient has 7 mm of ptosis on the right side, and there is minimal swelling. After appropriate evaluation of the globe, the best treatment is to
    a. Repair skin laceration and wait several months for ptosis to resolve
    b. Keep wound clean and wait for swelling to subside in 2–3 days before attempting repair
    c. Repair muscle layer and skin layer separately
    d. Explore the wound to examine the levator aponeurosis and attempt to reattach it if it is severed from the tarsus, after which the skin and muscle should be repaired
    e. Repair skin laceration and tape eyelid to brow for several days to promote healing

38. The management of rhabdomyosarcoma of the orbit usually involves
    a. Lumbar puncture to rule out central nervous system metastasis
    b. Exenteration of the orbit
    c. Enucleation and orbital radiation
    d. Systemic chemotherapy and orbital radiation
    e. Radical neck dissection if cervical lymph nodes are involved

39. Which of the following statements about medial canthal trauma is correct?
    a. It is always associated with a history of direct, sharp trauma to the medial canthal soft tissues.
    b. It occasionally involves the nasolacrimal duct but frequently spares the canalicular system.
    c. It must be repaired within 6 hours of injury.
    d. It may result in telecanthus if not repaired.
    e. Delayed lacrimal drainage repair (>6 months) would probably require a standard DCR.

40. Indications for repair of orbital blowout fracture include all of the following *except:*
    a. Cosmetically unacceptable enophthalmos
    b. Fractures involving more than half of the orbital floor
    c. Inferior rectus weakness
    d. Pain and oculocardiac reflex on upgaze
    e. Significant inferior rectus entrapment

41. The temporal pocket dissection for standard endoscopic brow lift is performed immediately below what layer?
    a. Deep temporal fascia
    b. Temporoparietal fascia
    c. Frontalis muscle
    d. Galea aponeurotica

42. In a subcutaneous rhytidectomy with SMAS, the tension of the lift is placed on which layer?
    a. Skin
    b. Osteocutaneous ligaments
    c. Superficial musculoaponeurotic system
    d. Periosteum

43. Cicatricial ectropion is generally associated with
    a. Trichiasis
    b. Anterior lamellar shortage
    c. Blepharospasm
    d. Symblepharon

44. All of the following are true regarding optic nerve tumors *except:*
    a. Optic nerve gliomas in children are associated with neurofibromatosis type 1.
    b. Optic nerve meningiomas in children are associated with neurofibromatosis type 2.
    c. Radiation therapy is an accepted therapy for optic nerve sheath meningiomas.
    d. Optic nerve gliomas of childhood can be malignant.

45. In cases of implant extrusion following enucleation or evisceration all of the following are true *except:*
    a. Early extrusion is associated with an implant that is too small.
    b. Early extrusion is associated with poor wound closure.
    c. Late implant extrusion can be associated with tumor recurrence.
    d. Late implant extrusion can be associated with a conjunctival cyst.

Answers

1. Answer—b. CN IV is the only nerve innervating an extraocular muscle that does not pass through the muscle cone on entering the orbit. CN IV passes over the levator muscle and enters the superior oblique muscle on its superior aspect at the junction of the posterior third and anterior two-thirds.
2. Answer—c. The optic canal is located immediately superior and lateral to the sphenoid sinus wall.
3. Answer—b. The zygomatic branch of the facial nerve is located between the temporal and buccal branches.
4. Answer—a. The parotidomasseteric fascia is generally a thin, wispy structure that overlies the facial nerve branches, which overlie the masseter muscle, which is therefore the deepest of the structures listed.
5. Answer—d. Whitnall's ligament extends horizontally across the levator muscle several millimeters above its tendon. Lockwood's ligament is an analogous structure in the lower eyelid.
6. Answer—b. The lack of artifact from bone with MRI scanning provides better soft tissue contrast in viewing the structures of the orbital apex, intracanalicular optic nerve, and adjacent intracranial space.
7. Answer—b. Neurogenic blepharoptosis is due to a cranial nerve III palsy, not a cranial nerve VII (facial nerve) palsy. Patients with a total palsy of the facial nerve may have pseudoptosis secondary to an atonic, overhanging upper eyelid fold in the palpebral fissure.
8. Answer—c. Dermoid cysts are the most common congenital mass in the orbit. Dermoid cysts consist of skin elements trapped in a suture line during embryogenesis. The most common location is at the frontozygomatic suture. None of the other lesions listed is usually present at birth. Rhabdomyosarcoma, Ewing sarcoma, and capillary hemangioma show growth that can often be rapid.
9. Answer—b. The history and appearance of this mass are suggestive of a lymphoproliferative lesion. Approximately 80% of orbital lymphoproliferations will prove monoclonal, suggesting a diagnosis of lymphoma; while 20% are polyclonal, suggesting reactive lymphoid hyperplasia.
10. Answer—c. Eyelid retraction is the most common clinical feature of Graves ophthalmopathy (and Graves ophthalmopathy is the most common cause of eyelid retraction).
11. Answer—c. Orbital abscesses in adults are more likely to arise from chronic sinusitis. These infections are more likely to be mixed polymicrobial infections of aerobic and anaerobic bacteria.
12. Answer—d. In upper eyelid trauma, identification of the preaponeurotic fat pad will assist in orientation of the disrupted tissues. The levator aponeurosis is immediately posterior to the fat pad, and the anterior lamella of the eyelid (skin and orbicularis muscle) is anterior to the fat pad.
13. Answer—d. Although Graves ophthalmopathy occurs most commonly in association with hyperthyroidism (and treatment of hyperthyroidism is important in the overall care of the Graves patient), the course of the ophthalmopathy does not necessarily parallel the activity of the thyroid gland or the treatment of thyroid abnormalities. In some patients, the characteristic eye findings occur in the absence of objective evidence of thyroid abnormalities (euthyroid Graves disease).

14. Answer—d. The lack of sympathetic innervation at birth in congenital Horner syndrome leads to a relative lack of pigmentation of the ipsilateral iris.

15. Answer—c. Up to 50% of orbital lymphoproliferative lesions arise in the lacrimal fossa.

16. Answer—b. Although systemic steroids are useful in idiopathic orbital inflammatory syndrome (orbital pseudotumor), they are not recommended in the treatment of lymphoproliferative lesions. Radiotherapy is the treatment of choice for patients with localized ocular lymphoproliferative disease. A surgical cure usually cannot be attained because of the infiltrative nature of lymphoid tumors. Patients must be monitored indefinitely for development of additional lymphoproliferative lesions.

17. Answer—c. In more than 90% of cases, orbital cellulitis occurs as a secondary extension of acute or chronic sinusitis. Infection in adults is most often caused by multiple organisms, and drainage of the infected sinus is usually indicated. In contrast, orbital cellulitis in children is more often caused by a single organism and is less likely to require drainage, especially in patients under age 9.

18. Answer—e. At 4 days after injury with exophthalmos and restricted motility, additional observation is necessary to allow traumatic edema to subside. This subsidence may be enhanced by the administration of oral prednisone, 1 mg/kg per day for 1 week. Urgent exploration of orbital blowout fractures is necessary only if there is radiographic evidence of gross extraocular muscle entrapment beneath the fracture fragments. It is generally preferable to allow 10–14 days for swelling to resolve and motility to be reevaluated before proceeding with surgical repair.

19. Answer—a. See Figures 4-6 and 4-7. Although extraocular muscle enlargement is fusiform, it typically spares the tendons.

20. Answer—c. The amount of levator function is the most important determinant from both a diagnostic and therapeutic standpoint when dealing with blepharoptosis. In those cases in which levator function is good, innervation and strength of the muscle are usually normal, and the problem is usually one of mechanical disinsertion of the attachment of the muscle or loss of supporting sympathetic tone (Horner syndrome). In either situation, surgical correction would be directed toward strengthening the effective action of the levator muscle by shortening its insertion to the eyelid. Patients in whom levator function is reduced are more likely to have a problem with the innervation to the levator muscle (third nerve palsy), a problem at the myoneural junction (myasthenia gravis), or a problem within the levator muscle itself (congenital ptosis). If levator function is significantly reduced, procedures to strengthen the levator muscle will be ineffective in raising the eyelid and may also result in significant lagophthalmos. In these cases, the surgeon may consider slinging of the eyelid to the frontalis muscle so that the frontalis function can be used to elevate and depress the eyelid, bypassing the dysfunctional levator muscle.

21. Answer—c. This patient presents with typical clinical signs of levator aponeurosis dehiscence of the right upper eyelid. This may be idiopathic or may be related to previous ocular surgery with manipulation of the eyelids. The 1 mm of left upper eyelid retraction is secondary to a compensatory increased innervation of both levator muscles to clear the visual axis on the right side. Frequently, after levator muscle repair of the ptotic eyelid, the compensatory contralateral eyelid retraction will spontaneously resolve. The amount of ptosis (4 mm) cannot be easily corrected with either a moderate internal tarsoconjunctival resection or a standard müllerectomy. A frontalis muscle suspension is not needed in a patient with normal levator function.

22. Answer—c. Excessive sun exposure in the first two decades of life, history of smoking, and light skin and iris pigmentation are all risk factors for development of basal cell carcinoma. In addition, individuals with Celtic ancestry (Irish or Scottish) have an increased incidence. Approximately 90% of basal cell carcinomas occur in persons with blue, green, or gray irides.

23. Answer—e. Capillary hemangioma is the most common benign primary orbital tumor among children. Orbital cellulitis is the most common cause of unilateral exophthalmos in children. Metastatic neuroblastoma is the most common metastatic cancer of the orbit in children. Neurofibromas are rarely malignant and are uncommon orbital tumors in children. Graves ophthalmopathy is very rare in children.

24. Answer—a. Adenoma sebaceum is associated with tuberous sclerosis, another phakomatosis.

25. Answer—a. Unilaterality is characteristic of hemifacial spasm, not essential blepharospasm. Essential blepharospasm occurs most frequently over the age of 50 and causes visual incapacitation related to involuntary episodic total bilateral eyelid closure secondary to involuntary episodic spasm of the orbicularis muscles. The etiology is still unknown.

26. Answer—e. Skin grafting is used to correct cicatricial *ectropion*. The skin graft vertically lengthens the anterior lamella of the eyelid, allowing the eyelid margin to rotate posteriorly into a normal anatomic position.

27. Answer—a. In addition to acute fulminant fungal sinusitis with orbital invasion, aspergillosis can cause chronic indolent infection resulting in slow destruction of the sinuses and adjacent structures.

28. Answer—b. Apocrine hidrocystomas, which develop from the glands of Moll, are common clear cystic structures that occur along the eyelid margin. They tend to enlarge slowly. In contrast, epidermal inclusion cysts are not clear but contain white keratin material. Syringomas arise from the eccrine sweat glands and thus do not appear at the eyelid margin.

29. Answer—c. Generally speaking, traumatic eyelid margin flaps should always be saved and carefully reapproximated in order to preserve the eyelid margin architecture and lashes as much as possible and to avoid more involved closure techniques.

30. Answer—d. Basal cell carcinomas occur approximately 40 times more often than either sebaceous carcinomas or squamous cell carcinomas. Even though both sebaceous cell carcinomas and squamous cell carcinomas occur more often in the upper eyelid than they do in the lower and basal cell carcinoma occurs more often in the lower lid than in the upper, the far greater frequency of basal cell carcinoma results in its still being the most common malignant neoplasm of the upper eyelid.

31. Answer—d. The majority of histologically malignant lymphoid lesions of the orbit are relatively indolent or low-grade lymphomas.

32. Answer—e. The levator palpebrae muscle fibers are sparse and are usually replaced by fibrofatty tissue in most cases of congenital ptosis. The lacrimal gland is divided by the lateral expansion of the aponeurosis, and the orbital septum fuses with the aponeurosis just above the upper tarsal margin. Whitnall's ligament serves as a check ligament to the muscle to change its vector of force from anteroposterior to a more vertical direction to elevate the eyelid.

33. Answer—c. Sudden pain associated with tense, ecchymotic eyelids following blepharoplasty is indicative of a postoperative orbital hematoma. If there is no decreased vision, altered pupillary response, or other indication of decreased optic nerve function, the patient may be managed conservatively with close observation. If there is any evidence of optic nerve or ocular compromise, the wounds should be opened immediately and drains inserted to decompress a possible orbital hemorrhage. A lateral canthotomy and inferior cantholysis should be performed next if the above is not effective.

34. Answer—b. This is a typical presentation of primary acquired nasolacrimal duct obstruction. Mucopurulent discharge with compression of the sac or with irrigation is typical. If the common canaliculus were blocked, there would not be discharge and the irrigation would not enter the sac to cause a mucopurulent reflux. Medical management does not offer a long-term cure. The appropriate treatment is dacryocystorhinostomy.

35. Answer—c. A child with congenital tearing is likely to have a nasolacrimal duct problem. Other abnormalities, such as punctal agenesis or lacrimal sac fistulas, are rare but should be ruled out. Dye disappearance testing is usually markedly asymmetric. Jones tests are not necessary to make the diagnosis in the typical case. In general, the problem should be treated with massage and antibiotic drops until the child is 12 or 13 months old. Nasolacrimal probing is usually curative and, in severe cases, may be undertaken at an earlier age.

36. Answer—c. Blepharophimosis syndrome usually includes telecanthus, epicanthus inversus, and ptosis with poor levator function. Ectropion occurs less often. Distichiasis is not associated with the syndrome.

37. Answer—d. If ptosis is present, the wound should be explored. If orbital fat (preaponeurotic fat pad) is visible, exploration of the deeper orbital structures should be undertaken. Repair of the levator aponeurosis is indicated as a primary procedure.

38. Answer—d. Rhabdomyosarcoma is not treated by surgery but rather by systemic multiagent chemotherapy and by orbital radiation therapy (4000–4500 rads) that begins about 2 weeks after the initiation of chemotherapy.

39. Answer—d. Medial canthal trauma usually results from tangential (lateral) forceful traction on the lower eyelid causing an avulsion type of injury at the weakest point of the eyelid, the medial canthal tendon. This frequently involves the canalicular system. Repair can be easily delayed 12–24 hours. Delayed lacrimal repair (>6 months) will require a CJDCR with Jones tube.

40. Answer—c. In blowout fractures, the presence of significant restrictive defects on upgaze due to entrapment of the inferior rectus indicates surgical repair. However, inferior rectus weakness is generally caused by a contusive injury to the inferior rectus muscle and is more likely to worsen after surgical repair.

41. Answer—b. The temporal dissection occurs in the potential space between the temporoparietal fascia superficially and the deep temporal fascia. The frontalis muscle and surrounding galea are superficial to the central subperiosteal dissection.

42. Answer—c. The superficial musculoaponeurotic system (SMAS) is a fibromuscular layer that provides excellent long-term support for the face. Facelifts that rely on the skin for tension fail early and can cause a "surgical" appearance; they also tend to be associated with more obvious scarring and earlobe deformities.

43. Answer—b. Cicatricial shortening of the anterior lamella (skin and muscle) relative to the posterior lamella (tarsus and conjunctiva) of the eyelid produces an outward rotation of the lid margin and retraction of the lid away from the globe, leading to exposure keratopathy.

44. Answer—d. Optic nerve gliomas are uncommon, usually benign, tumors that occur predominantly in children in the first decade of life. Malignant optic nerve gliomas (glioblastomas) are very rare and most often occur in middle-aged males. About 25%–50% of optic nerve gliomas are associated with neurofibromatosis.

45. Answer—a. Early implant extrusion is typically associated with either poor wound closure or an implant that is too large.

Index

(i = image; t = table)

Abducens nerve. *See* Cranial nerve VI
Abscesses, orbital, 42–44, 45i
Accessory lacrimal glands
    of Krause, 140i, 145, 253
    of Wolfring, 140i, 145, 253
ACE. *See* Angiotensin-converting enzyme
Acetylcholine receptor antibody tests, for myasthenia gravis, 213
Acrocephalosyndactyly (Apert syndrome), 38
Acrochordons (skin tags), 163, 164i
Acropachy, in Graves ophthalmopathy, 53
Acrospiroma, eccrine (clear cell hidradenoma), 167
Actinic (solar) keratosis, 172i, 172–173
Actinomyces israelii, canaliculitis caused by, 276
Acute lymphoblastic leukemia, orbital involvement in, 94–95
Adenocarcinoma, sebaceous, 180–182, 180i, 181i
    medial canthal/lacrimal sac involvement and, 284
Adenoid cystic carcinoma (cylindroma)
    of eyelid, 168
    of lacrimal glands, 90–91
Adenoma
    pleomorphic (benign mixed tumor)
        of eyelid, 167
        of lacrimal gland, 89
    sebaceous (sebaceum), 167
Adnexa. *See* Ocular adnexa
Advancement flaps
    for canthal repair, 192
    for eyelid repair, 190i, 192
Afferent pupillary defects, in traumatic optic neuropathy, 107
Aging
    extrinsic, 236
    facial changes caused by
        cosmetic surgery and, 235–248. *See also specific procedure*
        pathogenesis of, 236
        physical examination of, 236
    intrinsic, 236
AIDS. *See* HIV infection
Albright syndrome, 81
Allergic aspergillosis, sinusitis and, 46–47
Alpha (α) interferon, for capillary hemangioma, 66
Alveolar rhabdomyosarcoma, 80
Amblyopia, in congenital ptosis, 211
Ampullectomy, 274
ANA/ANCA. *See* Antinuclear (antineutrophil) antibodies
Anesthesia (anesthetics)
    for blepharoplasty, 231
    for eyelid surgery, 150–151
Angiography, in orbital evaluation, 34
    for arteriovenous fistulas, 70
    magnetic resonance, 34
Angiotensin-converting enzyme (ACE), in sarcoidosis, 36
Angular artery, 255
    eyelids supplied by, 147

Angular vein, 255
    eyelids drained by, 147
Animal bites, eyelid injuries caused by, 187
Ankyloblepharon, 154–156, 155i
Annulus of Zinn, 14, 14i, 15
Anophthalmic ectropion, 126–127
Anophthalmic ptosis, 127
Anophthalmic socket, 119–129. *See also specific aspect*
    complications and treatment of, 124–127, 124i, 125i, 126i
    contracted, 125–126, 126i
    enucleation and, 119–122
    evisceration and, 119, 123–124
    exenteration and, 119, 127–129, 128i
Anophthalmos (anophthalmia), 37
Anterior orbitotomy, 109–114
    inferior approach for, 110–111, 112i, 113i
    medial approach for, 111–114
    superior approach for, 109–110
Antinuclear (antineutrophil) antibodies, in Wegener granulomatosis, 36, 60–61
Antiviral therapy, before laser skin resurfacing, 238
Antoni A pattern/Antoni B pattern, in schwannomas, 79
Apert syndrome (acrocephalosyndactyly), 38
Apocrine glands of eyelid, 166
    tumors arising in, 167–168, 169i
Aponeurotic ptosis, 215, 216i, 217t
Arcus marginalis, 12
Argon laser therapy
    for punctal occlusion, 274
    for trichiasis, 208
Arteriography. *See* Angiography
Arteriovenous fistulas, orbital, 70, 71i
Arteriovenous malformations, orbital, 69–70
Arteritis, giant cell (temporal), 59–60
Asian eyelid, epicanthus tarsalis and, 156
Aspergillus (aspergillosis), 46–47
Auscultation, in orbital disorders, 27
AVM. *See* Arteriovenous malformations
Axial displacement of globe, in orbital disorders, 23

B-cell lymphomas, marginal zone, 85, 86t
Bacteria, orbital infections caused by
    cellulitis, 42–43
    necrotizing fasciitis, 44–45
Balloon catheters, in dacryocystorhinostomy, 283
Balloon dacryoplasty (balloon catheter dilation), for congenital tearing/nasolacrimal duct obstruction, 264–265
Basal cell carcinoma
    of eyelid, 174–179, 175i
    medial canthal/lacrimal sac involvement and, 284
Basal cell nevus syndrome (Gorlin syndrome), 174
Basal skull fracture, arteriovenous fistula caused by, 70
BEB. *See* Benign essential blepharospasm
Benign essential blepharospasm, 226
Benign mixed tumor (pleomorphic adenoma)
    of eyelid, 167

of lacrimal gland, 89
Beta (β)-hemolytic group A streptococci (*Streptococcus pyogenes*), orbital necrotizing fasciitis caused by, 44–45
Betamethasone, for capillary hemangioma, 66
Bick procedure, 198
Bites, eyelid injuries caused by, 187
Blepharochalasis, 228–229
Blepharophimosis syndrome, 153, 154*i*, 212
    with congenital ectropion, 154
    with epicanthus, 156
Blepharoplasty, 229–234
    complications of, 232–234, 233*i*
        eyelid retraction, 224, 233, 233*i*
    infraciliary incision for, for anterior orbitotomy, 110–111
    laser resurfacing as adjunct to, 237
    techniques for, 230–232
Blepharoptosis. *See* Ptosis
Blepharospasm
    botulinum toxin for, 226
    essential, 226
Blindness. *See also* Visual loss
    after blepharoplasty, 232
Blowout fractures
    of medial orbital wall, 101–102
    orbital cellulitis following, 42
    of orbital floor, 21, 102–106, 103*i*
    surgery for, 104–106
Blue nevus, 171
Blunt trauma
    eyelid, 184
    ptosis caused by, 219
Bone, unifocal and multifocal eosinophilic granuloma of, 88
Botox. *See* Botulinum toxin
Botryoid rhabdomyosarcoma, 80
Botulinum toxin
    for acute spastic entropion, 202
    for blepharospasm, 226
    cosmetic uses of, 239
    for hemifacial spasm, 226
    ptosis caused by, 219
Bowen disease, 173
Bowman probe, 262, 263*i*
Breast cancer, eye/orbital metastases of, 95*i*, 96
Bronchogenic carcinoma, orbital metastases in, 96
Brow and forehead lift, 239–241, 240*i*
Brow lift, 241
Brow ptosis, 234–235, 234*i*
Browpexy, 235
Bruits, in orbital disorders, 27
Buccal mucous membrane graft
    for eyelid repair, 187
    for symblepharon, 207
Bupivacaine, for blepharoplasty, 231
Burns, eyelid, 187

Café-au-lait spots, in neurofibromatosis, 75
Canal
    nasolacrimal, 11, 256
        balloon catheter dilation of, for congenital tearing/nasolacrimal duct obstruction, 264–265
    optic, 11–12
        decompression of, for traumatic visual loss, 108
    zygomaticofacial, 11
    zygomaticotemporal, 11
Canaliculi, lacrimal, 254, 255*i*
    congenital abnormalities of, 257–258
    infection or inflammation of, 268*i*, 276, 276*i*
    obstruction of, 271*i*, 275
        irrigation in evaluation of, 270–271, 270*t*, 275
    trauma to, 186, 276–277
Canaliculitis, 268*i*, 276, 276*i*
Canaliculodacryocystorhinostomy, for canalicular obstruction, 275
Canaliculotomy, for canaliculitis, 276
Canthal reconstruction, 188–193. *See also* Eyelids, reconstruction of
Canthal tendons, 146
    lateral, 146
    medial, 146
    trauma involving, 186
Canthal tissues, trauma involving, 186
Canthal tumors, 277–278
Cantholysis
    for traumatic visual loss, 107
    for trichiasis, 208
Canthotomy
    lateral, for lateral orbitotomy, 114
    for traumatic visual loss, 107
Capillary hemangiomas
    of eyelid, 158
    of orbit, 26, 64–66, 66*i*
Capsulopalpebral fascia, 140–141, 145
Carbon dioxide laser
    for orbital lymphangioma, 69
    for skin resurfacing, 237–238
Carcinoma
    adenoid cystic (cylindroma)
        of eyelid, 168
        of lacrimal glands, 90–91
    basal cell
        of eyelid, 174–179, 175*i*
        medial canthal/lacrimal sac involvement and, 284
    squamous cell
        of eyelid, 179–180, 179*i*
            in situ (Bowen disease), 173
        medial canthal/lacrimal sac involvement and, 284
        of orbit, secondary, 92*i*, 93
Carotid arteries
    eyelids supplied by, 147
    orbit supplied by, 15
Carotid cavernous fistula, 70, 71*i*
Carotid system, eyelids supplied by, 147
Cautery, thermal
    for involutional ectropion, 197
    for involutional entropion, 204
Cavernous carotid fistula, 70, 71*i*
Cavernous hemangioma, of orbit, 67, 68*i*
Cavernous sinus thrombosis, septic, orbital infections causing, 42, 44
Cellulitis, 41–44
    orbital, 20, 42–44, 43*i*, 44*t*, 45*i*
        fungal (mucormycosis), 45–46
            exenteration in management of, 45–46, 128
    preseptal, 41–42

in children, 41
Haemophilus causing, 41
Central surgical space (intraconal fat/surgical space), 12–13, 109, 110*i*
Chalazion, 158–159, 160*i*
Cheek advancement flap (Mustardé flap), for eyelid repair, 191*i*, 192
Cheek elevation, in eyelid repair, 192
Chemotherapy (cancer)
   for lacrimal gland tumors, 91
   for optic nerve glioma, 75
   for rhabdomyosarcoma, 80
Children
   enucleation in, 121
   orbital cellulitis in, 42
   orbital metastatic disease in, 94, 94*i*
   preseptal cellulitis in, 41
Chloasma, of eyelids, 170
Chloroma (granulocytic sarcoma), 94–95
Chocolate cyst, of orbit, 68
Chondrosarcoma, of orbit, 81
Choristomas, of orbit, 63
Choroid, melanoma of, enucleation for, 120
Cicatricial ectropion, 196*i*, 200–201
   after blepharoplasty, 233
Cicatricial entropion, 205–207, 205*i*, 206*i*
Cigarette smoking, thyroid disease and, 53–54
Cilia. *See* Eyelashes
Ciliary margin, 146
Ciliary nerves, long and short, 15
CJDCR. *See* Conjunctivodacryocystorhinostomy
Clear cell hidradenoma (eccrine acrospiroma), 167
Cleft syndromes, 38–39, 38*i*, 39*i*
   lacrimal outflow disorders and, 258, 258*i*
CO_2 laser. *See* Carbon dioxide laser
Cocaine, in Horner syndrome diagnosis, 212, 212*i*
Collagen plugs, for dry eye, 274
Colobomas, eyelid, 157–158, 157*i*
Colobomatous cyst (microphthalmos with cyst), 37–38
Compartment syndrome, visual loss after orbital trauma and, 104
Compound nevi, 170–171
Computed tomography (CT scan)
   in acquired tearing evaluation, 272
   in orbital evaluation, 29
      MRI compared with, 31–33, 32*i*, 33*t*
Concave (minus) lenses, anophthalmic socket camouflage and, 127
Conchae (turbinates), nasal, 20
   infracture of, for congenital tearing/nasolacrimal duct obstruction, 263, 265*i*
Congenital anomalies. *See also specific type*
   craniofacial malformations, 38–39, 38*i*, 39*i*
   of eyelid, 153–158
   of orbit, 38–39, 38*i*, 39*i*
Congenital ptosis. *See* Ptosis
Conjunctiva, 140*i*, 141*i*, 142*i*, 145
   epithelium of, evaluation of, in pseudoepiphora, 273
Conjunctival flaps, for symblepharon, 207
Conjunctivodacryocystorhinostomy
   for canalicular obstruction, 275–276
   after canthal repair, 193
   for punctal agenesis and dysgenesis, 265
Connective tissue disorders, vasculitis associated with, 60

Contracted fornices, anophthalmic socket and, 125
Contracted socket, 125–126, 126*i*
Convex (plus) lenses, anophthalmic socket camouflage and, 127
Cornea, epithelium of, evaluation of, in pseudoepiphora, 273
Coronal scalp flap, for anterior orbitotomy, 110
Corrugator muscle, 140, 143*i*
Corticosteroids (steroids)
   for eyelid hemangioma, 158
   for idiopathic orbital inflammation, 58
   in orbital surgery, 114–115
   for traumatic visual loss, 104, 108
Cosmetic facial surgery, 235–248. *See also specific procedure*
Cosmetic optics, for anophthalmic socket, 127
Cranial fossa, middle, 21
Cranial nerve II. *See* Optic nerve
Cranial nerve III (oculomotor nerve), 13, 14
   aberrant regeneration of, synkinesis in, 211, 215–217
   congenital palsy of, ptosis caused by, 215–217
Cranial nerve IV (trochlear nerve), 13, 14
Cranial nerve V (trigeminal nerve)
   V_1 (ophthalmic nerve), 14, 15
      facial innervation and, 137
      in reflex tear arc, 253
   V_2 (maxillary nerve), 15
      facial innervation and, 137
Cranial nerve VI (abducens nerve), 13, 14
Cranial nerve VII (facial nerve), 15, 136, 136*i*, 137–139, 138*i*
   aberrant regeneration of, synkinesis in, 211, 227–228
   in hemifacial spasm, 227–228
   palsy of, paralytic ectropion and, 199
   in reflex tear arc, 253
   surgical ablation of, for benign essential blepharospasm, 227
Cranial nerves
   eyelids supplied by, 147
   orbit supplied by, 14*i*, 15, 19*i*
Craniofacial cleft syndromes, 38–39, 38*i*, 39*i*
   lacrimal outflow disorders and, 257–258, 258*i*
Craniofacial dysostosis (Crouzon syndrome), 38, 39*i*
Craniofacial malformations, 38–39, 38*i*, 39*i*
   Apert syndrome (acrocephalosyndactyly), 38
   craniosynostosis, 38
   Crouzon syndrome, 38, 39*i*
   mandibulofacial dysostosis (Treacher Collins–Franceschetti syndrome), 38, 38*i*
Craniosynostosis, 38
Creases, eyelid. *See* Eyelids, creases of
Crigler massage, for nasolacrimal duct obstruction, 261
Crouzon syndrome (craniofacial dysostosis), 38–39, 39*i*
Cryotherapy
   for basal cell carcinoma of eyelid, 179
   for congenital distichiasis, 157
   for trichiasis, 208
Cryptophthalmos, 158, 159*i*
CT scan. *See* Computed tomography
Cutaneous horn, 164
Cutler-Beard procedure, 189, 190*i*
Cylindroma (adenoid cystic carcinoma)
   of eyelid, 168
   of lacrimal glands, 90–91

Cystadenoma (apocrine hidrocystoma), of eyelid, 167–168, 169*i*
Cystic carcinoma, adenoid (cylindroma)
  of eyelid, 168
  of lacrimal glands, 90–91
Cysticercosis, orbital involvement and, 47

Dacryocystectomy, for lacrimal sac tumors, 284
Dacryocystitis, 278–283
  acute, 279*i*, 278–279
  chronic, 279
  tumor associated with, 283–284
Dacryocystocele/dacryocele, 260–261, 260*i*
Dacryocystography
  for acquired tearing evaluation, 272, 273*i*
  for dacryolith evaluation, 284
  for lacrimal sac tumor evaluation, 284
Dacryocystorhinostomy, 279–283, 281*i*, 282*i*
  for congenital tearing/nasolacrimal duct obstruction, 266–267
  for dacryocystitis, 279–283, 281*i*, 282*i*
Dacryoliths, 283
Dacryoplasty, balloon (balloon catheter dilation), for congenital tearing/nasolacrimal duct obstruction, 264–265
DCR. *See* Dacryocystorhinostomy
DDT. *See* Dye disappearance test
Decompression
  optic canal, for traumatic visual loss, 108
  orbital, 115, 116*i*
    complications of, 117
    for Graves ophthalmopathy, 54, 115
    for lymphangioma, 69
    for traumatic visual loss, 107, 108
Deep mimetic muscles, 135–137, 138–139
Deep plane rhytidectomy, 241*i*, 245
Deep superior sulcus deformity, anophthalmic socket and, 124, 124*i*
Deep temporalis fascia, 138
Depression of eye (downgaze)
  disorders of, in blowout fractures, 102–104
    surgery and, 104
  ptosis exacerbation in, 208–209
  ptotic eyelid position in, 211
Dermal melanocytosis, 171–172. *See also* Oculodermal melanocytosis
Dermatochalasis, 228, 228*i*
  pseudoptosis and, 220*i*, 219
Dermis-fat grafts
  for anophthalmos, 37, 121
  for exposure and extrusion of orbital implant, 125
  for superior sulcus deformity, 124
Dermoids (dermoid cysts/tumors), orbital, 63–64, 65*i*
Dermolipomas (lipodermoids), of orbit, 64, 65*i*
Dermopathy, thyroid, in Graves ophthalmopathy, 53
Diffuse soft-tissue histiocytosis. *See* Histiocytosis
Diplopia
  after blepharoplasty, 233
  in blowout fractures, 102–104
    surgery and, 104
Distichiasis
  acquired, 147
  congenital, 147, 157
Dog bites, eyelid injuries caused by, 187

Dog tapeworm (*Echinococcus granulosus*), orbital infection caused by, 47
Doppler imaging, in orbital evaluation, 34
Double convexity deformity, 236
Double elevator palsy/paresis (monocular elevation deficiency), 214
Downgaze. *See* Depression of eye
Dry eye
  in blepharospasm, 226, 227
  punctal occlusion for, 274
Duane syndrome, synkinesis in, 211, 217
Dural sinus fistula, 70
Dye disappearance test, 268, 269*i*
Dysthyroid ophthalmopathy. *See* Graves disease/ophthalmopathy
Dystonia, facial, 226–228

Eccrine sweat glands of eyelid, 167
  tumors arising in, 167, 168*i*
Echinococcus granulosus (echinococcosis), orbital infection caused by, 47
Ectropion, 195–201, 196*i*
  anophthalmic, 126–127
  cicatricial, 196*i*, 200–201
    after blepharoplasty, 233
  congenital, 154, 155*i*
  involutional, 195–198, 196*i*, 197*i*
  mechanical, 196*i*, 201
  paralytic, 196*i*, 199–200, 200*i*
  tarsal, 198
Edema, eyelid, 160
Edrophonium, in myasthenia gravis diagnosis, 213
Electrolysis, for trichiasis, 207
Elevated intraocular pressure, orbital trauma and, 107–108
Elevation of eye (upgaze)
  disorders of, in blowout fractures, 102–104, 103*i*
    surgery and, 104
  monocular deficiency of (double elevator palsy), 214
Embryonal rhabdomyosarcoma, 80
Emphysema (ocular), of orbit and eyelids, in blowout fractures, 101–102, 104
Encephaloceles, 38
Endocanalicular laser dacryocystorhinostomy, 281–282
Endophthalmitis, evisceration for, 123
Endoscopic brow and forehead lift, 239–241, 240*i*
Endoscopic brow lift, 241
Endoscopic dacryocystorhinostomy, 282–283, 282*i*
Endoscopic midface lift, 243*i*, 248–249
Endoscopy, nasal, for acquired tearing evaluation, 271
Enophthalmos, 24, 25
  in blowout fractures, 102, 103
    surgery and, 105
  orbital varices and, 70
Entropion, 201–207
  acute spastic, 201–202, 202*i*
  cicatricial, 205–207, 205*i*, 206*i*
  congenital, 156–157
  involutional, 202–205, 203*i*
  lash margin, in anophthalmic socket, 127
Enucleation, 119–122
  in childhood, 121
  complications of, 123
  definition of, 119

guidelines for, 120–121
ocular prostheses after, 122
orbital implants after, 121–122
for prevention of sympathetic ophthalmia, 119–120
removal of wrong eye and, 123
Eosinophilic granuloma of bone, unifocal and multifocal, of orbit, 88
Ephelis (freckle), of eyelid, 171
Epiblepharon, 155*i*, 156
Epicanthus, 155*i*, 156
  inversus, 156
  palpebralis, 156
  supraciliaris, 156
  tarsalis, 156
Epidermal cysts, of eyelid, 164–166, 165*i*
Epidermis, eyelid, neoplasms of
  benign, 164–166, 165*i*
  premalignant, 172–173, 172*i*, 173*i*
Epidermoid cysts, of orbit, 63
Epilation, mechanical, for trichiasis, 207
Epimyoepithelial islands, 92
Epinephrine, with local anesthetic
  for blepharoplasty, 231
  for eyelid surgery, 150
Epiphora. *See* Tearing
Episcleral surgical space, 109
Epithelial cysts, of eyelids, benign, 164–166, 165*i*
Epithelial hyperplasias, of eyelids, 163–164, 164–165*i*
Epithelial tumors, of lacrimal glands, 89–91, 90*i*
  exenteration for, 128
Epithelium
  conjunctival, evaluation of, in pseudoepiphora, 273
  corneal, evaluation of, in pseudoepiphora, 273
  eyelid, hyperplasia of, 163–164, 164*i*, 165*i*
Essential blepharospasm, 226
Ethmoid air cells, 20, 20*i*
Ethmoidal bone (lamina papyracea), 7, 8*i*, 9, 9*i*
Ethmoidal foramen, anterior/posterior, 9*i*, 11
Euryblepharon, 154, 155*i*
Evisceration, 123–124
  definition of, 119, 123
Excisional biopsy, 176*i*, 177
Excretory lacrimal system, 253–256, 255*i*, 256*i*. *See also* Lacrimal drainage system
Exenteration, 127–129, 128*i*
  definition of, 119, 127
  histopathology findings and, 114
  for lacrimal gland tumors, 90, 128, 284
Exophthalmometry, 25
Exophthalmos, 24. *See also* Proptosis, in Graves ophthalmopathy (thyrotoxic)
Exorbitism, 24–25. *See also* Proptosis
External dacryocystorhinostomy, 280–281, 281*i*
External hordeolum (stye), 160
Extraconal fat/surgical space (peripheral surgical space), 12–13, 109, 110*i*
Extraocular muscles, 12–13
  damage to
    during blepharoplasty, 233
    in blowout fractures, 102–104
      surgery and, 104–105
    during enucleation, 123
  in Graves ophthalmopathy, 48, 50*i*, 53
  innervation of, 12–13

in ptosis, 211–212
tumors of, eye movements affected by, 26
Extraocular myopathy, restrictive, in Graves ophthalmopathy, 48, 53
Extraperiosteal route
  for inferior anterior orbitotomy, 111
  for superior anterior orbitotomy, 109–110
Exuberant hyperkeratosis (cutaneous horn), 164
Eye, removal of. *See* Anophthalmic socket; Enucleation; Evisceration; Exenteration
Eye movements
  disorders of
    in blowout fractures, 102–104, 103*i*
      surgery and, 104–105
    conditions causing, 26
    in Graves ophthalmopathy, 26
    after orbital surgery, 117
  extraocular muscles controlling, 12–13
Eyebrows
  direct elevation of, 235
  drooping of (brow ptosis), 234–235, 234*i*
Eyelashes (cilia), 146–147
  entropion/ptosis of, in anophthalmic socket, 127
  in epiblepharon, 155*i*, 156
  misdirection of. *See* Trichiasis
Eyelid crutches, for ptosis, 220
Eyelid imbrication syndrome, 161
Eyelid-sharing techniques, in eyelid repair, 189–192
Eyelid springs, for paralytic ectropion, 199–200
Eyelid weights, for paralytic ectropion, 199
Eyelids
  anatomy of, 139–147, 140*i*, 142*i*, 144*i*
  basal cell carcinoma of, 174–179, 175*i*
  biopsy of, 176–177, 176*i*
  canthal tendons and, 146
  coloboma of, 157–158, 157*i*
  congenital anomalies of, 153–158
  conjunctiva of, 140*i*, 141*i*, 142*i*, 145
  creases of, 139, 143
    in ptosis, 210, 210*i*
  disorders of, 153–193. *See also specific type*
    acquired, 158–161
    congenital, 153–158
    in Graves ophthalmopathy, 26, 48–51, 48*i*, 53. *See also* Graves disease/ophthalmopathy
    neoplastic, 162–184
    traumatic, 184–188
  ectropion of, 195–201, 196*i*. *See also* Ectropion
  edema of, 160
  emphysema of, in blowout fractures, 101–102, 104
  entropion of, 201–207. *See also* Entropion
  eversion of. *See* Ectropion
  floppy, 160–161, 161*i*
  fusion of (ankyloblepharon), 154–156, 155*i*
  glands of. *See also specific type*
    benign tumors of, 167
  horizontal shortening/tightening of
    for cicatricial ectropion, 200–201
    for involutional ectropion, 198
    for involutional entropion, 204
  inversion of. *See* Entropion
  keratosis of
    actinic (solar), 172–173, 172*i*
    inverted follicular, 163

seborrheic, 163, 165*i*
lacerations of
  lid margin involved in, 185, 185*i*
  lid margin not involved in, 184–185
  ptosis caused by, 219
  repair of, 184–187, 185*i*
    secondary, 186–187
lower
  blepharoplasty on, 229–230, 231–232
    laser resurfacing as adjunct to, 237–238
    visual loss after, 232–233
  crease of, 139
  entropion of, 200–202. *See also* Entropion
  horizontal laxity of, in involutional ectropion, 197–198
  reconstruction of, 189–192, 191*i*
  retraction of, treatment of, 224–225
  retractors of, 141*i*, 144*i*, 145
    in involutional ectropion, repair of, 198, 202–203
    in involutional entropion, 202–203
      repair of, 203*i*, 204–205
    vertical elevation of, for paralytic ectropion, 199–200
malpositions of, 195–234. *See also specific type*
margin of, 142*i*, 146
  lacerations of, 185, 185*i*
  repair of defects in, 189–192, 190*i*, 191*i*
nerve supply of, 147
orbital septum and, 140–141, 140*i*, 141*i*
orbital tumors originating in, 92
protractors of, 139–140, 143*i*
reconstruction of, 188–193
  after basal cell carcinoma surgery, 178–179
  for blepharophimosis syndrome, 153
  for defects involving eyelid margin, 189–192, 190*i*, 191*i*
  for defects not involving eyelid margin, 188–189
  for epicanthus, 156
  for euryblepharon, 154
  general principles of, 188
  after Mohs' micrographic surgery, 178–179
retraction of, 223–225, 224*i*
  after blepharoplasty, 224, 233, 233*i*
  in Graves ophthalmopathy, 26, 48, 48–51, 48*i*, 53, 223–224, 224*i*
    proptosis differentiated from, 223–224
  after strabismus surgery, 224
  treatment of, 224–225
retractors of, 141*i*, 142–145, 144*i*
  in involutional ectropion, repair of, 198, 202–203, 204–205
  in involutional entropion, 202–203
    repair of, 203*i*, 204–205
skin of, 139, 140*i*, 141*i*
subcutaneous tissue of, 139
suborbicularis fat pads and, 141*i*, 145–146
  midface rejuvenation surgery and (SOOF lift), 241–242, 242*i*
surgery of
  anesthesia for, 150–151
  for basal cell carcinoma, 177–179
  for blepharophimosis syndrome, 153
  blepharoplasty, 229–230

  for epicanthus, 156
  for euryblepharon, 154
  for eyelid retraction, 54, 225
  for Graves ophthalmopathy, 54
  patient preparation for, 149
  principles of, 149–151
  for ptosis repair, 220–223, 221*i*
symblepharon and, 207
tarsus of, 140*i*, 141*i*, 145
trauma to, 184–188
  blunt, 184
  penetrating, 184–186
  ptosis caused by, 219
  repair of, 184–187, 185*i*
tumors of, 162–184
  basal cell carcinoma, 174–179, 175*i*
  benign, 163–166
  biopsy in evaluation of, 176–177, 176*i*
  clinical evaluation/diagnostic approaches to, 162–163
  epidermal
    benign, 164–166, 165*i*
    premalignant, 172–173, 172*i*, 173*i*
  malignant, 174–184
  masquerading neoplasms and, 184
  mechanical ptosis caused by, 219
  melanocytic, 169–172
    benign, 169–170, 170*i*, 172*i*
    malignant (melanoma), 182–183
    premalignant, 174
upper
  blepharoplasty on, 229–230, 231
  congenital eversion of, 154, 155*i*
  crease of, 139, 140*i*, 143
    in ptosis, 210, 210*i*
  entropion of, 200–201. *See also* Entropion
  reconstruction of, 188–189, 190*i*
  retractors of, 142–144, 144*i*
vascular supply of, 147
vertical splitting of, for anterior orbitotomy, 110

Face. *See also under* Facial
  aging affecting, cosmetic/rejuvenation surgery and, 235–248
    lower face and neck surgery, 244–247, 245*i*, 246*i*, 247*i*
    midface surgery (suborbicularis oculi fat/midface lift), 241–242, 242*i*, 243*i*
    upper face surgery (brow and forehead lift), 239–241, 240*i*
  anatomy of, 135–139, 136*i*, 137*i*, 138*i*
Facelift, 244–245, 245*i*, 246*i*
Facial artery, orbit supplied by, 15
Facial clefts, 38–39, 38*i*, 39*i*
  lacrimal outflow disorders and, 258, 258*i*
Facial dystonia, 226–228
Facial muscles, 135–137, 137*i*, 138*i*
Facial nerve. *See* Cranial nerve VII
Facial paralysis/weakness, paralytic ectropion and, 199
Facial surgery, 235–248. *See also specific procedure*
  anesthesia for, 150–151
  cosmetic, 235–248
  patient preparation for, 149
  principles of, 149–151

Facial vein, eyelids drained by, 147
Fasanella-Servat procedure (tarsoconjunctival müllerectomy), for ptosis correction, 222
Fascia lata, autogenous and banked, for frontalis suspension, 222
Fascia lata sling, for paralytic ectropion, 199
Fasciitis, necrotizing, of orbit, 44–45
Fat
　orbital, 12, 141
　sub-brow, 146
　suborbicularis oculi (SOOF/suborbicularis fat pads), 135, 141i, 145–146
　　midface rejuvenation surgery and (SOOF lift), 241–242, 242i
Fat-suppression techniques, in magnetic resonance imaging, 31
Fibrosarcoma, of orbit, 81
Fibrosing (morpheaform) basal cell carcinoma, 175, 175i
Fibrous dysplasia of orbit, 81, 82i
　secondary, 93
Fibrous histiocytoma (fibroxanthoma), orbital, 81
Fine-needle aspiration biopsy (FNAB), of orbit, 35, 116–117
Fissures
　orbital, 10i, 11, 21–22
　　inferior, 10i, 11, 21–22
　　superior, 11, 21
　palpebral
　　congenital widening of (euryblepharon), 154, 155i
　　vertical height of, in ptosis, 206i, 209
Fistulas
　arteriovenous, of orbit, 70, 71i
　carotid cavernous, 70, 71i
　dural sinus, 70
　lacrimal, congenital, 258, 258i, 266–267
Flaps
　for canthal repair, 192–193
　coronal scalp, for anterior orbitotomy, 110
　for eyelid repair, 189–193, 190i
　for symblepharon, 207
"Flesh-eating disease." See Necrotizing fasciitis
Floppy eyelid syndrome, 160–161, 161i
Fluorescein
　for dye disappearance test, 268
　for Jones I and Jones II tests, 264–266
　for lacrimal irrigation, 263, 264i
FNAB. See Fine-needle aspiration biopsy
Foramen (foramina)
　ethmoidal (anterior/posterior), 9i, 11
　oculomotor, 14
Forced ductions, in blowout fractures, 103
　surgery and, 103
Foreheadplasty, 239–240
Foreign bodies, intraorbital, 106
Fornices, contracture of, anophthalmic socket and, 125
Fossae
　infratemporal, 22
　middle cranial, 21
　orbital, 21–22
　pterygopalatine, 21
Frames (spectacle), anophthalmic socket camouflage and, 127
Freckle, of eyelid, 171

Frontal bone, 7, 8i, 9i
Frontal nerve, 14
Frontal sinuses, 9i, 20, 20i
Frontalis sling, for blepharophimosis syndrome correction, 153
Frontalis suspension, for ptosis correction, 217, 221i, 222
Frontoethmoidal incision, for anterior orbitotomy, 112
Full-thickness eyelid biopsy, 176i, 181–182
Fungi, orbital infections caused by
　aspergillosis, 46–47
　exenteration in management of, 128
　mucormycosis/phycomycosis, 45–46
　　exenteration in management of, 45–46, 128

General anesthesia, for eyelid surgery, 150
Giant cell (temporal) arteritis, 59–60
Glands of Moll, 166. See also Apocrine glands of eyelid
　hidrocystoma arising in, 167–168
Glands of Zeis, sebaceous adenocarcinoma arising in, 180
Glioblastomas, optic nerve (malignant optic nerve gliomas), 72
Gliomas, optic nerve, 72–75, 73i
　malignant (glioblastomas), 72
　in neurofibromatosis, 72–74, 76
Globe
　displacement of, in orbital disorders, 23, 24
　orbital tumors originating in, 92
　ptosis of, in blowout fractures, 103
Goblet cells, mucin tear secretion by, 253
Gold eyelid weights, for paralytic ectropion, 199
Goldenhar syndrome (oculoauricular/oculoauriculovertebral dysplasia), 38
GORE-TEX, for frontalis suspension, 222
Gorlin syndrome (basal cell nevus syndrome), 174
Grafts
　for canthal repair, 193
　for cicatricial ectropion, 200–201
　for cicatricial entropion, 207
　dermis-fat
　　for anophthalmos, 37, 121
　　for exposure and extrusion of orbital implant, 125
　　for superior sulcus deformity, 124
　for eyelid repair, 187, 190i, 191i
　for symblepharon, 207
　tarsoconjunctival
　　for cicatricial entropion, 207
　　for eyelid repair, 187, 190i, 191i, 192
Granulocytic sarcoma (chloroma), 94–95
Granulomas, eosinophilic, of orbit, 88
Granulomatosis, Wegener, 60–61, 61i
　diagnosis of, 36, 60–61
Granulomatous disease, nasolacrimal obstruction caused by, 278
Graves disease/ophthalmopathy (thyroid ophthalmopathy, dysthyroidism, thyroid orbitopathy), 48–56, 48i, 49–50i
　clinical presentation and diagnosis of, 48–51, 51i, 53
　epidemiology of, 52–53
　euthyroid, 48
　eye movements affected in, 26
　eyelid disorders and, 26, 48–51, 48i, 53
　　retraction, 26, 48–51, 48i, 53, 223–225, 224i

myasthenia gravis and, 53
pathogenesis of, 51–52
prognosis of, 53–55
proptosis and, 26
  eyelid retraction differentiated from, 224
thyroid function tests in, 35–36
treatment of, 53–55
Gray line (intermarginal sulcus), 142*i*, 146
Group A beta-hemolytic streptococci *(Streptococcus pyogenes),* orbital necrotizing fasciitis caused by, 44–45
Guerin (maxillary) fracture, 98*i*

H zone, basal cell carcinoma in, 177
Haemophilus influenzae, cellulitis caused by, 41, 42
Hair follicles, of eyelid (lash follicles), 142*i*
  tumors arising in, 168–169, 169*i*
Hamartomas, of orbit, 63
Hand-Schüller-Christian syndrome, orbital involvement in, 88
Hard palate composite grafts, for eyelid repair, 187
Hashimoto thyroiditis, in Graves ophthalmopathy, 53
Hasner, valve of, 255*i*, 256
  nasolacrimal duct obstruction and, 257, 261
Hemangiomas (hemangiomatosis)
  of eyelid, 158
  of orbit
    capillary, 26, 64–66, 66*i*
    cavernous, 67, 68*i*
Hemangiopericytoma, of orbit, 67
Hemifacial spasm, 227–228
Hemorrhages
  orbital, 72, 106
    after blepharoplasty, visual loss and, 232–233
    from orbital lymphangioma, 67–68
  retrobulbar, after blepharoplasty, visual loss and, 232–233
Hering's law, eyelid retraction and, 224
Herpes simplex virus, skin infection after laser resurfacing caused by, 238
Hertel exophthalmometer, 25
Hidradenoma, clear cell (eccrine acrospiroma), 167
Hidrocystoma
  apocrine, 167–168, 169*i*
  eccrine, 167
Histiocytic disorders, of orbit, 88
Histiocytoma, fibrous (fibroxanthoma), orbital, 81
Histiocytosis, Langerhans cell (histiocytosis X/diffuse soft tissue histiocytosis), orbital involvement in, 88
HIV infection/AIDS, Kaposi sarcoma in, 183, 183*i*
Hordeolum
  external (stye), 160
  internal, 158–159, 160. *See also* Chalazion
Horizontal eyelid shortening/tightening
  for cicatricial ectropion, 200–201
  for involutional ectropion, 198
  for involutional entropion, 204
Horner syndrome
  congenital, 217
  in neuroblastoma, 94, 94*i*
  pharmacologic testing for, 212–213, 212*i*
Horner's muscle, 255, 256*i*
Horner's tensor tarsi, 140
Hughes procedure/modified Hughes procedure, in eyelid repair, 191*i*, 192

Human bites, eyelid injuries caused by, 187
Hutchinson's melanotic freckle (lentigo maligna/precancerous melanosis), 174
Hydatid cyst, orbital infection caused by rupture of, 47
Hydroxyapatite orbital implants, 122
  exposure and extrusion of, 125*i*
Hyperkeratosis, exuberant (cutaneous horn), 164
Hyperpigmentation, after laser skin resurfacing, 238
Hyperplasia
  epithelial, of eyelid, 163–164, 164*i*, 165*i*
  lymphoid, of orbit, 81–89. *See also* Lymphomas, orbital
  pseudoepitheliomatous, 164
  sebaceous, of eyelid, 166–167
Hypertelorism (telorbitism), 25
  clefting syndromes and, 38
Hyperthyroidism, ophthalmopathy and, 48. *See also* Thyroid ophthalmopathy
  treatment of, 54
Hypoesthesia, in infraorbital nerve distribution, in blowout fractures, 21, 104
Hypothyroidism, ophthalmopathy and, 53

Ice-pack test, for myasthenia gravis, 213
Idiopathic orbital inflammation (orbital inflammatory syndrome/orbital pseudotumor), 56–59, 57*i*
  plasma cell–rich, 88
Idiopathic sclerosing inflammation of orbit, 57, 58. *See also* Idiopathic orbital inflammation
Implants, orbital, 121–122
  in children, 121
  exposure and extrusion of, 125, 125*i*
  for superior sulcus deformity, 124
Incisional biopsy, 176, 176*i*
Incisions
  for orbital surgery, 109, 111*i*
  for rhytidectomy, 244
Inclusion cysts, epidermal, of eyelid, 164–166, 165*i*
Inferior oblique muscles, 13, 141*i*
Inferior orbital fissure, 10*i*, 11, 22
Inferior rectus muscles, 13
Inferior tarsal muscle, 145
Inferolateral displacement of globe, in orbital disorders, 23
Inferomedial displacement of globe, in orbital disorders, 23
Infraciliary blepharoplasty incision, for anterior orbitotomy, 110–111
Infracture of turbinates, for congenital tearing/nasolacrimal duct obstruction, 263, 265*i*
Infraorbital nerve, hypoesthesia in distribution of, in blowout fractures, 21, 104
Infratemporal fossa, 22
Inspection, in orbital disorders, 24–26
Interferon-α, for capillary hemangioma, 66
Intermarginal sulcus (gray line), 142*i*, 146
Intermuscular septum, 12
Interpalpebral fissure, vertical, height of, in ptosis, 209, 210*i*
Intraconal fat/surgical space (central surgical space), 12, 109, 110*i*
Intradermal nevus, 170
Intraocular pressure, elevated, orbital trauma and, 107
Intraocular tumors
  enucleation for, 119–122

exenteration for, 128–129, 128*i*
Intraorbital foreign bodies, 106
Intraorbital portion of optic nerve, 12
   length of, 7*t*, 12
Intraorbital pressure, in traumatic optic neuropathy, 107
Intubation, silicone
   for acquired nasolacrimal obstruction, 278
   for canalicular constriction, 275
   for canalicular trauma, 277
   for congenital lacrimal duct obstruction/tearing, 263–264, 266*i*
Inverted follicular keratosis, 163
Involutional ectropion, 195–198, 196*i*, 197*i*
Involutional entropion, 202–205, 203*i*
Involutional stenosis, nasolacrimal obstruction caused by, 278
Iodine, radioactive, for Graves disease, 54
Irrigation, of lacrimal drainage system
   for acquired tearing evaluation, 270–271, 270*t*
   for canalicular obstruction, 270–271, 270*t*, 271*i*, 275
   for congenital tearing management, 262–263, 264*i*

Jaw winking, in ptosis, 217, 218*i*
Jones I and Jones II tests, 268–270, 269*t*
Junctional nevus, 170–171
Juvenile xanthogranuloma (nevoxanthoendothelioma), of orbit, 88–89

Kaposi sarcoma, of eyelid, 183, 183*i*
Kasabach-Merritt syndrome, 66
Keratoacanthoma, 173, 173*i*
Keratosis
   actinic (solar), 172–173, 172*i*
   inverted follicular, 163
   seborrheic, 163, 165*i*
Krause, glands of, 140*i*, 145, 253

Lacerations
   canalicular, 277
   eyelid
      lid margin involved in, 185, 185*i*
      lid margin not involved in, 184–185
      ptosis caused by, 219
      repair of, 184–187, 185*i*
      secondary, 186–187
Lacrimal bone, 7, 8*i*, 9*i*
Lacrimal canaliculi. *See* Canaliculi, lacrimal
Lacrimal–cutaneous fistula, congenital, 258, 258*i*, 266–267
Lacrimal drainage system, 253–256, 255*i*, 256*i*. *See also* Nasolacrimal duct
   developmental abnormalities of, 257–258
   diagnostic tests for evaluation of, 268–274
   irrigation of
      for acquired tearing evaluation, 270–271, 270*t*, 271*i*
      for canalicular obstruction, 270–271, 271*i*, 275
      for congenital tearing management, 262–263, 264*i*
   obstruction of. *See also* Tearing
      acquired, 268–284
      congenital, 258, 261–265
Lacrimal ducts, 253
Lacrimal glands, 16, 253, 254*i*. *See also* Lacrimal system
   accessory, 140*i*, 145, 253

sarcoidosis involving, 59
tumors of, 89–92, 90*i*
   epithelial, 89–91, 90*i*
   exenteration for, 90, 128
   nonepithelial, 91–92
Lacrimal nerve, 14
Lacrimal probing
   for congenital nasolacrimal duct obstruction, 261, 262–265, 263*i*
   diagnostic, for acquired nasolacrimal duct/canalicular obstruction, 271, 275
Lacrimal pump, 256, 257*i*
Lacrimal sac (tear sac), 255, 255*i*
   cast formation in (dacryoliths), 283
   distension of, in dacryocystitis, 278, 279*i*
   trauma to, 284
   tumors of, 283–284
Lacrimal scintigraphy, for acquired tearing evaluation, 272, 273*i*
Lacrimal system. *See also specific structure*
   anatomy of, 253–256
   disorders of. *See also* Tearing
      acquired, 267–284
      congenital, 259–267
      developmental abnormalities, 257–258, 258*i*
      lower system abnormalities, 278–284
      upper system abnormalities, 274–278
   excretory apparatus of, 253–256, 255*i*, 256*i*. *See also* Lacrimal drainage system
   physiology of, 256–257, 257*i*
   secretory apparatus/function of, 253, 254*i*. *See also* Lacrimal glands
   silicone intubation of
      for acquired nasolacrimal obstruction, 278
      for canalicular constriction, 275
      for canalicular trauma, 277
      for congenital lacrimal duct obstruction/tearing, 263–264, 266*i*
   tumors of, 277–278, 283–284
Lagophthalmos
   after blepharoplasty, 233
   in paralytic ectropion, 199
      gold weight loading for, 199
   after ptosis repair, 217, 223
Lamellar deficiency, surgery for eyelid retraction and, 225
Lamina papyracea (ethmoidal bone), 7, 8*i*, 9*i*, 11
Langerhans cell histiocytosis (histiocytosis X), orbital involvement in, 88
Laser dacryocystorhinostomy, 281–282, 282*i*
Laser skin resurfacing, 237–238
Laser therapy (laser surgery)
   for capillary hemangioma, 66
   for orbital lymphangiomas, 69
   for punctal occlusion, 274
   for skin resurfacing, 237–238
   for trichiasis, 208
   for xanthelasmas, 166
Lash follicles, 142*i*
   tumors arising in, 168–169, 169*i*
Lash margin entropion, in anophthalmic socket, 127
Lateral canthal defects, repair of, 192
Lateral canthal tendon, 146
Lateral orbitotomy, 114–115

Lateral rectus muscles, 13
Lateral tarsal strip operation
   for cicatricial ectropion, 200–201
   for involutional ectropion, 197–198, 197i
   for involutional entropion, 205
Le Fort fractures, 97, 98i
Lentigo (lentigines)
   maligna (Hutchinson's melanotic freckle/
      precancerous melanosis), 174
   senile (liver spots), 171
   simplex (simple lentigines), 171
   solar, 171
Lentigo maligna melanoma, 182
Letterer-Siwe disease. See also Histiocytosis
   orbital involvement in, 88
Leukemia, orbital involvement in, 94–95
Levator aponeurosis, 140, 140i, 142–143, 144, 144i
   lacrimal gland development and, 253
   ptosis and, 215, 216i, 217t, 219
   repair of, for ptosis correction, 222
Levator muscle (levator palpebrae superioris)
   anatomy of, 140i, 142
   external (transcutaneous) advancement of, for ptosis
      correction, 221
   function of, in ptosis, 210–211, 210i
   innervation of, 12
   internal (conjunctival) resection of, for ptosis
      correction, 221
   in myogenic ptosis, 214–215
   in traumatic ptosis, 219
Lid margin. See Eyelids, margin of
Lidocaine, for blepharoplasty, 231
Ligaments
   Lockwood's suspensory, 145
   superior transverse (Whitnall's), 140i, 142–143, 144i,
      253
Lipodermoids (dermolipomas), of orbit, 64, 65i
Liposarcomas, of orbit, 81
Liposuction, neck, 245–246, 246i
Liver spots, 171
Local anesthesia
   for blepharoplasty, 231
   for eyelid surgery, 150
Lockwood's suspensory ligament, 145
Longitudinal/spin-lattice relaxation time (T1), in
      magnetic resonance imaging, 30–31
Lower eyelid. See Eyelids, lower
Lymphangiomas, orbital, 67–69
Lymphatics, eyelid, 147
Lymphoid hyperplasia of orbit, 81–89. See also
      Lymphomas, orbital
Lympholysis, radiotherapy for Graves ophthalmopathy
      and, 54
Lymphomas, orbital, 81–89, 83i, 86t
   clonality of, 84
   identification and classification of, 82–85, 83i
   lacrimal gland origin and, 89, 92
   MALT-type (marginal zone), 85–87, 86t
   management of, 87
Lymphoproliferative lesions
   of lacrimal glands, 89, 91
   of orbit, 81–89, 83i, 86t
      lymphoid hyperplasia/lymphomas, 82–87
      plasma cell tumors, 88

   histiocytic disorders, 88
   juvenile xanthogranuloma, 88–89
Lynch incision, for anterior orbitotomy, 112

Magnetic resonance angiography (MRA), in orbital
      evaluation, 34
Magnetic resonance imaging (MRI), in orbital
      evaluation, 30–31, 30i
   CT scanning compared with, 31–33, 32i, 33t
Malignant melanoma. See Melanomas
MALT-type tumors. See Mucosa-associated lymphoid
      tissue (MALT) lymphoma
Mandibulofacial dysostosis (Treacher
      Collins–Franceschetti syndrome), 38, 38i
Marcus Gunn jaw-winking ptosis/syndrome, 217, 218i
   synkinesis in, 211, 217, 218i
Margin
   ciliary, 146
   lid. See Eyelids, margin of
Margin–reflex distance, in ptosis, 209–210, 210i
Marginal rotation, for cicatricial entropion, 206, 206i
Marginal tear strip (tear meniscus), in pseudoepiphora
      evaluation, 273
Marginal zone B-cell lymphoma, 85
Masquerade conditions
   eyelid tumors and, 184
   orbital tumors and, 69–70, 71i, 72i
Maxilla/maxillary bone, 7, 8i
   fracture of, 97, 98i
Maxillary nerve. See Cranial nerve V (trigeminal
      nerve), V$_2$
Maxillary sinuses, 20–21, 20i
Mechanical ectropion, 196i, 201
Mechanical ptosis, 219
Medial canthal tendon, 146, 255, 256i
   trauma involving, 186
Medial canthal tumors, 277–278
Medial orbital fractures, 101–102, 101i
Medial rectus muscles, 12
Medial spindle procedure, 197, 197i
Meibomian glands, 142i, 147, 166
   chalazion caused by obstruction of, 158
   sebaceous adenocarcinoma arising in, 180
   in tear film lipids/tear production, 253
Melanocytic tumors of eyelid
   benign, 169–170
   premalignant, 174
Melanocytosis
   dermal, 171–172
   oculodermal (nevus of Ota/congenital
      oculomelanocytosis), 171–172, 172i
Melanomas
   enucleation for, 119–120
   exenteration for, 128
   of eyelid, 182–183
   lentigo maligna, 182
   nodular, 182–183
Melanosis, precancerous (lentigo maligna/Hutchinson's
      melanotic freckle), 174
Melasma, of eyelids, 170
Meningiomas, 77–79, 77–78i
   optic nerve sheath, 77
   orbital, 77–79, 77–78i, 93
Meningoceles, 38

Meningoencephaloceles, 38, 38*i*
Mesenchymal tumors, orbital, 79–81, 79*i*, 82*i*
Metastatic disease of orbit, 94–96
 in adults, 95–96, 95*i*
 in children, 94, 94*i*
 management of, 96
Methicillin, for *Staphylococcus aureus* preseptal cellulitis, 42
Methimazole, for Graves disease, 54
Methylprednisolone, for traumatic visual loss, 108
MG. *See* Myasthenia gravis
Micrographic surgery, Mohs'
 for canthal tumors, 193
 for neoplastic disorders of eyelid
  basal cell carcinoma, 178–179
  sebaceous adenocarcinoma, 182
  squamous cell carcinoma, 178–179
Microphthalmos (microphthalmia), 37–38
 with cyst (colobomatous cyst), 37–38
Middle cranial fossa, 21
Midface lift, 241–242
Midfacial fractures, 97, 98*i*
Mikulicz syndrome, 91
Milia, 164–166
Mimetic muscles, 135–137, 138*i*
 facial nerve supplying, 137–138
Minus (concave) lenses, anophthalmic socket camouflage and, 127
Mitomycin C, for dacryocystitis, 283
Mixed tumor
 benign (pleomorphic adenoma)
  of eyelid, 167
  of lacrimal gland, 89–90
 malignant, of lacrimal gland, 90
Mohs' micrographic surgery
 for canthal tumors, 193
 for neoplastic disorders of eyelid
  basal cell carcinoma, 178–179
  sebaceous adenocarcinoma, 182
  squamous cell carcinoma, 178–179
Moll, glands of, 166. *See also* Apocrine glands of eyelid
 hidrocystoma arising in, 167–168
Molluscum contagiosum, of eyelid, 166
Morpheaform (fibrosing) basal cell carcinoma, 175, 175*i*
Motility disorders. *See* Ocular motility, disorders of
MRA. *See* Magnetic resonance angiography
MRD. *See* Margin–reflex distance
MRI. *See* Magnetic resonance imaging
Mucoceles
 congenital, 260
 in dacryocystitis, 278
 orbital invasion by, 92–93, 93*i*
Mucopyoceles, orbital invasion by, 92–93, 93*i*
Mucor (mucormycosis), orbit involved in, 45–46
 exenteration in management of, 45–46, 128
Mucosa-associated lymphoid tissue (MALT) lymphoma, of orbit, 85–87, 86*t*
Muir-Torre syndrome, eyelid manifestations of, 167
Müllerectomy, tarsoconjunctival (Fasanella-Servat procedure), for ptosis correction, 222
Müller's muscle (superior tarsal muscle), 140*i*, 144
 in congenital Horner syndrome, 217
 internal (conjunctival) resection of, for ptosis correction, 222

Muscle relaxants, for benign essential blepharospasm, 227
Mustardé flap, for eyelid repair, 189, 191*i*, 192
Myasthenia gravis, 218
 diagnosis of, edrophonium in, 213
 Graves ophthalmopathy and, 54
 ptosis in, 213, 218
Myectomy, for benign essential blepharospasm, 227
Myogenic ptosis, 214–215, 214*i*, 217*t*
Myopathies, restrictive extraocular, in Graves ophthalmopathy, 48, 53

Nasal cavity, 20
Nasal conchae (turbinates), 20
 infracture of, for congenital tearing/nasolacrimal duct obstruction, 263, 265*i*
Nasal endoscopy, for acquired tearing evaluation, 271
Nasal septum, 20
Nasociliary nerve, 15
Nasolacrimal canal, 11, 256
 balloon catheter dilation of, for congenital tearing/nasolacrimal duct obstruction, 264–265
Nasolacrimal duct, 20, 255*i*, 256
 irrigation of
  for acquired tearing evaluation, 270–271, 270*t*, 271*i*
  for congenital tearing management, 262–263, 264*i*
 obstruction of. *See also* Tearing
  acquired, 278
   examination in evaluation of, 267–268, 268*i*
   irrigation in evaluation of, 270–271, 270*t*, 271*i*
   probing in evaluation of, 271
  congenital, 258, 261–265
   balloon catheter dilation (balloon dacryoplasty) for, 264–265
   in dacryocystocele, 260–261, 260*i*
   irrigation for, 262–263, 264*i*
   probing for, 261, 262–265, 263*i*
   silicone intubation for, 263–264, 266*i*
   turbinate infracture for, 263, 265*i*
  in dacryocystitis, 278–279
 trauma to, 284
Naso-orbital-ethmoidal fractures, 101, 101*i*
Nd:YAG laser therapy, for orbital lymphangioma, 69
Neck, cosmetic/rejuvenation surgery on, 244–247, 245*i*, 246*i*, 247*i*
 liposuction, 245–246, 246*i*
Necrotizing fasciitis, of orbit, 44–45
Neural tumors of orbit, 72–79, 73*i*, 76*i*, 77–78*i*. *See also specific type*
Neurilemoma. *See* Schwannoma
Neuroblastoma, of orbit, 94, 94*i*
Neurofibromas
 discrete, 75
 of orbit, 26, 75, 76*i*
Neurofibromatosis type 1 (von Recklinghausen disease), 75
 optic nerve gliomas and, 72–74, 75
 orbital involvement in, 75
Neurogenic ptosis, 215–219, 218*i*
Neuropathy, optic. *See* Optic neuropathy
Nevoxanthoendothelioma (juvenile xanthogranuloma), of orbit, 88–89
Nevus
 blue, 171

compound, 170
of eyelid, 170, 170*i*
intradermal, 170
junctional, 170
of Ota (oculodermal melanocytosis/congenital oculomelanocytosis), 171, 172*i*
Nevus cells, tumors arising from, 170–171. *See also* Nevus
Nodular basal cell carcinoma, 174–175, 175*i*
Nonaxial displacement of globe, in orbital disorders, 23
Nose, 20–21. *See also under* Nasal
orbital tumors originating in, 92–93

Oblique muscles, 12, 140*i*, 141*i*
Ocular adnexa
benign lesions of, 166–169
definition of, 166
Ocular motility
disorders of
in blowout fractures, 102–104, 103*i*
surgery and, 104–105
conditions causing, 26
in Graves ophthalmopathy, 26
after orbital surgery, 117
after evisceration, 123
extraocular muscles controlling, 12
Ocular movements. *See* Eye movements
Ocular myasthenia gravis, 218. *See also* Myasthenia gravis
Ocular prostheses, 122
Oculoauricular dysplasia (Goldenhar syndrome), 38
Oculodermal melanocytosis (nevus of Ota), 171, 172*i*
Oculomotor foramen, 14
Oculomotor nerve. *See* Cranial nerve III
Oculomotor nerve palsy. *See* Third nerve (oculomotor) palsy
Oil glands, of eyelid, lesions of, 166–167
Ophthalmia, sympathetic, enucleation for prevention of, 119–120
Ophthalmic artery, 14*i*, 15
eyelids supplied by, 147
Ophthalmic nerve. *See* Cranial nerve V (trigeminal nerve), V$_1$
Ophthalmic pathology, of orbit, 35
Ophthalmic vein, 15
Optic canal, 11–12
decompression of, for traumatic visual loss, 108
Optic nerve (cranial nerve II)
in Graves ophthalmopathy, 48, 53
intraorbital portion of, 12
length of, 7*t*, 12
trauma to, 107
Optic nerve glioblastoma (malignant optic glioma), 72
Optic nerve glioma, 72–75, 73*i*
malignant (glioblastoma), 72
in neurofibromatosis, 72–74, 75
Optic nerve sheath meningioma, 77
Optic neuropathy
in Graves ophthalmopathy, 48, 53
traumatic, 107
Optical pocket, for endoscopic brow and forehead lift, 239
Optics, cosmetic, for anophthalmic socket, 127
Orbicularis oculi muscle, 139–140, 141*i*, 142*i*, 143*i*
tear flow pumped by, 256, 257*i*

Orbit
anatomy of, 7–22
anophthalmic socket and, 119–129
apertures in walls of, 8*i*, 9*i*, 10*i*, 11–12
basal cell cancer involving, 177–178
cellulitis affecting. *See* Orbital cellulitis
congenital disorders of
anomalies, 37–39, 38*i*, 39*i*
tumors, 63–64, 65*i*
cysts of
chocolate, 68
dermoid, 63–64, 65*i*
epidermoid, 63
with microphthalmos (colobomatous cyst), 37–38
dimensions of, 7, 7*t*
disorders of. *See also specific type*
evaluation of, 23–36
globe displacement and, 23, 24
imaging studies in
primary, 27–34, 28*i*
secondary, 34
laboratory studies in, 35–36
pain and, 23
palpable masses and, 24, 26–27
periorbital changes and, 24, 25*t*
proptosis and, 23–24
pulsation and, 24, 26–27
rate of progression of, 24
emphysema of, in blowout fractures, 101–102, 104
fissures of, 10*i*, 11, 21–22
floor of, 10, 10*i*
fractures of, 21, 102–106, 103*i*
foreign bodies in, 106
fossae of, 21–22
fractures of, 97–106, 99*i*, 101*i*, 103*i*
hemorrhages in, 72, 106
after blepharoplasty, visual loss and, 232–233
from orbital lymphangioma, 67–68
infection/inflammation of, 41–61
idiopathic. *See* Idiopathic orbital inflammation
lacrimal gland neoplasia and, 89–92, 90*i*
lateral wall of, 8–9
lipodermoids of, 64, 65*i*
lymphoproliferative lesions of, 81–89, 83*i*, 86*t*
medial wall of, 9–10, 9*i*
fracture of, 101–102, 101*i*
length of, 7*t*
nerves of, 14*i*, 15, 19*i*
optic nerve in, 12
length of, 7*t*, 12
paranasal sinuses and, 7, 20–21, 21*i*
periorbital structures and, 12, 20–22, 21*i*
roof of, 8
fractures of, 100
septum of, 7, 140–141, 140*i*, 141*i*
lacerations of, 184–185
soft tissues of, 12–19
surgery of, 109–117. *See also specific procedure*
for blowout fractures, 105–106
indications for, 104–105
complications of, 117
incisions for, 109, 111*i*
postoperative care and, 116
special techniques in, 116–117

surgical spaces and, 12–13, 109, 110*i*
teratomas of, 64
tight, 107
topography of, 7–10, 8*i*, 9*i*, 10*i*
trauma to, 97–108
    foreign bodies, 106
    hemorrhages, 72, 106
    midfacial (Le Fort) fractures, 97, 98*i*
    orbital fractures, 97–106, 99*i*, 101*i*, 103*i*
    septal disruption and, 12–13
    visual loss with clear media and, 106–108
tuberculosis affecting, 47
tumors of, 63–96
    congenital, 63–64, 65*i*
    enucleation for, 119–122
    exenteration for, 127–129, 128*i*
    lymphoproliferative, 81–89, 83*i*, 86*t*
    mesenchymal, 79–81, 79*i*, 82*i*
    metastatic, 94–96
      in adults, 95–96, 95*i*
      in children, 94, 94*i*
      management of, 96
    neural, 72–79, 73*i*, 76*i*, 77–78*i*
    palpable, 24, 26–27
    pathologic examination of, 35
    secondary, 92–93, 92*i*
      eyelid carcinoma and, 177–178
    vascular, 64–69, 66*i*, 68*i*
      masquerading conditions and, 69–70, 71*i*, 72*i*
vascular system of, 15, 16–18*i*
volume of, 7*t*
Orbital apex fractures, 100
Orbital apex syndrome
    in orbital cellulitis, 42
    in phycomycosis, 45–46
Orbital cellulitis, 20, 42–44, 43*i*, 44*t*, 45*i*
    fungal (mucormycosis), 45–46
      exenteration in management of, 45–46, 128
Orbital decompression, 115, 116*i*
    complications of, 117
    for Graves ophthalmopathy, 54, 115
    for lymphangioma, 69
    for traumatic visual loss, 107, 108
Orbital fat, 13, 141
    aging affecting, 236
    dermatochalasis and, 228
    eyelid lacerations and, 184–185
Orbital fissures, 21–22
    inferior, 10*i*, 11, 21–22
    superior, 11, 21
Orbital implants, 121–122
    in children, 121
    exposure and extrusion of, 125, 125*i*
    for superior sulcus deformity, 124
Orbital inflammatory syndrome (idiopathic orbital inflammation/orbital pseudotumor), 56–59, 57*i*
    plasma cell–rich, 88
Orbital orbicularis muscles, 140, 140*i*, 143*i*
Orbital pseudotumor. *See* Orbital inflammatory syndrome
Orbital septum, 6, 140–141, 140*i*, 141*i*
Orbital varices, 70–71, 72*i*
Orbital vein
    eyelids drained by, 147
    thrombophlebitis of, 61
Orbitectomy, for lacrimal gland tumors, 91
Orbitotomy
    anterior, 109–114
      inferior approach for, 110–111, 112*i*, 113*i*
      medial approach for, 111–114
      superior approach for, 109
    for cavernous hemangioma, 67
    lateral, 114–115
    in orbital evaluation, 35
Osteocutaneous ligaments, 135
Osteoma, of orbit, 81
    secondary, 93
Osteosarcoma, of orbit, 81
Ota, nevus of (oculodermal melanocytosis), 171, 172*i*

Pain, orbital, 23
    in blowout fractures, 102
    in idiopathic orbital inflammation, 56–57
Palatine bone, 7, 8*i*, 10*i*
Palpation, orbital, 24, 26–27
Palpebral fissures
    congenital widening of (euryblepharon), 154, 155*i*
    vertical height of, in ptosis, 209, 210*i*
Papillomas
    eyelid, 163–164, 164*i*
    lacrimal sac, squamous cell, 284
Paralytic ectropion, 196*i*, 199–200, 200*i*
Paranasal sinuses, 7, 20–21, 21*i*
    Aspergillus causing infection of, 46–47
    orbital cellulitis caused by infections of, 42, 44*t*
    orbital tumors originating in, 92–93, 93*i*
    preseptal cellulitis caused by infection of, 41–42
    tuberculous infection of, orbital involvement and, 47
Parasites, orbital infection caused by, 47
Parasympathetic nerves/pathway, orbit supplied by, 15
Parinaud syndrome, eyelid retraction in, 224
Parotidomasseteric fascia, 137
Patching, orbital surgery and, 116
Pedicle flap, for canthal repair, 192
Penetrating injuries, eyelid, 184–186. *See also* Lacerations, eyelid
Pentagonal resection, for trichiasis, 208
Periocular hemangiomas, 66
Periorbita (periorbital structures), 12, 20–22, 21*i*. *See also specific structure*
    capillary hemangiomas involving, 65
    cellulitis affecting, 41–44. *See also* Orbital cellulitis; Preseptal cellulitis
    innervation of, 14*i*, 15–16, 19*i*
    involutional changes in, 228–229
    orbital diseases causing changes in, 24, 25*t*
Peripheral surgical space (extraconal fat/surgical space), 13, 109, 110*i*
Phleboliths, orbital varices and, 70
Phycomycetes (phycomycosis), orbit involved in, 45–46
    exenteration in management of, 45–46, 128
Pigmentations, after laser skin resurfacing, 238
Pilar (trichilemmal) cyst, 166
Pilomatrixomas, 169
Plasma cell tumors, of orbit, 88
Plasmacytoma, of orbit, 88
Platysmaplasty, 247, 247*i*
Pleomorphic adenoma (benign mixed tumor)
    of eyelid, 167

of lacrimal gland, 89–90, 90*i*
Pleomorphic rhabdomyosarcoma, 80
Plexiform neurofibromas, of orbit, 26, 75–76, 76*i*
Plus (convex) lenses, anophthalmic socket camouflage and, 127
Polyarteritis nodosa, 60
Polytetrafluoroethane, for frontalis suspension, 222
Pork tapeworm, orbital infection caused by, 47
Posttarsal venous drainage, of eyelid, 147
Precancerous melanosis (lentigo maligna/Hutchinson's melanotic freckle), 174
Preperiosteal SOOF lift, 241, 242*i*
Preseptal cellulitis, 41–42
Preseptal orbicularis muscles, 140, 140*i*, 143*i*
Preseptal tissues, 139
Pretarsal orbicularis muscles, 139–140, 143*i*
Pretarsal tissues, 139, 140*i*
  venous drainage of, 147
Pretrichial brow lift, 241
Primary dye test (Jones I test), 268, 269*t*
Prisms, anophthalmic socket camouflage and, 127
Probing of lacrimal system
  for congenital nasolacrimal duct obstruction, 261, 262–265, 263*i*
  diagnostic, for acquired nasolacrimal duct/canalicular obstruction, 271, 275
Procerus muscle, 140, 143*i*
Proptosis (exophthalmos/exorbitism), 23–24
  bilateral, 23–24, 26
  evaluation checklist for, 27
  in Graves ophthalmopathy (thyrotoxic), 26, 48, 48*i*, 53
    eyelid retraction differentiated from, 223–224
  in orbital phycomycosis, 45–46
  in orbital tumors, 23–24
  unilateral, 26
Prostate cancer, orbital metastases in, 95*i*, 96
Prostheses, ocular, 122
Proton density, in magnetic resonance imaging, 30
Protractors, eyelid, 139–140, 143*i*
Pseudoepiphora, 274
Pseudoepitheliomatous hyperplasia, 164
Pseudoproptosis, 26
Pseudoptosis, 219, 220*i*
Pseudostrabismus, in epicanthus, 156
Pseudotumor, orbital. *See* Orbital inflammatory syndrome
Pterygoid venous plexus, eyelids drained by, 147
Pterygopalatine fossa, 21
Ptosis (blepharoptosis), 208–223
  acquired, 208
    aponeurotic, 215, 216*i*
      eyelid position in downgaze and, 211–212
    myogenic, 214
    neurogenic, 217–218
  anophthalmic, 127
  aponeurotic, 215, 216*i*, 217*t*
  apparent (pseudoptosis), 219, 220*i*
  in blowout fractures, 103
  brow, 234–235, 234*i*
  classification of, 208–209, 213–219
  congenital, 208, 214
    amblyopia in, 211
    aponeurotic, 215

  eyelid position in downgaze and, 211–212
  myogenic, 214, 214*i*, 217*t*
  neurogenic, 215–218, 218*i*
  enucleation and, 123
  evaluation of, 208–209
  in Horner syndrome, 217
    pharmacologic testing for, 212–213, 212*i*
  lower eyelid, 217
  Marcus Gunn jaw-winking, 217, 218*i*
    synkinesis in, 211, 217, 218*i*
  mechanical, 219
  in myasthenia gravis, 213, 218
    edrophonium chloride (Tensilon) test and, 213
  myogenic, 214, 214*i*, 217*t*
  neurogenic, 215–219, 218*i*
  physical examination of patient with, 209–213, 211*i*, 212*i*
  surgical repair of, 220–223, 221*i*
  synkinesis in, 211
  traumatic, 219
  treatment of, 187, 220–223, 221*i*
  visual field testing in, 212
Ptosis data sheet, 210, 210*i*
Pulsation, orbital, 24, 26–27
Pulsed-dye laser therapy, for capillary hemangiomas, 66
Punch (incisional) biopsy, 171, 176*i*
Puncta, 254, 255*i*
  disorders of
    acquired, 274
    congenital, 257–258
      agenesis and dysgenesis, 257–258, 265–267
    malposition of, 274
Punctal occlusion, for dry eye, 274
Pupillary defects
  afferent, in traumatic optic neuropathy, 107
  in ptosis, 212
Pupils, examination of, in ptosis, 212
Pyoceles, orbital invasion by, 93

Quickert sutures, for involutional entropion, 204

Radiation therapy
  for basal cell carcinoma of eyelid, 179
  for capillary hemangiomas, 66
  for Graves ophthalmopathy, 54–55
  for lacrimal gland tumors, 91
  for lacrimal sac tumors, 284
  for lymphoproliferative lesions of orbit, 87
  for optic nerve glioma, 74–75
  for optic nerve sheath meningioma, 78
  for rhabdomyosarcoma, 80
Radioactive iodine, for Graves disease, 54
Radiography, in orbital evaluation, 27–28, 28*i*
Radionuclide scintigraphy/scans, for acquired tearing evaluation, 272, 273*i*
Reactive lymphoid hyperplasia, of orbit, 82. *See also* Lymphoproliferative lesions
REAL classification, for ocular adnexal lymphoma evaluation, 85, 86*t*
Reconstructive surgery
  eyelid, 188–193
    after basal cell carcinoma surgery, 178–179
    for blepharophimosis syndrome, 153

Index • 321

for epicanthus, 156
for euryblepharon, 154
for eyelid defects involving eyelid margin, 189–192, 191*i*
for eyelid defects not involving eyelid margin, 188–189
for lower eyelid defects, 189–192, 191*i*
after Mohs' micrographic surgery, 178–179
for upper eyelid defects, 188–190, 190*i*
socket, 126
Rectus muscles, 13, 140*i*
Reflex tear arc, 253
Refraction, in ptosis, 211
Rejuvenation surgery, facial, 237–248. *See also specific procedure*
Relaxation time, in magnetic resonance imaging, 30
Retinoblastoma
enucleation for, 120
exenteration for, 128
Retraction, eyelid, 223–225, 224*i*
after blepharoplasty, 224, 233, 233*i*
in Graves ophthalmopathy, 26, 48–51, 48*i*, 53, 223–224, 224*i*
proptosis differentiated from, 223–224
after strabismus surgery, 224
treatment of, 224–225
Retractors, eyelid, 141*i*, 142–145, 144*i*
lower eyelid, 140*i*, 144*i*, 145
in involutional ectropion, repair of, 198
in involutional entropion, 202–203
repair of, 203*i*, 204–205
upper eyelid, 142–144, 144*i*
Retrobulbar hemorrhage, after blepharoplasty, visual loss and, 232–233
Retro-orbicularis oculi fat (ROOF), 134
Rhabdomyosarcoma, of orbit, 79–80, 79*i*
Rhizopus, infection caused by, orbital, 45–46
Rhytidectomy, 244–245, 245*i*, 246*i*
Ring sign, in idiopathic orbital inflammation, 58
ROOF. *See* Retro-orbicularis oculi fat
Rosengren-Doane tear pump, 256, 257*i*
Rosenmüller, valve of, 254
Rotational flap, for eyelid repair, 190*i*, 191*i*, 192

Sarcoidosis, orbit affected in, 59
Sarcoma
granulocytic (chloroma), 94–95
Kaposi, of eyelid, 183, 183*i*
orbital
exenteration for, 128
secondary, 94–95
Scalp flap, coronal, for anterior orbitotomy, 110
Schirmer test, type I, in pseudoepiphora, 274
Schwannoma (neurilemoma/neurinoma), of orbit, 79
Scintigraphy, lacrimal, for acquired tearing evaluation, 272, 273*i*
Sclerosing inflammation of orbit, idiopathic, 57, 58. *See also* Idiopathic orbital inflammation
Sebaceous adenomas, 167
Sebaceous carcinoma/adenocarcinoma, 180–182, 180*i*, 181*i*
medial canthal/lacrimal sac involvement and, 284
Sebaceous cysts (epidermal inclusion cysts), of eyelid, 164–166, 165*i*

Sebaceous glands of eyelid, 166–167
tumors arising in. *See* Sebaceous adenomas; Sebaceous carcinoma/adenocarcinoma
Sebaceous hyperplasia, of eyelid, 166–167
Seborrheic keratosis, 163, 165*i*
Sedatives, for benign essential blepharospasm, 227
Semicircular flap, for eyelid repair, 189, 190*i*, 191*i*, 192
Senile lentigo (liver spots), 171
Seventh nerve palsy/paralysis, paralytic ectropion and, 199
Shave biopsy, 176*i*, 181
Silastic rods, for frontalis suspension, 222
Silicone intubation
for acquired nasolacrimal obstruction, 278
for canalicular constriction, 275
for canalicular trauma, 277
for congenital lacrimal duct obstruction/tearing, 263–264, 266*i*
Silicone suspension sling, for paralytic ectropion, 199
Simple lentigines (lentigo simplex), 171
Sinuses
ethmoid, 20, 21*i*
frontal, 9*i*, 20, 21*i*
maxillary, 20–21, 21*i*
paranasal, 7, 20–22, 21*i*
Aspergillus causing infection of, 46–47
orbital cellulitis caused by infection of, 42, 44*t*
orbital tumors originating in, 92–93, 93*i*
preseptal cellulitis caused by infection of, 41–42
tuberculous infection of, orbital involvement and, 47
sphenoid, 10*i*, 20, 21*i*
Sinusitis
allergic aspergillosis, 46–47
orbital cellulitis caused by, 42, 44*t*
preseptal cellulitis caused by, 41–42
tuberculous, orbital infection and, 47
Skin
eyelid, 139, 140*i*, 141*i*
laser resurfacing of, 237–238
tumors of, medial canthal/lacrimal sac involvement and, 284
Skin grafts. *See* Flaps; Grafts
Skull fracture, arteriovenous fistula caused by, 70
SMAS. *See* Superficial musculoaponeurotic system
Smoking, thyroid disease and, 53
Snapback test, 202
Socket contraction, 125–126, 126*i*. *See also* Anophthalmic socket
Soft tissue histiocytosis. *See* Histiocytosis
Solar (actinic) keratosis, 172–173, 172*i*
Solar lentigo, 171
SOOF (suborbicularis oculi fat). *See* Suborbicularis fat pads
SOOF lift, 241, 242*i*
Spasms
benign essential blepharospasm, 226
hemifacial, 227–228
Spastic entropion, 201–202, 202*i*
Spectacle lenses/frames, anophthalmic socket camouflage and, 127
Sphenoethmoidal recess, 20
Sphenoid bone, 7, 8*i*, 9*i*, 10*i*
Sphenoid sinuses, 10*i*, 20, 21*i*

Spin-lattice/longitudinal relaxation time (T1), in magnetic resonance imaging, 30
Spiradenoma, eccrine, 167
Spiral computed tomography, in orbital evaluation, 29
Squamous cell carcinoma
    of eyelid, 179–180, 179*i*
        in situ (Bowen disease), 173
        medial canthal/lacrimal sac involvement and, 284
    of orbit, secondary, 92*i*, 93
Squamous cell papillomas
    of eyelid, 163, 164*i*
    lacrimal sac involvement and, 284
Stallard-Wright incision, for lateral orbitotomy, 114
Staphylococcus aureus, preseptal cellulitis caused by, 42
Steatoblepharon, 228
Stent placement, for canalicular trauma, 277
Strabismus surgery, for Graves ophthalmopathy, 54
Streptococcus pyogenes (group A beta-hemolytic streptococcus), orbital necrotizing fasciitis caused by, 44–45
Stye (external hordeolum), 160
Sub-brow fat pads, 146
Subcutaneous rhytidectomy, 244
Subcutaneous tissue
    of eyelid, 139
    of face, 135
Suborbicularis fat pads (suborbicularis oculi fat/SOOF), 135, 141*i*, 145–146
    midface rejuvenation surgery and (SOOF lift), 241, 242*i*
Subperiorbital surgical space, 109, 110*i*
Subperiosteal midface lift, 241–242
    endoscopic, 242–243, 243*i*
Sudoriferous cysts, of eyelid (apocrine hidrocystoma), 168, 169*i*
Superficial mimetic muscles, 135, 138–139
Superficial musculoaponeurotic system (SMAS), 135, 136*i*
    subcutaneous rhytidectomy with, 244–245, 245*i*
Superior displacement of globe, in orbital disorders, 23
Superior oblique muscles, 12–13, 140*i*
Superior orbital fissure, 11, 21
Superior rectus muscles, 12–13, 140*i*
Superior sulcus deformity, anophthalmic socket and, 124, 124*i*
Superior tarsal muscle of Müller, 140*i*, 144
    in congenital Horner syndrome, 217
    internal (conjunctival) resection of, for ptosis correction, 222
Superior transverse ligament (Whitnall's ligament), 140*i*, 142–143, 144*i*, 253
Supraorbital ethmoids, 20
Surgical spaces, orbital, 12–13
Suspensory ligament of Lockwood, 145
Sutures (surgical), Quickert, for involutional entropion, 204, 205
Sweat glands of eyelid, 167
    tumors arising in, 167, 168*i*, 169*i*
Symblepharon, 207
Sympathetic nerves/pathway, orbit supplied by, 15–16
Sympathetic ophthalmia, enucleation in prevention of, 119–120
Synkinesis, 211
    in Marcus Gunn jaw-winking ptosis, 211, 217, 218*i*

Syringomas, 167, 168*i*

T1 (longitudinal/spin-lattice relaxation time), in magnetic resonance imaging, 30
Taenia solium, orbital infection caused by, 47
Tapeworms, ocular infection caused by, 47
Tarsal ectropion, 198
Tarsal fracture operation, for cicatricial entropion, 206, 206*i*
Tarsal kink, 157
Tarsal muscles
    inferior, 145
    superior (Müller's), 140*i*, 144
        in congenital Horner syndrome, 217
        internal (conjunctival) resection of, for ptosis correction, 222
Tarsal plates/tarsus, 140*i*, 141*i*, 145
    internal (conjunctival) resection of, for ptosis correction, 222
Tarsal strip procedure
    for cicatricial ectropion, 200–201
    for involutional ectropion, 197–198, 197*i*
    for involutional entropion, 205
Tarsoconjunctival grafts
    for cicatricial entropion, 207
    for eyelid repair, 187, 190*i*, 191*i*, 192
Tarsoconjunctival müllerectomy (Fasanella-Servat procedure), for ptosis correction, 222
Tarsorrhaphy, for paralytic ectropion, 199, 200*i*
Tarsotomy, for cicatricial entropion, 206, 206*i*
Tarsus. *See* Tarsal plates/tarsus
TBUT. *See* Tear breakup time
Tear breakup time, in pseudoepiphora evaluation, 273
Tear film (tears), composition of, 253
Tear meniscus (marginal tear strip), in pseudoepiphora evaluation, 272
Tear pump, 256, 257*i*
Tear sac. *See* Lacrimal sac
Tearing (epiphora), 251, 259–284. *See also specific cause*
    acquired, 267–284
        evaluation of, 267–274
        management of, 274–284
    congenital, 259–267
        evaluation of, 259
        management of, 259–267
    definition of, 272
    diagnostic tests for evaluation of, 268–274
Telecanthus, 25
Telorbitism (hypertelorism), 25
    clefting syndromes and, 38
Temporal (giant cell) arteritis, 59–60
Temporal artery, eyelids supplied by, 147
Temporal vein, eyelids drained by, 147
Temporalis fascia, deep, 138
Tensilon test, for myasthenia gravis diagnosis, 213
Tenzel semicircular rotation flap/modified Tenzel flap, in lower eyelid repair, 192
Teratomas, orbital, 64
Thermal cautery
    for involutional ectropion, 197
    for involutional entropion, 204
    for punctal occlusion, 274
Third nerve (oculomotor) palsy, congenital, ptosis in, 217–218

Three-dimensional computed tomography, in orbital evaluation, 29
Thrombocytopenia, capillary hemangiomas and (Kasabach-Merritt syndrome), 66
Thrombophlebitis, of orbital vein, 61
Thyroid-associated ophthalmopathy. *See* Thyroid ophthalmopathy
Thyroid dermopathy, in Graves ophthalmopathy, 53
Thyroid disease, screening/testing for, in thyroid ophthalmopathy, 35–36
Thyroid eye disease. *See* Thyroid ophthalmopathy
Thyroid ophthalmopathy (Graves disease/ophthalmopathy, dysthyroidism, thyroid orbitopathy), 48–56, 48*i*, 49–50*i*
 clinical presentation and diagnosis of, 48–51, 51*i*, 53
 epidemiology of, 52–53
 euthyroid, 48
 eye movements affected in, 26
 eyelid disorders and, 26, 48–51, 48*i*, 53
  retraction, 26, 48–51, 48*i*, 53, 223–225, 224*i*
 myasthenia gravis and, 54
 pathogenesis of, 51–52
 prognosis of, 53–55
 proptosis and, 26
  eyelid retraction differentiated from, 224*i*
 thyroid function tests in, 35–36
 treatment of, 53–55
Thyroid orbitopathy/ophthalmopathy. *See* Thyroid ophthalmopathy
Thyroiditis, Hashimoto, in Graves ophthalmopathy, 53
Thyrotoxic exophthalmos. *See* Thyroid ophthalmopathy
Thyrotropin (thyroid-stimulating hormone/TSH), receptor for, antibodies to, in Graves disease, 49, 51–52
Thyroxine (T$_4$), in block-and-replace therapy, for Graves disease, 54
Tight orbit, 107
Tolosa-Hunt syndrome, idiopathic orbital inflammation presenting as, 56
Tomography
 computed. *See* Computed tomography
 in orbital evaluation, 27–28, 28*i*
Topography, orbital, 7–10, 8*i*, 9*i*, 10*i*
Transcaruncular route, for anterior orbitotomy, 113–114
Transconjunctival route
 for blepharoplasty, 232
 for inferior anterior orbitotomy, 112*i*, 113, 113*i*
 for medial anterior orbitotomy, 113
 for ptosis repair, 222
 for superior anterior orbitotomy, 113
Transcutaneous routes
 for inferior anterior orbitotomy, 112–113
 for medial anterior orbitotomy, 112–113
 for ptosis correction, 222
 for superior anterior orbitotomy, 109–110
Transnasal laser dacryocystorhinostomy, 281–282, 282*i*
Transposition flaps, for lateral canthal defects, 192
Transseptal route, for anterior orbitotomy, 109
Transverse ligament, superior (Whitnall's), 140*i*, 142–143, 144*i*, 253
Transverse relaxation time, in magnetic resonance imaging, 31

Trauma
 blunt, eyelid, 184
 canalicular, 276–277
 eyelid, 184–188
  repair of, 184–187, 185*i*
  secondary, 186–187
 lacrimal sac and nasolacrimal duct, 284
 penetrating
  canthal soft tissue, 184–186
  eyelid, 184–186, 185*i*
 ptosis caused by, 219
Traumatic visual loss with clear media, 106–108
Treacher Collins–Franceschetti syndrome (mandibulofacial dysostosis), 38, 38*i*
Triamcinolone, for capillary hemangioma, 66
Trichiasis, 207–208
 in anophthalmic socket, 127
Trichilemmal (pilar) cyst, 166
Trichilemmoma, 168–169
Trichinella spiralis (trichinosis), orbital infection caused by, 47
Trichoepithelioma, 168, 169*i*
Trichofolliculoma, 168
Trigeminal nerve. *See* Cranial nerve V
Tripod (zygomatic-maxillary complex) fractures, 97–100, 99*i*
Trochlear nerve. *See* Cranial nerve IV
TSH receptor antibodies, in Graves disease, 49
Tuberculosis, orbital involvement and, 47
Turban tumors, 168
Turbinates (conchae), nasal, 20
 infracture of, for congenital tearing/nasolacrimal duct obstruction, 263, 265*i*
Turkey gobbler defect, 236

Ultrasonography, in orbital evaluation, 33–34
Upgaze. *See* Elevation of eye
Upper eyelid. *See* Eyelids, upper

Valve of Hasner, 255*i*, 256
 nasolacrimal duct obstruction and, 257, 261
Valve of Rosenmüller, 254
Varices, orbital, 70–71, 72*i*
Vascular system
 of eyelids, 147
 of orbit, 15, 16–18*i*
Vascular tumors, of orbit, 64–69, 66*i*, 68*i*
 masquerading conditions and, 69–70, 71*i*, 72*i*
Vasculitis. *See also specific type and* Arteritis
 connective tissue disorders associated with, 60
 orbital vessels involved in, 59–61
Venography, in orbital evaluation, 34
Verruca vulgaris (wart), eyelid, 164, 165*i*
Vertical diplopia, in blowout fractures, 102–104
 surgery and, 104
Vertical eyelid splitting, for anterior orbitotomy, 110
Vertical interpalpebral fissure height, in ptosis, 209, 210*i*
Vertical traction test, in blowout fractures, 103
 surgery and, 104
Visual acuity
 periorbital trauma affecting, 106–108
 in ptosis, 211–212
Visual field testing, in ptosis, 212

Visual loss/impairment
    after blepharoplasty, 232–233
    in blepharoptosis, 208
    in blowout fractures, 102–105
    after orbital surgery, 117
    traumatic, with clear media, 106–108
von Recklinghausen disease. *See* Neurofibromatosis type 1

Wart (verruca vulgaris), eyelid, 164, 165*i*
Wegener granulomatosis, 60–61, 61*i*
    diagnosis of, 36, 60–61
Whitnall's ligament (superior transverse ligament), 140*i*, 142–143, 144*i*, 253
Wies repair
    for involutional entropion, 204, 204*i*
    for lash margin entropion of anophthalmic socket, 127
Wolfring, glands of, 140*i*, 145, 253

Xanthelasma, of eyelid, 166
Xanthogranuloma, juvenile (nevoxanthoendothelioma), of orbit, 88–89

Xanthomas, fibrous (fibrous histiocytoma), orbital, 81
Xeroderma pigmentosum, 174

Y-V-plasties, for blepharophimosis syndrome, 153

Z-plasties
    for blepharophimosis syndrome, 153
    for eyelid repair, 187
    for symblepharon, 207
Zeis, glands of, 166
    sebaceous adenocarcinoma arising in, 180
Zinn, annulus of, 14, 14*i*, 15
ZMC fractures. *See* Zygomatic-maxillary complex (tripod) fractures
Zygomatic bone, 7, 8*i*, 10*i*
    fractures of, 97–100, 99*i*
Zygomatic-maxillary complex (tripod) fractures, 97–100, 99*i*
Zygomatic nerve, in reflex tear arc, 253
Zygomaticofacial canal, 11
Zygomaticotemporal canal, 11
Zygomaticotemporal nerve, in reflex tear arc, 253